NURSING LEADERSHIP GLOBAL STRATEGIES

International Nursing Development for the 21st Century

Claire M. Fagin

University of Pennsylvania School of Nursing

National League for Nursing • New York

Pub. No. 41–2349

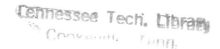

Cover photo: Approaching the waterfront at
Bellagio, Italy, by ferry on Lake Como. Bellagio
was the site of the 1989 conference on International
Nursing Development for the 21st Century.
Photo credit: Craig H. Little.

This book was set in Times Roman by Better Graphics.
The editors were Barbara J. Barnum and Sally J. Barhydt.
The cover was designed by Lillian Welsh.
The printer and binder was Automated Graphic Systems.
Project management was done by The Total Book.

ISBN 0-88737-496-4

The views expressed in this book reflect those of the
authors and do not necessarily reflect the official views
of the National League for Nursing.

Printed in the United States of America.

Contents

Contributors   v

Preface   vii
Claire M. Fagin

Foreword   ix
Constance Holleran

Conference Overview   xiv
Claire M. Fagin

SECTION 1   MANPOWER NEEDS

1. An Analysis of the U.S. Experience   3
   Linda H. Aiken

2. Planning for Nursing Manpower Needs in New Zealand   15
   Marion R. Clark

3. Manpower Needs: Womanpower Demands   29
   Christine Hancock

4. The Greek Nursing Workforce: Present Needs and Future
   Predictions   39
   Dimitri Monos and John Yfantopoulos

5. Health Manpower in Korea: Demands, Supply, and Education   49
   Mo-Im Kim

SECTION 2   EDUCATIONAL GOALS AND IMPLEMENTATION

6. Nursing Educational Goals for the 21st Century: Canada   67
   Jean Innes, Judith Oulton, Marianne Lamb, Shirley Stinson

7. Nursing in the 21st Century in Latin America   75
   Esperanza de Monterrossa, Ilta Lange, Roseni Rosangela Chompré

8. Nursing Education in China   85
   Dai Yu-Hua

9. Nursing Education in Korea   89
   So Woo Lee

10. Educational Goals and Implementation in Pakistan   99
    Patricia Scott

11. Some Thoughts on Education in Hungary   111
    Klára Sövényi

SECTION 3   CHALLENGES TO PRACTICE

12. Midwifery and Safe Motherhood   119
    Barbara Kwast

13. The Challenges of the Practice of Nursing in Latin America   135
    Esperanza de Monterrossa, Ilta Lange, Roseni Rosangela Chompré

14. Challenges to Practice: Midwifery   145
    Margaret Brain

15. Challenges to Practice in France   155
    Genevieve Dechanoz

16. Challenges to Practice in Geriatrics   163
    James Williamson

SECTION 4   POLICY ISSUES

17. Improving Health Status through Health Policy:
    An Agenda for Nursing Leaders   181
    David Mechanic

18. Health and Social Policy in Australia: The Role and
    Professionalism of Nursing   189
    Paul Gross

19. The Case for Nursing's Preeminence in International Health   209
    Pamela Maraldo

20. Political Challenges for Nursing in Latin America:
    The Next Century   221
    Esperanza de Monterrossa, Ilta Lange, Roseni Rosangela Chompré

21. The Future Role of Nursing in Health Policy-Making in
    Colombia   229
    Jaime Arias

Contributors

Conference Director and Chair of Planning Committee

CLAIRE M. FAGIN, PhD, RN, FAAN
Professor and Margaret Bond Simon Dean
University of Pennsylvania School of Nursing
Philadelphia, Pennsylvania, United States

Conference Participants

LINDA H. AIKEN, PhD, RN
Professor of Nursing and Sociology
University of Pennsylvania School of Nursing
Philadelphia, Pennsylvania, United States

JAIME ARIAS, MD
Representativo a la Camara
Bogota, Colombia

MARGARET BRAIN, OBE, SRN, SCM, MTD, FBIM
International Confederation of Midwives
London, United Kingdom

ROSENI ROSANGELA CHOMPRÉ, RN, MS
Escola de Enfermagem
Universidade Federal de Minas Gerais
Belo Horizonte, Brazil

MARION R. CLARK, RN
Nurse Advisor—Work Force Development
Department of Health
Wellington, New Zealand

DAI YU-HUA, MD
Professor, Vice President
Peking Union Medical College
Chinese Academy of Medical Sciences
Beijing, China

GENEVIEVE DECHANOZ
Infirmiere Generale—Nursing Director
Director of WHO Collaborating Center for Nursing
  in France
Lyons, France

HELEN GRACE, PhD, RN, FAAN
Program Director
W. K. Kellogg Foundation
Battle Creek, Michigan, United States

PAUL GROSS
Chairman of the Board
Institute of Health Economics and Technology
  Assessment
North Sydney, Australia

CHRISTINE HANCOCK
General Secretary
The Royal College of Nursing of the United
  Kingdom
London, United Kingdom

CONSTANCE HOLLERAN, RN, FAAN
Executive Director
International Council of Nurses
Geneva, Switzerland

JEAN INNES, RN, MScN
Associate Professor
University of Alberta Faculty of Nursing
Edmonton, Alberta, Canada

MO-IM KIM, RN, DrPH
President, Korean Nurses Association
Seoul, Korea

v

BARBARA KWAST, MTD, MCOMMH, PhD
Public Health Nurse/Midwife Educator/
  Epidemiologist
Division of Family Health
World Health Organization
Geneva, Switzerland

MARIANNE LAMB, RN, MN, PhD candidate
Department of Health Administration
Division of Community Health
University of Toronto
Toronto, Ontario, Canada

ILTA LANGE, RN, MS
Prof. Aux. Escuela de Enfermeria
CEDIUC
Santiago, Chile

SO WOO LEE, PhD
Professor, Department of Nursing
College of Medicine
Seoul National University
Seoul, Korea

PAMELA MARALDO, PhD, RN, FAAN
Executive Director
National League for Nursing
New York, New York, United States

DAVID MECHANIC, PhD
Rene Dubos Professor of Behavioral Science
Institute of Health, Rutgers University
New Brunswick, New Jersey, United States

DIMITRI MONOS, PhD
Associate Professor of Sociology of Nursing
School of Health Sciences, Faculty of Nursing
University of Athens
Athens, Greece

ESPERANZA DE MONTERROSSA, RN, MS
Unidad Camilo Torres
Universidad Nacional de Colombia
Bogota, Colombia

JUDITH OULTON, RN
Executive Director
Canadian Nurses Association
Ottawa, Ontario, Canada

PATRICIA SCOTT, DNSC, RN
Department of Nursing and Health Visiting
University of Ulster at Jordanstown
Newtownabbey, County Antrim, Northern Ireland
Formerly Professor and Director, Degree Program
Faculty of Health Sciences, School of Nursing
The Aga Khan University
Karachi, Pakistan

KLARA SÖVÉNYI
Chief Nursing Officer
Department of Preventive and Curative Care
Ministry of Social Affairs and Health
Budapest, Hungary

SHIRLEY STINSON, RN, EdD, LLD
Professor, Faculty of Nursing and Faculty of
  Medicine
University of Alberta
Edmonton, Alberta, Canada
Adjunct Professor, Faculty of Nursing
University of Calgary
Calgary, Alberta, Canada

JAMES WILLIAMSON, CBE, FRCPE, D.SC
  (Hon.)
Department of Geriatric Medicine
City Hospital
University of Edinburgh
Edinburgh, Scotland, United Kingdom

JOHN YFANTOPOULOS, PhD
Assistant Professor of Health Economics
Department of Nursing
School of Health Sciences
University of Athens
Athens, Greece

Preface

This book represents the thoughts of a selected group of international leaders in nursing/midwifery and other disciplines.[1] The group was brought together at the Rockefeller Foundation Conference Center in Bellagio, Italy, to focus on long-term planning for effective preparation and utilization of nursing/midwifery personnel in the coming decade.

Several years ago Constance Holleran, executive director of the International Council of Nurses, Amelia Maglacas, then chief nurse scientist of the World Health Organization, and I talked about the need for an international "think tank" on nursing which would bring together a small group of leaders, chosen on the basis of individual distinction rather than solely as organization representatives—leaders who would be free to think creatively about nursing development for the twenty-first century. A planning committee was formed which selected potential participants and alternates based on their reputations in the areas of concern: manpower, educational goals and implementation, challenges to practice, and nursing and health policy issues. These potential participants came from a variety of countries, represented several disciplines, and were able to be in Bellagio for the week given to the group by the Foundation. The meeting was organized as follows:

- Nineteen participants wrote papers on one of the four areas.
- These participants presented a version of this paper or a related one.
- Large group discussions followed the presentations and panel discussions.

[1]The term *nursing/midwifery* will be used throughout the introductory and summarizing sections of this publication. This decision was made by the participants in their consensus discussion.

• Consistent small group discussion took place daily and went beyond the papers presented.

• Summaries of the group's thinking in each area were prepared and shared with the entire group at the meeting and by mail for consensus.

All these papers are presented here, preceded by an introductory chapter in which I will present and discuss the major issues and solutions summarizing the group's consensus.

The group discussions were enriched by the sharing of papers and thoughts and by the excellent environment. Acknowledgements must be made to the Rockefeller Foundation, to Roberto Celli, director of the center, to Mrs. Celli for her immense hospitality, and to the excellent staff who contributed to the achievement of the conference goals with services and cordiality.

Claire M. Fagin

Foreword

International nursing leadership is no different from any other leadership, although it may vary in the amount available or extent exerted or in methods used since culture is such an important factor.

Those of you here come from a broad spectrum of cultures and political systems. How you exert leadership is probably quite different from how I do.

We all know how many mistakes we have made with people from different backgrounds. Tensions occur because of misunderstanding. What I might consider to be time-efficient another might find curt and brusque. Meeting deadlines can be a problem among some groups.

When we designed our new offices I had the reception area very open, light, and with lots of windows. One secretary we had hated it.

She always closed all the doors to the board room and sat with a shawl around her although she was really not cold. When we talked about it she said she hated all that open space. It made her feel insecure, as she was used to houses with smaller rooms and doors to close off each room. We had different cultural backgrounds, and we needed to make adjustments.

Therefore, working in a situation such as the International Council of Nurses (ICN), where we deal with nurses from more than 110 countries, it is essential that we be culturally sensitive and adaptable.

Political differences cannot be ignored. Private-health and all-government employees have differences in approach and outlook. People who must sit low on the floor for their royal family cannot be expected to want to stand and address the health ministers of the world at the World Health Assembly (WHA) or even of the region. They have their own ways, and we must learn and listen.

In one Asian country, the chief nurse had been trying for years to get land from the government for a college of nursing. The land was often promised but never delivered. So one day at a public dedication of a hospital unit she approached the President's car and asked again about the unmet promise. He turned to his aide and said it must be done right away.

It was allocated that week, and the nurses now have that college building. Unfortunately the President was assassinated later the same month. In that nurse's country her action was an accepted type of leadership behavior.

In another Asian country several years ago, the association president had tried without success during my visit to have a meeting with the minister of health. She was blocked by his aides, who kept saying call back. She knew the minister fairly well, knew when and how he traveled to his office, so she stopped his car along the road to ask for an appointment. He said come in one hour. I got a rush call, and we had a very successful meeting with that minister of health. In my country if I approached the car of the President or a minister I would probably be arrested if not shot. Again, there are culturally acceptable ways for leaders to act.

Leadership, mentorship, and networking are hardly new ideas for any of us here, yet the words today are used almost as what Hayakawa would call "jargon on jargon."

Nursing and the other health fields are not alone in emphasizing leadership today. Every management or professional journal is calling for, even crying for, leaders.

Why? Is cost-effectiveness the only reason? No, of course not, but it is one of the important reasons. Others are limited resources, including demands for service and technology. Technology, although able to handle many of

the old routine tasks, makes the need for effective leaders and managers even greater.

Nurse leaders in every country must be prepared to project future needs, to budget well, to document facts, and to understand and practice good human resources management.

Everyone in this room is considered a leader (at least by someone, if not universally). Why? Because we have the ability to bring about change, to make things happen if not directly then through others.

This is a great responsibility, as we know in particular when we do our personal year-end reviews and develop our long- and short-term program plans. Where to start? What can wait? What haven't we taken into account? Will the resources be there when needed? [These October stock market crises or major fluctuations in exchange rates such as a decrease of 90 percent in the official exchange rate in the USSR or rampant inflation (20 to 2000 percent) are a little hard on the heart, have you noticed?]

Vance, in 1977, said "the movement, growth, and values of a profession, are inextricably tied to its leadership."[1] Her contention was that leadership resided in "influentials," the sources of influence being "political activity, access to funds, expertise, work position, scholarly publications, mobilization of groups, superior abilities, intellectual stature, personality, charismatic qualities and a few other items."[2]

Ross Perot in 1989 said in his foreword to *Tough Minded Leadership,* "Success or failure will depend on the leaders' ability to motivate the people, keep a results-oriented climate, build a unified team that builds the highest quality products in the field, and looks forward to taking on all competitors in fair, open competition—and beating them soundly."[3] So there we have the nonprofit and the profit-making views, and really they do not conflict. Only the emphasis varies.

In some of the countries where I have

worked, I have been amazed that the nurses accomplish as much as they do. One director of nursing at a large teaching hospital in Africa told me when we were talking about precautions needed in caring for AIDS patients: "It is hard for a nurse who, with one assistant, is responsible for 100 patients at night to ensure that any type of precaution is carried out." How true. Especially when there is little water, erratic electricity, and *no* equipment.

It was the leadership of that nursing director that kept those nurses going and kept them coming back to work every night. As president of the association, she even started projects based wholly on nurse volunteers of immunizing children out in the rural areas. Yes, I would say this nursing director had leadership skills.

One of our staff, in visiting a large hospital in a capital city of another African country, saw nurses coping with overwhelming burdens. A ward of eighty patients, forty with AIDS. Again, no water, no linen, no food for patients, and, of course, no dressings, gloves, or disposable needles. Yes, nursing leadership was in that institution too. Perhaps the leader was not high enough up the chart to influence budget allocation, however.

We all think we face problems, and of course we do, but really the inequity in today's world, and how little is being said or done about it, is quite shocking.

International nursing leadership from my perspective requires an ability to mobilize resources, identify needs, and set priorities, to listen and to learn and to change as the situation requires. It is also important to assist others to bring about the changes needed.

It is difficult when perhaps chief nurses are appointed because they are cousins of the minister or the spouse of a politician. But even in those circumstances, if they have the position, they have to be helped to do an overwhelming job.

Demb and Derr point out that "The management of future leadership and succession may be among the most important issues facing any company."[4] We can substitute institution or organization for "company," I am sure.

One aspect of leadership that is rarely done well is succession planning. That is a statement you may disagree with. But it is a difficult thing to do. Search committees and boards of directors may have very specific ideas of what type of leadership is needed for the next phase of an organization or school. It may not be what the one retiring would propose. Some studies show that if we select our own replacements either we may pick one set to fail (thus making us look good in retrospect) or someone very like ourselves who may be wrong for the future.

Yet career development, mentoring, and succession planning are important responsibilities for any leader in any country. In nursing, in many countries, this is a great lack. It is especially noticeable in those countries where the current leaders are not as well prepared as are some of the younger people. So instead of giving the young the chance to develop (such as preparing reports, representing the unit at meetings, developing budgets), current leaders hold youth back. Again culture is a factor. If you spend your whole life showing deference to anyone even slightly older than you are, then of course it will be hard not to hold onto receiving deference and exercising authority once it is yours.

Leadership is developed, whether in the family (in which instances people often say "a born leader"), in school, or in the workplace. Today's leaders must prepare and assist tomorrow's. Better role models are badly needed in many places. They exist in great numbers in others.

The role of women in any society has had a great influence on the development of nursing. Poor education from childhood is one obvious problem area as is the role of women in the home and in the workplace. The international news has been pointing out the sudden move forward of women in Japan, for example, where it has been very difficult to have a professional career.

If nursing leadership is to be improved, then potential leaders must be given the push and the support to meet their potential. It is very hard for those who go away to study to come back and be accepted by their peers. I once met a nurse who had gone abroad to study for a BSc, and 25 years later her colleagues were still bitter that she had not gone up the same ladder they had, earning certificates in a variety of nursing courses.

Faculty in educational settings must be aware of the situations their students will face, even more so if the student will be returning to another country. Discussions of what awaits them at work, what expectations others will have of them, and of what they expect of themselves may be helpful.

Leadership development is a continuous process. Klara Sövényi and I were at a meeting recently for chief nurses in Europe. It was the *first* time they had such an opportunity. Why? Maybe they had not asked or had not asked the right people, or maybe "the money is not available. Only the physicians and ministers meet." Ways must be found to keep people in key nursing positions up to date and prepared for future changes.

At ICN, association management and leadership development are among our high priorities. It is a difficult area. Goals are different, methods are different, but the needs are very similar and quite obvious worldwide.

One nurse said to me "I realize that our association is like a ladies' tea party when I see what others are doing." Perhaps that was the first step for her. She is now her association's president, and she is doing many good things.

I recently came across some mega trends identified by Jan Peter Paul[5] for business educators that nursing leadership needs to be aware of. Those trends are:

From strategy to structure
From centralization to decentralization
From function to systems
From hierarchy to horizontal networks (this one has special significance for the health system)
From hands to brains (also important to nursing)
From individuals to teams
From a soft culture to a hard culture (the culture of "success"—results and profits, again especially important for nursing)
Laissez-faire to social accountability (the growing importance of ethics)

If these trends are as significant for the health system and for nursing as I feel they are, then we must provide appropriate basic and continuous learning opportunities for those with leadership potential. They must be found when young enough, pushed a bit if needed, assisted in career planning, supported during their growth period, and exposed early to the inside working of the "corporate" life of health governments and educational institutions. Then they must be given the chance to perform before it is too late.

I was given such a push, several times, exposed to "internal" politics, allowed to learn from many real leaders, and then thrown in the pool. I survived. At least so far.

Preluncheon talks should not be long or heavy, but to help stimulate the digestion they should rumble things up a bit just to get those flitting ideas moving around.

Leaders of the future, according to a recent international survey, will need to be:

• People capable of inspiring managers to implement their optimistic views
• Ultimate communicators
• Ethical gurus who can set standards for their organizations and keep them out of trouble

- Master strategists, able to anticipate and sidestep conflicts before they become crises

To close I will just say if health care in the future is to come close to meeting the demands, then development of nursing leadership must be made a higher priority worldwide. This must be done by governments, organizations, educational institutions, funding agencies and by everyone here tonight, because in the year 2010 we will need to have health services of a high quality for ourselves.

Constance Holleran

REFERENCES

1 Vance, Connie Nicodemus, *Group Profile of Contemporary Influentials in American Nursing*, Ph.D. diss., Teachers College, Columbia Univ., N.Y., 1977.
2 Ibid., pp. 230–231.
3 Bitter, Joe D., *Tough Minded Leadership*, American Management Association, N.Y., 1989.
4 Demb, A., and Derr, C. B., "Managing Strategic Human Resources Leadership for the 21st Century," *European Management Journal*, June 1989, pp. 150–158.
5 Paul, Jan Peter, "The Consequences of Management—Trends on Business Education," *European Management Journal*, September 1989, pp. 284–285.

Conference Overview: International Nursing Development: Consensus on Solutions

Claire M. Fagin

The University of Pennsylvania School of Nursing convened the Bellagio Conference on International Nursing Development in the 21st Century to take stock of current world health problems and the challenges they present to nursing. The conferees considered changing health and illness profiles around the world in the next century and set out to develop the beginnings of a consensus on what nursing's international agenda should be to promote the health and well-being of the world's population. Of overall importance is the rapid implementation of the resolution of the forty-second World Health Assembly (42.27), which recommends greater participation of nurse/midwifery personnel at all levels and strengthened education and practice. All the recommendations which follow rest on the commitments implied by this resolution.

PRIORITY POLICY RECOMMENDATIONS

Nursing and midwifery are proven cost-effective investments in improving health outcomes. Many countries in the world are underinvesting in nursing/midwifery relative to other options and are thus not achieving as much healthcare as would be possible under present spending levels. Every country should undertake a systematic reappraisal of the relative resources invested in nursing/midwifery as compared to investments in physician training, hospitals, and acquisition of high technology.

The intuitive solution to cyclical nursing shortages that are plaguing every country in the world—increasing the supply of nurses—has not worked, not without other changes. Nurse-to-population ratios vary by a hundredfold between countries, but nursing shortages still persist. New solutions must be pursued that focus on controlling excess demand for nurses through better use of nurses and midwives.

International trade in nurses should be discouraged. It is clear that developed countries cannot solve their shortages by importing nurses in the absence of controlling excess demand for nurses. Moreover, the majority of countries that export large numbers of nurses have substantial health problems in their own countries that could be addressed by retention of more nurses. The conferees recognize the rights of any individual nurse to travel and seek employment internationally, but organized efforts to import significant numbers of nurses from countries that have a shortage of nurses and/or poor health indicators should be discouraged within the international community. Specifically, World Health Organization (WHO) and other private and public nursing education funds should be used cautiously in countries which engage in international trade in nurses.

Nurses and midwives are poorly compensated around the world relative to other professionals and relative to their contributions to health care. Poor wages and working conditions encourage poor retention of nurses, discourage qualified and talented young people from choosing nursing as a career, and lead to inappropriate utilization of nurses/midwives. Improvement in compensation, working conditions, and professional recognition of nurses and midwives is critical to maintaining an adequate pool of nurses worldwide.

In many parts of the world, families do not allow their children to elect nursing as a career due to cultural taboos as well as the perception of the profession's poor status. National governments in these countries should undertake educational programs to overcome these cultural biases and to educate families about nursing's record of promoting social mobility.

All countries must invest more resources in the education and strengthening of nursing/midwifery leadership. Leaders must be knowledgable in health economics and health policy development to help solve the human resource problems of their countries and to serve in policy, advisory, and management roles in the highest levels of government and the private sector. Regional or cross-country collaboration among nursing leaders (particularly in developing countries where leadership groups may be small and relatively isolated) is an efficient and effective strategy to develop nurse leaders in developing countries.

Efforts must be made to develop regional multi-institutional collaboration among nursing leaders, particularly in developing countries where leadership groups may be small and relatively isolated.

Educational programs in all countries should prepare students to work with and supervise those "nursing helpers" participating in formal, traditional, and informal caring, i.e., support personnel, healers and herbalists, family and friends.

Consultants brought in by ministries or international agencies to assist with curriculum development and preparation of licensing exams should be appropriate to the task, knowledgeable about the country and its needs and resources, and able to target their consultation at problems identified by the local nurses/midwives and governments.

Basic education in nursing should prepare generalists. Educational advancement through clinical specialization at the postbasic level provided in traditional graduate programs and through "distance" educational methods is crucial for both teachers and practitioners. Continuing education should be available in all countries, using on-site traditional methods as well as off-site "distance" educational methods to update knowledge in specific fields.

Nurses worldwide are dissatisfied with conditions of professional nursing practice in hospitals. To enhance recruitment and retention of nurses and improve outcomes, the organization and policies of hospitals must be reshaped to use nurses more effectively and to provide appropriate levels of support services and resources.

Every WHO regional office should have at least one highly qualified nurse/midwife, in addition to current nurse advisers.

It is futile to formulate solutions to health care problems affecting all peoples in the world today without the active involvement of a prepared, knowledgeable, respected nursing group. Nurses/midwives cannot achieve the necessary outcomes for their own development and that of their country's health care systems without marked change in governmental priorities, attitudes toward women and nursing, strategic planning, and respect for the body of practice that is commonly defined as "nursing." The papers prepared for the University of Pennsylvania Bellagio Conference speak eloquently to the current activities and potential of nurses/midwives. It is time to move on with the agenda of change.

The following is a distillation of the discussion of the conferees at the University of Pennsylvania Conferences on International Nursing Development held at the Rockefeller Conference Center in Bellagio, Lake Como, Italy. The following issues were identified at the outset of the conference; they shaped the conference discussion and recommendations:

Poor health outcomes are common in many parts of the world despite existing knowledge about how to improve health.

Maternal and infant mortality remain unacceptably high in much of the world.

The world's population is aging. Even developing countries are experiencing a dramatic growth in the number of elderly persons. Very few countries have adequately planned for the changing health services needs of an aging population.

AIDS has become a major threat to world health and requires both national and international intervention to control its spread and to care for those already infected.

Chronic illness has emerged as a major problem affecting populations in most countries. Yet resources continue to be disproportionately placed in the acute sector.

All countries of the world face growing demands for health care in a context of limited resources.

Nurses and/or midwives are cost-effective providers with proven records of accomplishment in all the above areas. Yet, nurses/midwives are in short supply around the world, and access to their service is limited. A major purpose of the conference was to explore why.

As mentioned, nurse-to-population ratios vary a hundredfold between countries. Yet, almost all countries experience cyclical or persistent nursing shortages, even those with high nurse-to-population ratios. Since increasing the supply of nurses, in the absence of other changes, has not prevented recurrent shortages in any part of the world, should nursing rethink its strategies to solve the shortage of nursing personnel from an international perspective?

How much of the shortage of nurses worldwide actually results from underinvestment in nursing/midwifery relative to investments in other kinds of health resources? Countries around the world appear to be making decisions about resource allocations within healthcare that are not justifiable in terms of marginal benefits. Nurse-to-physician ratios vary widely, and a substantial number of countries have more doctors than nurses, a distribution of resources that would not appear to be in the best interests of the health of the populations given constrained resources and unmet needs.

What are feasible strategies for educating

and positioning nursing/midwifery leaders so that they can educate and influence decision makers about national resource allocations?

The appropriate use of ancillary workers as extensions/assistants to nurses/midwives is a topic of debate around the world in both developed and developing countries. To what extent could ancillary personnel, appropriately organized and deployed, ameliorate nursing/midwifery shortages?

What are the appropriate nursing/midwifery education models for different parts of the world? The fact that the illness profile, resources, and educational standards vary so substantially from country to country suggests that no single nursing education model will apply around the world. How can countries be helped to develop a program of health professional education that meets their needs?

The remainder of this section will explore these issues from the perspective of four dimensions: health personnel, education, practice, and health policy. Chapters that follow discuss in considerable detail each of these dimensions from a country or regional standpoint. Those chapters represent the authors' perspective to a greater or lesser extent.

HEALTH PERSONNEL

There appears to be a worldwide shortage of nurses/midwives. The few countries reporting no present nursing shortage, e.g., New Zealand, have experienced a shortage within the past 5 years. Thus the problem of cyclical or long-lasting shortages of nurses seems to be a shared dilemma around the world. Paradoxically, nursing shortages persist across countries with widely varying nurse-to-population ratios. In the developed world, the shortage appears to be demand driven, resulting in large part from the growth of technology and from inappropriate use of nurses. In developing countries, the shortage of nurses is real

and acute and is a result of an insufficient number of qualified nurses plus too few budgeted positions. Increasing the supply of nurses, in the absence of other changes, has not been effective in eliminating the worldwide nurse shortage, and other solutions should be sought.

Data on nurses/midwives and other health workers are difficult to compare across countries. Countries define nurses/midwives differently; often little information exists on the work histories of those originally trained as nurses/midwives, so many countries cannot estimate retention rates; finally, many countries do not keep records of the number of nurses working in various settings, i.e., hospital versus community care. It is thus not surprising that few countries even attempt to plan for health personnel needs, since so little information is available on present supply and demand. One recommendation was to improve national data on nurse/midwives and other health care personnel. At the very least each country should establish a registration system that periodically requires each nurse/midwife to complete a minimal data sheet.

The international trade in nurses is of increasing concern as developed countries continue to use more nurses than are available domestically. Developed countries should not recruit nurses from countries that are themselves experiencing shortages. Complicating the situation is that in some of the countries claiming shortages, budgeted positions for qualified nurses are so limited or wages are so substandard as to make it unrealistic for qualified nurses to remain in their home countries. A better option for all countries of the world would be for developed countries to utilize their existing supply of domestic nurses more effectively and to reduce reliance on foreign-trained nurses. Countries that now export nurses, often educated at public expense, should be encouraged to fund enough positions to enable their nurses to stay in nursing and to help improve health outcomes in their own countries. Educational exchanges should be encouraged, but countries should be cautioned against "pirating" the trainees. WHO and other fellowship-granting institutions are asked to review the process by which fellowships are granted so that nations that engage consistently in international trade of nurses/midwives are not subsidized by the fellowship programs.

Nurse/midwife shortages have an important political dimension. Many countries have not defined nursing/midwifery as a priority within health care despite much evidence on its cost-effectiveness. To educate policy makers, nurses are needed in the highest levels of government as advocates for a more appropriate distribution of health resources, which would include nursing/midwifery support.

In many countries there is concern about the inappropriate substitution of others for qualified nurses/midwives and of insufficient numbers of nurses/midwives to supervise and receive referrals from ancillary workers. On the one hand, in developing countries, much of the front line care is delivered by untrained and unsupervised persons. This results in poor outcomes, including high maternal and infant mortality. On the other hand, in developed countries, the lack of access to qualified nurses/midwives often leads to more expensive care of questionable quality. One example is the high rate of cesarean sections in the United States (1 out of 4 births). Access to midwives in the United States is limited compared to the United Kingdom, where 85 percent of deliveries are by midwives. Clearly this issue must be addressed in examining health personnel supply and policies governing practice.

In subsequent chapters specific national or regional human resource issues will be considered more fully by Aiken, Clark, Hancock,

and Dai. In discussion the conferees agreed that solving shortages of nurses/midwives must start with government priorities in allocation of resources. In some countries additional funds for health care are essential to improve health outcomes of the population. However, even without a larger investment, those funds currently available need to be distributed differently to meet the health needs of the country where they exist.

This recommendation might include a better balance between the numbers of physicians and nurses. Most agree that there should be at least two qualified nurses for every physician at a minimum, and a more cost-effective ratio in developing countries with large rural populations would be more on the order of four or more nurses per physician.

The question of money is an essential part of the solution. In many countries nurses' wages are not commensurate with their education and responsibilities, making recruitment and retention of qualified persons to careers in nursing/midwifery extremely difficult. Directly connected with financial reward, although with somewhat different connotations, is the question of the status of nursing within countries. Although equitable pay would improve the status of nurses, often cultural beliefs and values associated with the practice of nursing deter women and men from entering the field. Here the solution lies in educating families about the legitimacy of nursing/midwifery and in making nursing an attractive career opportunity.

To solve human resource problems in nursing/midwifery, global, regional, and national goals must reevaluate the distribution of national health care resources and effect change that would yield the greatest benefits to the population and develop appropriate opportunities for advancement and compensation to make nursing more attractive as a career option.

EDUCATIONAL GOALS AND IMPLEMENTATION

The differences in standards and methods for educating nurses/midwives throughout the world are enormous. Currently, work is underway to standardize definitions and set regulations for practice which will bring some measure of comparability to the definition of *nurse* or *midwife* and to the education of these individuals. Nonetheless the conferees chose to acknowledge differences existing at this time and to be flexible and consultative rather than prescriptive in their recommendations. Despite differences in educational requirements, recruitment of students is a problem in most countries. This problem was viewed as very serious now and with dangerous future implications. Further, the problem cannot be solved without the changes described above dealing with personnel resource issues and other changes affecting currently practicing nurses/midwives to be discussed below. The current student recruitment and personnel resources problems cannot be solved by downgrading nursing education or entry requirements to nursing programs. Rather the needs of all the countries represented indicated the importance of careful selection of students because of the priority for autonomous practice in the community and supervision of untrained personnel. Although the conferees were not prescriptive in stating educational requirements, we agreed that such requirements should be both appropriate to the country and comparable to other professions. As the level of general education rises for other groups, so should that of nursing.

It was agreed that education must reflect a view of the future demography of the country where education is occurring. All countries, including the developing world, are experiencing a rapid increase in the number of older people and people with chronic, debilitating conditions. Attention must be given to the continuing development of technology and acute care, but the increasing chronicity in health care problems of our world population requires comparably increasing attention to maintenance of function as well as primary care. Nursing education in all countries must include content on HIV infection with emphasis on how nurses can contribute to controlling transmission as well as caring for those with HIV-related illnesses. Nursing/midwifery education requires a balance between tertiary (high-technology) care and primary health care, but the present almost singular emphasis on acute, episodic, and disease-oriented care is increasingly a mismatch for the needs of developed and developing countries with their growing aging and chronically ill populations.

Efforts must be made to develop regional multi-institutional collaboration among nursing leaders, particularly in developing countries, under the auspices of governments, nongovernment organizations, bilateral and multilateral aid agencies, and regional groupings of states. Superb examples of such regional collaboration were provided at the meeting by the three participants from Latin America—Esperanza de Monterrossa, Ilta Lange, and Roseni Chompré—and by Helen Grace of the Kellogg Foundation.

The question of nurses/midwives working with untrained staff in auxiliary roles or in direct patient care received a great deal of attention. There was strong agreement that educational programs in all countries should integrate content, helping students learn how to work with and supervise those "nursing helpers" participating in formal, traditional, and informal caring, e.g., assistants, healers and herbalists, family and friends.

The need for standards was discussed at length. There was also discussion about the problem of irrelevancy of examinations in some countries, standards of professional excellence, contemporary trends of care, and quality of care. Advice on curriculum, standards, and examinations should be available from the professional nursing and midwifery organizations in the country and/or worldwide. Although much work is going on at present in examining credentialing, regulation, and standards, licensing examinations for entry into practice should be consistent with the curricula offered, and countries should be encouraged to ensure the congruence of curricula and exams. Where consultants are brought in to augment the formal structure, those brought in through the help of international agencies should be appropriate to the task, knowledgeable about the country and its needs and resources, and able to target their consultation at problems identified by the local nurses and governments.

It was clear to the conferees that educational programs should be based on the health needs of the population and should present content aimed at developing cost-effective strategies for providing high-quality care in rural areas, marginal urban areas, and to the seriously ill in hospitals. Students must be prepared for working where there are serious restraints in resources and technology.

There was great concern about the quality of clinical teaching. The conferees recommended that clinical faculty of schools of nursing/midwifery must maintain current, relevant clinical experience and be clinically competent. Although basic education in nursing/midwifery should prepare generalists, teaching clinical nursing content requires faculty who have sufficient knowledge and experience about the practice area. As mentioned, educational advancement through clinical specialization at the post-basic level provided in traditional graduate programs and through "distance" educational methods is crucial for both teachers and practitioners. Students must be taught by such specialized practice teachers and experience advanced practice in clinical settings. Continuing education should

be available in all countries, again using on-site traditional methods as well as off-site "distance" educational methods to update knowledge in specific fields.

Finally, the group recommended that all countries invest more resources in the education and strengthening of nursing/midwifery leadership. Leaders must be prepared to help solve the human resource problems of their countries and to serve in policy, advisory, and management roles in the highest levels of government and the private sector. Without such preparation countries cannot expect to answer the serious questions in health care and education of health care workers with which we are all grappling.

CHALLENGES TO PRACTICE

The Bellagio Conference agreed that there is an urgent need to implement resolution WHA 42.27 of the forty-second World Health Assembly (Appendix 1). This resolution requests the director-general:

1 To increase support to member states to strengthen the planning, implementation, and evaluation of the nursing/midwifery component of national health programs, in particular the development, utilization, and improvement of the qualifications of nursing/midwifery personnel
2 To strengthen the nursing/midwifery components of all WHO programs, increasing within available resources the number of nurses and midwives in senior positions at global and regional levels
3 To intensify support for the global network of WHO-collaborating centers for nursing development and, through these centers, promote the involvement of other institutions and agencies in extending WHO's work
4 To promote and support the training of nursing/midwifery personnel in research methodology to facilitate their participation in health research programs, including the development of information systems on nursing/midwifery

5 To develop tools for monitoring progress in this field and to report to the forty-fifth World Health Assembly on the progress made in the implementation of this resolution.

All nursing/midwifery professional organizations and policy makers, international organizations, and countries should undertake the planning necessary for rapid implementation of strategies for strengthening nursing/midwifery to achieve health for all by the year 2000.

The Bellagio Conference also recommends that every WHO regional office have at least one highly qualified nurse/midwife, in addition to current nurse advisers. Global experiences in infant and maternal mortality mandate such expertise throughout international health organizations. The Safe Motherhood Initiative (WHA 27) is an important program for reducing maternal mortality. Nurses/midwives must be more actively involved in this initiative through practice and in ensuring that necessary content is integrated in curricula worldwide.

Nursing/midwifery practice covers the spectrum of care from traditional, informal, and self-care through high- and low-technology nursing and medical care. Nursing/midwifery care is flexible in its orientations and implementations in that, providing a thorough generalist education, it can expand and contract in both directions in times of need.

Given this view of nursing/midwifery practice, several concerns emerge worldwide. One concern is the quality of clinical practice, particularly when many of the people giving direct care are unqualified or poorly qualified. Yet nursing/midwifery must be responsible for maintaining its standards of practice. Thus it was agreed that nurses/midwives must mobilize all informal careers, enhancing practices which are not harmful and identifying and eliminating those which are harmful. Although nurses/midwives must be in control of their practice, legal and moral problems of accountability occur when nurses/midwives feel responsible for the outcomes of care provided by untrained personnel under their supervision.

Experienced nurses/midwives have the knowledge to challenge problematic practices, participate in defining policy, publicly express needs, and respond to inappropriate outside advice. The opinions of informed nurses/midwives should be used to mold public attitudes about health and health care with prior regard for the opinions of the people served and their communities. An informed citizenry may have different ideas from professionals about how their health care needs should be met.

Primary health care in communities was the driving force in most of the discussion about education and practice. Many reasons explain this primary focus. First, the needs of our nations now and in the future militate for a major shift in resources from institutions to communities. Most of the very serious problems in our nations are not amenable to institutional care and are caused by poor education, unhealthy lifestyles, environmental problems, and the like. Demographic changes, poverty, lack of access to health care when it is needed, high infant mortality, maternal mortality, AIDS, and morbidity in vulnerable groups require a major focus of human and other resources in communities. Nursing/midwifery has its most powerful solutions to lend to the community, since nursing models of care include prevention, health teaching, health promotion, counseling and support of patients and families, and direct patient care. These models of care are congruent with community health needs in most of our countries.

Nonetheless, this focus on community primary health care should not exclude the need for nurses to continue to address the needs and problems of hospitals and the patients who are being treated in hospitals. A compelling commonality among the countries appeared with regard to nurses' attitudes about hospital work. There is a sense of extreme dissatisfaction, worldwide, with hospital practice because of rigidity; lack of autonomy for nurses; patient dissatisfaction; nurses' concern about quality of care; lack of resources such as supplies, equipment, and staff; overwork; stress; and nurses' perception that their work is not respected by physicians and administrators. Because of these conditions in most parts of the world, nurses may be perceived as turning their backs on hospital practice and on nursing itself; either outcome poses extreme danger to our communities. The conferees agreed that the philosophy of primary health care could be implemented in all settings and that nurses must assist others in reconceptualizing hospital care to be consumer centered. Primary health care is a strategy in such a goal.

Unfortunately, many developing countries are investing a large share of their resources in institutional care and western technology and drugs, emulating the developed countries and often disregarding the pressing needs of the majority of their citizenry. Insufficient attention is given to nursing in these countries as well. Clearly, strategies must be developed and implemented to recruit, retain, educate, reorient, and improve the qualifications of nurses/midwives to meet national health care needs wherever they occur.

Restraints to nursing practice come from such attitudes as well as absent or restrictive legislation, nurses' own limiting perspectives, and the constraints created by domination by other professionals, and, in some countries, their possibly limited education. At the very least the latter problem can be addressed internally as was indicated in the previous section. The conferees believe that major emphasis should be placed on examining and revising legislation. Nurses/midwives must be represented in formulating regulations affect-

ing health care, so that legislation is enabling of their effective practice in facilitating access to health care.

NURSING AND HEALTH POLICY ISSUES

Changing the policy agenda, changing the system of health care delivery, reorienting priorities, allocating resources more appropriately, and changing restrictive regulations are inherently health policy activities. The challenge for nurses and nursing/midwifery is to become effective participants in their countries' health systems and work with other health professionals and consumers, with common goals, to bring about necessary change. A well-developed, well-targeted health policy agenda based on nursing/midwifery's strengths and unique contributions will facilitate participation in the system. Obviously, nurses/midwives must be well educated and well positioned to advance this agenda in a competitive environment involving other interest groups.

As mentioned earlier, a greater investment in nursing/midwifery leadership is crucial to accomplish both the country's and nursing's goals for quality health care, improved nursing/midwifery education, strategies for supervision and teaching of auxiliary workers, and policy formulation. It is folly for countries to believe that plans for essential nursing/midwifery personnel can be achieved without the active involvement of nursing/midwifery leaders. Nurses must be well enough educated and positioned to be able to participate in a competitive environment involving other interest groups. Some countries have virtually no persons who meet any definition of *leaders* by virtue of education, experience, or placement in the system. For this reason and others, the Bellagio Conference recommends that the necessary nonnursing disciplines, such as economists, sociologists, demographers, physicians, and other scientists, be employed to collaborate with nurses/midwives in advancing the policy agenda.

The issue of shortage is extremely unclear, in part because data are inconsistent across countries; based on different definitions of nurses/midwives, the data give inadequate information on the profile of careers, they provide no indication of whether the numbers have anything to do with who is working or where, and they are often unrelated to health indicators of countries. Further there is little indication that needs for nursing/midwifery personnel have been defined; thus estimates of the need for nurses/midwives may be subjective and not based on real demand. Despite these data problems, the Bellagio conferees agreed that although the data may not be ideal, more exist than are currently used by nurses/midwives and country policy makers to advance the health policy agenda. Great and largely unutilized power results from the large numbers of nurses/midwives in many countries, and their largely positive public image, often more positive than that held by nurses/midwives themselves. Thus nurses/midwives do not capitalize on these assets in public forums. Nurses must make greater use of international comparisons and international collaboration and form alliances with other influential interests to advance their agenda to improve health care.

We know that economic development is related to improved health. However, education, particularly of women, has been the single most important indicator of improved health status, such as reducing infant and maternal mortality. We indicated above that nurses/midwives should build alliances with other health professionals and consumers; a concentrated effort must also be made to build alliances with educators and organizations of educators for the future health care of people. In coalition with educators and consumers,

using shared data, individual interests and skills can be actuated to change the policy agenda and implement rhetoric to improve health for the largest portion of the population. We recommend that nursing/midwifery organizations seek coalitions with local, regional, national, and international organizations of educators to fulfill our joint health agenda.

Policy implications for every country can be drawn from their demographic changes and the resulting health and illness needs:

- The increase in problems of health and function related to aging
- The dilemma of countries experiencing a discontinuity in population trends
- The increase of chronic health problems among children and adults

Nurses/midwives and others need to develop and utilize models for the prevention of secondary disability and restoration and maintenance of ability which emphasize quality of life. Given the same chronic disease state, there is great variability depending on the management of the condition. Nurses/midwives have the knowledge and experience to take on the challenge of managing direct care and the environment of patients with irreversible conditions to prevent secondary disability. Policy changes including legislation and education must liberalize nursing's potential to play these vital roles.

All the policy recommendations imply the importance of nursing research to understand and provide validity for nursing interventions. An important area of research where nurses should be playing an increasing role is that of technology assessment which often leads to the recommendation of policy. The Bellagio conferees suggest to nurses that they apply strong pressure to governments and non-government organizations to include nurses on national and regional policy-making bodies, including panels for technology assessment, reimbursement decisions, and related regulatory decisions. Necessary knowledge for leadership includes the understanding of the forces driving expenditures in their countries as well as the principles of technology assessment. National nursing organizations should identify nurses/midwives who are informed, articulate, and expert and publish a listing for reference to national and regional groups requiring nursing involvement in technology assessment. If they fail to achieve representation on policy-making bodies, nurses must form assessment groups of their own and publicize incidents of misuse of technology and lobby for changes in policy by publishing and disseminating their findings in the media and through coalitions with other health professionals.

One concluding comment seems relevant. The conference underscored the immense differences in educational preparation for nursing/midwifery around the world and the difference in resources and practice settings. Thus, it is truly remarkable that there is a common understanding among nursing leaders throughout the world as to what is nursing/midwifery, the core components of nursing/midwifery care, and a consensus on shared values and goals. The fact that we share a common language in this regard bodes well for our hopes to develop and implement an international agenda to improve world health.

Section One

Manpower Needs

Discussion points were prepared for each of the major themes of the conference. The presenters were asked to respond to these points so that areas of commonality and difference could be identified. An outline served to unify the chapters in the section without constraining authors from discussing other problems and issues relating to the topic.

For Section One, the presenters were asked to discuss the following:

1 Is there a shortage of nurses in your country or region? Do you have a method for forecasting nursing work force needs and supply? Please discuss data you have on this subject.

2 There is some evidence that the nursing shortage may be worldwide. Provide evidence from your country on the existence of a nursing shortage if this does exist.

3 Is your country a supplier (exporter) or an importer of nurses to or from other countries? Is this a problem for you? Do you have policies for dealing with this?

4 What is your national plan for balancing the "supply and demand" for nursing now and in the future?

5 If you are experiencing a nursing shortage, is this generalized or specific to certain practice areas? Please specify and describe any plan for meeting these specific supply problems.

6 If you have a shortage of nurses, is this related to shortages of other health personnel, such as physicians, aides, and allied health workers?

Chapter 1

An Analysis of the U.S. Experience

Linda Aiken

Most countries in the world are presently experiencing shortages of qualified nurses. Nursing shortages threaten to undermine access to quality health care and impede reaching the goal of health for all by the year 2000.[1]

Nursing shortages are commonly assumed to be the consequence of an insufficient supply of nurses. Thus, most policy initiatives to ameliorate nursing shortages focus on increasing the number of nurses. Such strategies include expanding enrollments to nursing schools, abbreviating the time required to educate nurses, using student nurses to offset shortages of graduate nurses, substituting persons with less training for nurses, and importing nurses from other countries.

However, supply-oriented policies alone will not solve nursing shortages. The case of

the United States demonstrates that in a developed country with a technologically sophisticated medical care system, vast increases in nurse supply have not satisfied national employer demand for nurses. Rather, a paradox exists where the more nurses there are, the more nurses are wanted.

Our research at this point has been limited to the United States, and thus we cannot draw inferences about nursing shortages in other countries. However, we suspect that other developed countries are experiencing similar problems of a demand-driven shortage. The nursing personnel issues in developing countries are sufficiently different to require a separate analysis. Hence, we will not here attempt to respond specifically to the issues of developing countries except to draw attention to the interrelationship between the growing demand for nurses in developed countries and the recruitment by these countries of nurses from the developing world.

We do need to think about health personnel policies differently. Specifically, we need to understand the factors affecting demand for nurses worldwide, and we need to develop strategies that influence demand as well as the supply of nurses in order to achieve a more appropriate balance between the two.

DETERMINING HOW MANY NURSES ARE NEEDED

Nurse-to-population ratios vary widely between countries and within single countries. Table 1-1 presents nurse-to-population ratios for selected countries as reported by the World Health Organization (WHO). These ratios vary from a low in Pakistan of 1.8 nurses per 10,000 population to 123.8 nurses per 10,000 people in New Zealand, a sixty-eight-fold difference. (Some representatives at the Bellagio conference questioned the accuracy of these ratios for their countries. However, absent any other international data, we use them here for illustrative purposes and assume that the relative differences between countries are roughly correct.)

Table 1-1 illustrates vividly that a greater supply of nurses has not solved nursing shortages. New Zealand, ranked by WHO as having one of the highest nurse-to-population ratios in the world, does not currently have a nursing shortage but had one as recently as 1985. Both Australia and the United States have high nurse-to-population ratios and are currently experiencing acute shortages of nurses in hospitals.

The United States has the largest number of nurses in the aggregate of any country in the world—over 2.1 million registered professional nurses (RNs) and another 900,000 licensed practical nurses (the latter would meet

Table 1-1 Nurse-to-Population Ratios for Selected Countries, 1984

	Absolute number	Rate per 10,000 population
Pakistan	20,295	1.8
Brazil	25,889	2.0
Chile	3,355	2.8
Columbia	9,800	3.5
Nigeria	37,112	4.3
Venezuela	8,914	5.3
China	759,485	7.2
Thailand	54,012	10.7
Israel	12,110	29.5
U.K.	182,897	32.5
West Germany	200,997	33.4
U.S.	1,943,700	83.0
Australia	139,434	93.4
New Zealand	40,950	123.8

Source: World Health Organization. *World Health Statistics Annual.* Geneva, 1988.

many countries' definition of qualified nurse). Yet, the United States has experienced two crippling nursing shortages within the past decade. Within the United States, the supply of nurses varies by geographic region from 44.1 registered nurses per 10,000 people in Louisiana to 116.6 in Massachusetts. However, hospitals in Boston, Massachusetts, where nurse-to-population ratios are among the highest, have experienced shortages as acute as anywhere in the country.

Nursing shortages have persisted in developed countries despite substantial increases in nurse-to-population ratios. The United States is an extreme example of this phenomenon. Between 1960 and 1988, the registered-nurse-to-population ratio in the United States increased from 28.2 to 66.8 RNs per 10,000 population, a 140 percent increase. Yet, there is continuing evidence of widespread and serious shortages of nurses across the United States, particularly in hospitals.[2] The intuitive solution to the nursing shortage, increasing the supply of nurses, has not worked thus far in the United States. The more nurses there are, the more nurses employers want to hire, and demand keeps growing at a faster rate than supply.[3]

The most common method of assessing the adequacy of nursing personnel for policy purposes is by use of nurse-to-population ratios, even though this method has serious limitations. Cross-national nursing personnel studies have relied primarily on nurse-to-population ratios because the majority of countries report the two relevant data elements to construct the ratio: the number of people trained as nurses and the size of the overall population. However, the accuracy of information on nurse supply is uneven, since many countries do not have a nurse registry which is periodically updated. Moreover, the definition of *nurse* varies widely across the world. Finally, nurses practice in a context that is shared with other personnel, particularly physicians. To evaluate the meaning of nurse-to-population ratios, information is also required on nurse-to-physician ratios and use of traditional healers.

Nurse-to-population ratios are most useful in assessing relative personnel resources, since an "ideal" ratio is difficult to establish. For example, nurse-to-population ratios are useful in comparing nurse resources across comparable countries or between geographic areas within a given country to estimate relative shortages or geographic maldistribution of current resources. Nurse-to-population ratios are also useful in forecasting future needs using current ratios and assumptions about expected population changes (such as age structure) and anticipated changes in the health care delivery system (such as increases in hospital bed supply).

One of the major limitations of nurse-to-population ratios in public policy and planning is the lack of a normative standard of what would be an acceptable ratio to seve as a goal by which progress could be measured. Need-based forecasting models for human resource planning have been developed to overcome this weakness. In need-based models, panels of experts set normative standards by defining how many nurses (or physicians, etc.) would be optimally required to meet the health care needs of a given population with specified characteristics. Estimates of the ideal are based on the prevalence of disease and disability, demographic characteristics of the population, and the types of health services available or desired.

Need-based measures of nursing personnel requirements have the advantage of setting a goal in which quality of care and reasonable access to services are implicit and against which progress can be measured. However, projections derived from need-based models are often so far in excess of what can be reasonably attained in countries with limited resources as to render them of limited utility in a policy context. In such cases, international comparisons of nurse-to-population ratios or nurse-to-physician ratios may be more useful.

Need-based models for estimating the nursing requirements in the developed world have been traditionally limited by insufficiently incorporated measures of demand for nurses. This is a major weakness since, as we will discuss in greater detail, shortages in the United States, and perhaps in many other developed countries, are now more driven by swings in demand than by changes in supply.

THE U.S. NURSING SHORTAGE: EXPLANATIONS AND SOLUTIONS

In the U.S. context, the term nurse usually refers to a registered professional nurse (RN). At present three kinds of educational programs qualify graduates to take the professional nurse licensing exam: 2-year associate degree community college programs, 3-year hospital diploma programs, and 4-year baccalaureate university programs. The United

States has another category of nursing personnel—the licensed practical or vocational nurse (LPN or LVN). LPNs usually having a high school education and complete a 1-year technical training program. LPNs in the United States have a more limited legal scope of practice and work under the supervision of an RN. Thus, in the U.S. context licensed practical nurses (LPNs) are considered to be ancillary personnel to nurses, although in an international context LPNs might be considered the equivalent of qualified nurses in some countries. In the following analysis of the U.S. nursing shortage, we will stay with the U.S. usage of the term *nurse* to refer only to RNs.

Vacancy rates for registered professional nurses in U.S. hospitals almost tripled between 1984 and 1987 (see Figure 1-1). Over three-quarters of all hospitals currently report a shortage of nurses; almost one in five describe their shortage as severe. Thirty percent of hospitals in urban areas and 15 percent of rural hospitals reported closing hospital beds in 1987 as a result of the nursing shortage.[2]

Cyclical shortages of RNs have occurred in the United States since World War II, but the current shortage is particularly perplexing, since the national supply of nurses has increased quite significantly in recent years (see

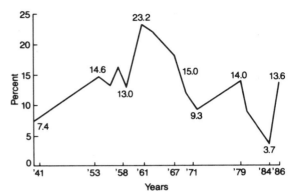

Figure 1-1 Nurse Vacancy Rates in Hospitals, 1941–1986.

Figure 1-2). Moreover, during the period in which the current shortage developed, hospital inpatient utilization declined significantly as a result of changing hospital reimbursement policy, efforts to reduce hospital utilization to control expenditures, and new technologies enabling many procedures formerly requiring an inpatient stay to be done on an outpatient basis. There were 51 million fewer inpatient hospital days in 1988 than in 1981. This scenario would suggest a surplus of nurses rather than a shortage. As recently as the fall of 1988, the Department of Health and Human Services in its report to the President and Con-

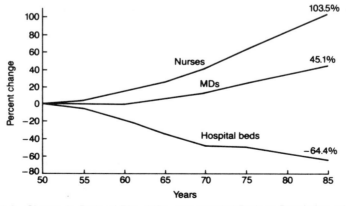

Figure 1-2 Change in Ratio of RNs, MDs, and Hospital Beds to Population, 1950–1985.

gress concluded that the supply of nurses was in balance with requirements until into the next century.[4]

Common Misconceptions about the Causes of the Nursing Shortage

Several misconceptions about the causes of the U.S. nursing shortage are common. These misconceptions are important to disclose because essays and press reports on nursing shortages in other developed countries often use these same explanations. Although we have data at this point only for the United States, we suspect that if these explanations were systematically investigated in countries such as Australia, New Zealand, Canada, and the United Kingdom, these explanations would no more provide plausible explanations for the nursing shortages in these countries than they do in the United States.

One commonly held misconception in the United States is that dissatisfied nurses are leaving their profession in large numbers. Although job dissatisfaction is common among U.S. nurses, approximately 80 percent are employed at any given time; this is a very high employment rate for a predominantly female occupation. Although the nurse turnover in hospitals averages about 20 percent a year, follow-up studies document that most of the resigning nurses are not lost to the hospital labor pool. Ninety percent obtain a job in another hospital, usually in the same local labor market.

About one-third of employed nurses in the United States work part-time, representing a potentially underutilized resource, although studies suggest that a large share of part-time nurses return to full-time employment as their children grow older. The high rate of part-time employment in nursing is consistent with the predominantly female character of the nursing work force, although some believe that these nurses would increase the hours they work if the economic rewards were great enough to offset the added costs of child care and domestic help associated with full-time employment.

Only about 5 percent of registered nurses in the United States work in nonhealth jobs, suggesting that the specialized nature of nursing education does not permit nurses to move easily into other occupations of comparable status without additional education. It has also been suggested that the growing number of jobs for nurses in ambulatory care and other nontraditional settings has siphoned nurses away from hospital practice. Quite to the contrary, hospitals have increased the number of nurses employed in the aggregate and the ratio of nurses to patients by more than 25 percent since 1982 (see Figure 1-3). It is true that more nurses work in ambulatory settings than ever before, but hospitals continue to employ two-thirds of an ever-increasing pool of RNs.

Enrollments in nursing schools have fallen significantly, 26 percent since 1983, causing great alarm as to the future supply of nurses. However, despite declining enrollments, still many more new graduates come into the employment pool each year than do nurses leave. Even if the trend in lower enrollments continues, the actual supply of nurses is expected to continue to increase until after the turn of the century. In any event, the recent decline in nursing school enrollments does not provide

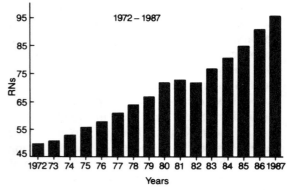

Figure 1-3 Hospital RNs Employed per 100 Average Adjusted Daily Patient Census.

an explanation for the current U.S. nursing shortage.

Explanations for Increased Demand

The current nursing shortage, then, has not been caused by a decline in the number of employed nurses but is due to an increase in the number of additional nurse positions offered by hospitals. In economic terms, the U.S. nursing shortage is demand driven and, specifically, hospital driven.

Demographic shifts, such as the aging of the population, and changing disease profiles, including the emergence of the AIDS epidemic, have contributed to the gradual increase in the demand for nurses in the United States and across many countries of the world. However, shifting age structure and changing disease and disability profiles do not occur rapidly enough to explain cyclical nursing shortages in a country as large as the United States. The increase in nursing supply over the past decade in the United States should have been more than enough to offset the increasing need for nurses as a result of these changes.

Unlike demographic changes that occur gradually, changes in financing of care in the U.S. context can effect rapid change in the utilization of hospitals and thus on the demand for nurses. Some of the recent increased employment of nurses by hospitals that is at the heart of the U.S. nursing shortage has been the result of dramatically altered patterns of hospital care resulting, in large part, from a major change in hospital reimbursement in 1983 known as the Medicare Prospective Payment System. The details of the change in hospital payment are not important for this discussion except that they included new financial incentives for hospitals to discharge patients as quickly as possible. And following the introduction of the new program, length of stay declined significantly. In addition, other public and private cost-containment initiatives lead to reduced hospital admissions made pos-

sible because of advances in surgical technology and innovations in noninvasive diagnostic testing.

On the one hand, the decline in hospital utilization reduced the demand for nurses, since there were far fewer inpatients in U.S. hospitals. On the other hand, the nursing care needs of the average hospitalized patient are reported to be greater. A scientific oversight committee appointed by the federal government to monitor the new hospital payment plan estimated that there was a "real case mix change" in U.S. hospitals of 14.2 percent between 1981 and 1988 as a result of the above changes.[5] Yet, the nurse-to-patient ratio over the same period increased by twice that rate—about 28 percent. Thus, the changing needs of hospitalized patients offer a partial explanation for the increased employment of nurses, but does not provide a convincing explanation for the entire increase since the reduced volume of patients should have offset, to some degree, the higher nursing care needs of the remaining patients.

In essence, employers have hired more nurses than can be accounted for solely on the basis of population need. This explains why federal manpower analysts conclude that the supply of nurses is in balance with national requirements in the midst of a perceived nursing shortage.[4] The federal nursing work force projection model is based on estimates of national requirements for nurses and does not take into account rapidly changing employer demand.

Labor Substitutions: The Preference for RNs

A major determinant of the demand for any worker is the cost of that worker compared to other possible alternatives. Cost to the employer is a function of wage rates and productivity. RNs are very versatile and productive in comparison to others in a hospital context; RNs perform a wide range of functions in addition to nursing care and require little supervision. Thus, when their wage rates are low compared to alternative kinds of workers, employers offer more nurse positions. For example, unless the wages of RNs are significantly higher than those of a ward clerk, it may be more economical for a hospital to employ an RN who is responsible for patient care and clerical duties than a clerk who is limited to clerical duties and who cannot pitch in to help care for patients if the nursing staff is overextended.

Unlike many other countries, nurses' wages in the United States are determined by competitive market forces, not by central decisions made by government or the hospital industry. Various factors can affect nurses' wage rates relative to others. The two historically important factors have been the unionization and resulting wage gains for ancillary nursing personnel in the United States, which narrowed the wage difference between RNs and others (LPNs and aides). And hospital cost-containment policies that have adversely affected the wages of RNs compared to those of other potential employees of hospitals such as administrative and clerical workers, housekeeping staff, dietary personnel, and other health professionals such as social workers, physical therapists, and pharmacists.

When there is a narrow difference between the market wage rates for nurses and those for other kinds of hospital employees, hospitals exhibit a preference for professional registered nurses (RNs). Over the past two decades, RNs have replaced large numbers of licensed practical nurses (LPNs) and aides in U.S. hospitals (see Figure 1-4). Between 1982 and 1987, U.S. hospitals reduced LPN employment by more than 67,000 full-time equivalent (FTE) positions, while increasing the employment of RNs. In 1989, more than 60 percent of nursing care personnel in U.S. hospitals were RNs, compared with only one-third in 1966. Many hospitals have only RNs providing patient care.

One important explanation for this shift toward more RNs was a narrowing of the wage differences between RNs, LPNs and aides.[6] The wages of LPNs, for example, are about 73 percent of those of RNs.[7] When costs of supervision and limitations of legal practice are factored in, at current wage rates RNs are a more economical choice for hospitals than LPNs or aides. Under the wage rates that have prevailed in the United States over the two past decades, it was cost effective for hospitals to move toward all-RN staffs.[8,9]

Also in response to pressures to contain

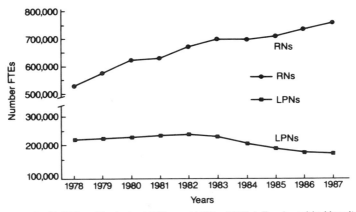

Figure 1-4 Full-Time Equivalent RNs and LPNs (FTEs) Employed in Hospitals

rapidly escalating costs, hospitals reduced the employment of nonnursing service support personnel such as clerks, technicians of all kinds, maintenance personnel, and patient transport couriers. Although the formal responsibilities of nurses did not change, in reality nurses had to take on more nonnursing responsibilities, particularly at night and on weekends. Between 1982 and 1985, the beginning of the present U.S. nursing shortage, the overall work force in hospitals was reduced by more than 300,000 positions, and positions for nurses increased by 40,000 over the same period. Now, nurses, on average, spend only about one-third of their time in direct patient care, apparently spending much of the remainder in activities that do not require the attention of a professional nurse but must be attended to for the comfort and/or safety of patients.[10,11]

Thus, a picture emerges of a restructuring of the work force in U.S. hospitals with greater reliance on RNs. As indicated in Figure 1-5, nurses' wages were seriously eroded by inflation throughout the decade of the seventies and the early eighties. Annual wage increases did not keep up with inflation. Thus, only now are nurses' real wages returning to what they were in the early 1970s. Thus, hospitals were able to replace aides and LPNs with RNs be-

cause RN relative wages were low compared to the cost of employing alternative personnel.[12] To prevent widespread substitution of nurses for others in a free market economy such as that in the United States, RN wages would probably have to be significantly higher than those of alternative workers, because nurses are viewed as contributing to good care, a matter of considerable value in an increasingly competitive hospital industry.[13]

The substitution of nurses for lower-level ancillary workers has not happened to the same extent in other health care settings in the United States. Ancillary nursing personnel are still much in evidence in all long-term care institutional settings such as nursing homes for the elderly and public mental hospitals and in home-based services. But it is the hospital system that drives the primary demand for nurses, regardless of whether this is the appropriate distribution of resources to meet population needs. Thus, as hospitals become more advanced technologically throughout the world, the demand for highly qualified nurses can be expected to escalate rapidly.

Potential Solutions to the U.S. Shortage

Wage Increases Hospital administrators generally do not believe that pay increases attract additional nurses into local labor mar-

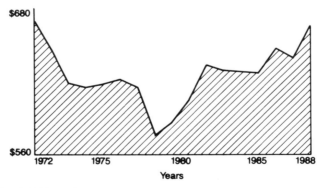

Figure 1-5 Hospital Nurses' Monthly Wages in 1982 Dollars, 1972–1988 *(Source: National Survey of Hospitals and Medical Schools, Galveston, TX: University of Texas Medical Branch, 1987.)*

kets, and the evidence suggests that this is correct, since 80 percent of nurses are already working.[14] The point that is often overlooked, however, is that raising nurses' wages significantly increases incentives to use nurses more appropriately. Increased salaries also encourage the more than 500,000 nurses who work part-time to increase the number of hours they work. In addition, trends over the past 25 years suggest there has been a wage impact on enrollments in nursing schools. Each major increase in nurses' relative wages has been accompanied by increased enrollments in nursing schools.

A major salary response to the current nursing shortage is likely to reduce or eliminate nursing vacancies, because hospitals would have a strong economic incentive to deliver care with fewer nurses. Even in the absence of economic incentives, hospitals should be restructured to enhance human resource utilization. There are simply not enough people who want to be nurses to continue to use nurses so indiscriminately.

Restructuring the Work Environment The objective of restructuring is to reduce the number of nurses required without reducing direct nursing care hours per patient day. This requires building a support system around nurses that enables them to increase the percentage of their time spent in direct patient care. The following changes would help accomplish this.

Clerical Administrative Support Personnel for Nurses It is hard to imagine another industry of the size and complexity of hospitals that has so few support personnel for the professional staff. The addition of a modest complement of secretaries and/or administrative assistants to nurses could go a long way in freeing nurses to spend their time with patients.

Unit Management Hospitals lack an administrative structure separate from nursing at the unit level with designated authority and responsibility for the effective operation of institutional support services. Nurses and physicians cannot take care of patients efficiently unless other departments meet reasonable performance standards. Yet nurses often have little recourse in cases of poor performance of support services but to take time away from nursing care to provide the services themselves. Providing fresh water, transporting patients to tests and therapy, preparing rooms for new admissions, handling food trays, obtaining drugs and supplies, providing directions and assistance to visitors are all examples of things that need to be done—but not by a nurse. At the very least, nurses must have more influence over the performance of hospital support services. Optimally, an improved management structure would be developed to take these responsibilities off the hands of nurses.

Assistants to Nurses New and creative strategies are needed for the effective use of ancillary nursing personnel in patient-care-related activities. Patients in U.S. hospitals today are too sick to have their care totally delegated to technical and informally trained staff, but careful delegation of tasks to assistants to nurses could enhance nurses' productivity and effectiveness and improve overall quality of care. Examples of tasks that might be delegated on a case-by-case basis include bed baths for those patients not needing professional nursing involvement, assistance with personal hygiene activities and eating, social interaction with anxious or disoriented patients, the execution of repetitious and routine procedures not requiring professional judgment or observation.

System Improvements Hospitals invest only 2.4 percent of their operating budgets on information technologies compared to 8 percent for banks and 11 percent for insurance companies.[15] Much of the existing computer capacity in hospitals is directed toward billing and third-party reimbursement, not clinical care. Nurses alone spend an estimated 40 percent of their time on paperwork, and much of the overtime paid to nurses is for charting. Greater investment in clinically based computer systems could lead to more cost-effective use of personnel in hospitals and could provide a more systematic data base on which to make clinical decisions and conduct research.

Nurse-physician Joint Practice Unsatisfactory relationships with physicians are a major source of dissatisfaction among nurses, and a common reason for nurse resignations.[16] Moreover, patient outcomes clearly depend on the nature and quality of nurse-physician communications. A recent multi-hospital study of the effectiveness of intensive care concluded that the differences in mortality rates between hospitals could be attributed in large part to the nature of the communications and decision-making partnerships between nurses and physicians.[17] This finding is not at all surprising when we consider how rapidly the condition of critically ill patients change and the importance of anticipating and preventing a catastrophic event rather than treating it under emergency conditions.

Nurses and physicians often do not fully appreciate the responsibilities and obligations that each hold for patients. This could be overcome by organizational arrangements for patient care in which specific nurses and physicians have longitudinal responsibility for the same groups of patients, as is the case in intensive care units, where the relationships between nurses and physicians are consistently better than on the general medical and surgical units. Nurses often let their respon-sibilities for "managing" the unit divert them from maintaining the kinds of longitudinal responsibilities that physicians usually have for patients.

INTERNATIONAL IMPLICATIONS

The recent cyclical shortages of nurses in the United States have been due primarily to factors affecting the demand for nurses not by changes in the number of nurses available for employment. The combination of low relative wages for nurses and increasingly complex medical technology in hospitals make nurses the most cost-effective workers, since nurses have greater versatility than other kinds of personnel. The U.S. experience suggests that as countries develop more technologically sophisticated hospitals, the demand for nurses will escalate dramatically. Hospitals have the capacity to employ very large numbers of nurses unless attention is given to how hospitals could use nurses more appropriately. All countries have needs for nursing care in settings other than hospitals. The U.S. experience suggests that unless attention is given to moderating demand for hospital nurses, the distribution of nurses in primary care roles and other out-of-hospital settings could be substantially eroded.

An important lesson here is that it is highly unlikely that any developed country will have enough people interested in becoming nurses to fully meet employer demand for nurses under conditions of low nurse wages. There are simply too many ways nurses can contribute to health care goals to control demand when their wages are low. Increasing the supply of nurses will simply not solve this problem. In fact, increasing the supply of nurses can exaggerate the demand problem by depressing wages even further.

Because the U.S. nursing shortage is one of excess demand not limited supply, it cannot be solved by supply solutions including recruitment of foreign-trained nurses. Foreign-trained nurses can have a negative rather than a positive effect on the domestic supply-demand balance in developed countries, because the addition of these nurses to the domestic pool depresses wages, which is often the underlying cause of excess employer demand. Yet, U.S. hospitals tend to look for short-term solutions to immediate problems rather than pursuing the necessary long-term strategies. Hence, the United States is an importer of nurses. In 1988, about 3.6 percent or 73,282 licensed registered nurses in the United States were foreign-trained. This included both permanent residents and foreign nurses with limited work visas.[18]

Although foreign-trained nurses make up a very small proportion of the total pool of U.S. nurses, in the aggregate the 73,000 foreign nurses represent a resource of much greater magnitude in relation to the nursing resources of other countries. Many countries in the world have nowhere near 73,000 nurses in their entire domestic supply. The 73,000 foreign-trained nurses have not solved the U.S. shortage and could potentially make important contributions to the health care needs of their countries of origin. However, many countries that export nurses do so because they cannot afford to support enough graduate nurse positions even for their own graduates. Hence, unless these countries can allocate more resources to health care, nurses will remain unemployed or underemployed. Also, some countries export nurses specifically as a strategy to gain hard currency to strengthen their national economies. Thus, the international trade in nurses is not as simple as it appears at first glance and should be studied further.

In summary, the evidence suggests that developed countries with highly technological health and medical care systems can and do consume an inordinate proportion of the world's nursing resources. This trend will only grow more serious in the years to come, since most technological advances in medicine have been nurse-intensive, and these advances are diffusing throughout the world in developing as well as developed countries. The developed world is not likely to solve its nursing shortages by supply-oriented strategies alone. Much more attention is required to moderating demand.

REFERENCES

1. World Health Organization. *Global Strategy for Health for All by the Year 2000*. Second Report on Monitoring Progress in Implementing Strategies for Health for All. March 10, 1989.
2. Secretary's Commission on Nursing. *Final Report*. Washington, DC: Department of Health and Human Services, July 1988.
3. Aiken, LH. The hospital nursing shortage: A paradox of increasing supply and increasing vacancy rates. *Western Journal of Medicine*, 151:87–92, 1989.
4. U.S. Department of Health and Human Services. *Sixth Report to the President and Congress on the Status of Health Personnel in the United States*. Bureau of Health Professions, Health Resources Administration, 1988.
5. Prospective Payment Commission. *Report and Recommendations*. Washington, DC: Office of Technology Assessment, March 1989, p. 64.
6. Aiken, LH, Blendon, RJ, Rogers, DE. The shortage of hospital nurses: A new perspective. *Annals of Internal Medicine*, 95:365–373.
7. National Survey of Hospital and Medical School Salaries. Galveston, TX: University of Texas Medical Branch, 1987.
8. Burt, ML. The cost of all RN staffing. In G. Alfano (ed.) *Nursing Resources*. Wakefield, MA, 1980.
9. Hinshaw, AS, Scofield, R, Atwood, JR. Staff, patient, and cost outcomes of all-registered nurse staffing. *Journal of Nursing Administration*. Nov.-Dec. 1981:30–36.
10. Misener, TR, Frelin, AJ, Twist, PA. Sampling nursing time pinpoints staffing needs. *Nursing and Health Care*, April 1978, pp. 233–237.
11. Rieder, KA, Leasing, SB. Nursing productiv-

ity: Evolution of a systems model. *Nursing Management,* 18:13–44, 1978.

12. Aiken, LH, Mullinix, CF. The nurse shortage: Myth or reality? *New England Journal of Medicine,* 317(10):641–646, 1987.

13. Robinson, JC. Hospital competition and hospital nursing. *Nursing Economics,* 6(3):116–124, 1988.

14. Gallup Poll. Reported in *Health Week,* August 8, 1988, p. 26.

15. Testimony by Ernst and Whinney, Inc., before the Secretary's Commission on Nursing, Washington, D.C., September 1988.

16. Mechanic, D., Aiken, LH. A cooperative agenda for medicine and nursing. *New England Journal of Medicine,* 307:747–750, 1982.

17. Knaus, WA, Draper, EA, Wagner, DP, Zimmerman, JE. An evaluation of outcome from intensive care in major medical centers. *Annals of Internal Medicine,* 104:410–418, 1986.

18. National Sample Survey of Nurses. Division of Nursing, DHHS, 1989; unpublished data from 1984 and 1988.

Planning for Nursing Manpower Needs in New Zealand

Marion Clark

INTRODUCTION

Chapter 2 discusses some of the key issues currently affecting the planning of nursing manpower in New Zealand. Examples are presented to illustrate the effects on nursing and highlight the implications for nursing leadership over the next few years.

BACKGROUND

New Zealand is a small country in the South Pacific and consists of several islands. Its area of 267,254 square kilometres (similar to that of Great Britain or Japan) contains a population of 3.3 million. The Maori people, of Polyne-sian origin, are the Tangata Whenua (people of the land) or original settlers and comprise 12 percent of the population. Of the total population, 25 percent are under 15 years old, and 10.5 percent are 65 years and over. Since 1983, political leadership has resulted in major economic, social, and political changes.

The state is the major funder and provider of health care. Through its district health development units, the Department of Health has been the main provider of environmental, health protection, and health promotion services. Curative (secondary and tertiary) services have been largely provided by locally elected hospital boards, funded by the government. The health sector also includes private services such as private hospitals and general practitioners and various voluntary organizations, some of which receive government funding subsidies.

The nation's health services have just been reorganized to integrate preventive and curative services and to rationalize service delivery on a regional basis. This includes the preventive services, referred to above, previously provided by the Department of Health, and the curative services provided previously by hospital boards. This reorganization took place in progressive stages and was completed in December 1989. The result is the formation of fourteen area health boards which also administer government funding by elected boards. The area health boards will be progressively responsible for the provision of all health care services in their area, which will encourage much greater coordination of health services and allow for greater community participation in the decision-making process.

The Nursing Workforce

The New Zealand qualified nursing workforce is made up of registered nurses (nurses who have been prepared in a 3-year course) and enrolled nurses (second-level nurses who have a 1-year practical training and practice under the supervision of registered nurses).

The nursing workforce has been steadily increasing as shown in Figure 2-1.

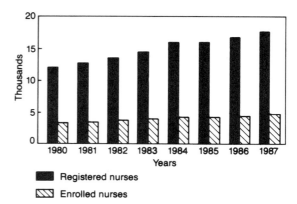

Figure 2-1   N.Z. Nursing Workforce (Full-Time Equivalent).

In 1989, there were 32,850 qualified nurses in active nursing employment in New Zealand. The majority of qualified nurses (82.7 percent) are employed in the three main types of hospitals: general and obstetric hospitals (62.5 percent), psychiatric and psychopaedic hospitals for the intellectually disabled (10.6 percent), and private hospitals (9.6 percent); 14.2 percent of the total qualified staff work in community health settings.[1] See Figure 2-2.

Historical Background

Before 1973, nursing preparation took place in hospital-based apprentice-type programs. The students met the service requirements of the hospital while filling their education needs. However, many problems were identified in this system of nursing training. There was a very high student attrition rate, general con-

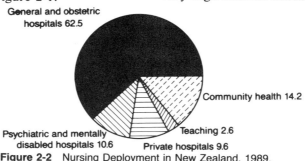

Figure 2-2   Nursing Deployment in New Zealand, 1989.

cern that the hospital-based training program was not adequate to meet the future requirements of the health service, and a strong belief that nursing care should be delivered by qualified nurses.

Pilot schemes for the first technical institute-based 3-year comprehensive courses were established in 1973. A gradual transfer, phased over 10 to 12 years, was proposed to minimize possible adverse effects on the nursing workforce.[2] It has taken 15 years to complete the transfer of nursing education. The last intake of hospital-based students for registration is now in training.

The comprehensive course produces nurses with a broad knowledge base, focused on health as well as illness, who can function effectively in a variety of settings. With the development of this course, nursing is taking the lead in New Zealand in producing a health care professional with a primary health care focus, who will be able to meet the needs of the rapidly changing health care delivery system.

The major impetus to develop national nursing workforce planning systems arose from the transition of nursing education from hospital-based programs to the general tertiary education system. Prior to this transfer, hospital boards monitored their own student intake levels to ensure adequate staffing. With the transfer to technical institutes, annual student intake numbers needed to be determined nationally. This was necessary for two reasons:

1 Careful planning of the timing and phases of the transfer was needed to avoid disruptions to nursing services.
2 As the government began to take over direct responsibility for the funding of these training schools, approval was required for each phase of the transfer in terms of student intake numbers and the necessary funding.

The phasing out of hospital-based programs highlighted the need for more information about numbers and levels of qualified nurses required as a "replacement factor" for the declining student numbers in hospitals, to provide efficient nursing service. From 1977 the Nursing Research Section of the Department of Health focused its attention on the preparation of a nursing workforce plan which would provide a basis for policy decisions such as student intake levels.

By 1980, the methodology for data collection was established. This initial research provided much useful information about the workforce, including the fact that nursing shortages were rather a maldistribution over geographical and service areas.

The accomplishment of a smooth transfer of nursing education can be attributed to the activities of the Department of Health in developing and maintaining an effective national nursing workforce information system. The accumulating historical database has given us the capacity to predict future workforce trends with greater accuracy. The database enabled the development of a model to determine future requirements for and supply of nurses. The planning model provides a focus for our nursing planning research, by identifying the specific information which is important for policy formulation, and the database has been the basis of decisions on intakes into nursing courses since 1983.

THE NURSING WORKFORCE PLANNING MODEL

Our planning model, which was developed and published in 1985, provides a tool for enabling projections on supply and requirements to be made. The model used here is based on the WICHE (Western Interstate Commission on Higher Education) forecasting model, developed in Colorado, in the United States. This model was based on estimating requirements for each category of nurse in a variety of service areas. However, it has been adapted to make it relevant for the New Zealand situation and to accommodate the available data.

The planning model contains two submodels: a requirements (demand) model and a supply model. It is a simulation model based on expert judgments on assumptions of future trends—a group of experts analyze trends and predict future scenarios based on a number of factors.

The requirements model (see Appendix 2-1) estimates requirements on the basis of "employment setting" (e.g., public general and obstetric hospital, psychiatric hospitals, or community, private hospital). The predictor used for nurses employed in hospital settings is nurse-to-average-occupied-bed, whereas for community settings it is nurse-to-population ratios. The model is based on employer demand, that is, nurses actually employed rather than ideal requirements. Projections are based on a number of assumptions about future trends and their effect on the predictors. These trends take into account:

- Demographic factors such as aging and fertility
- Economic factors such as the level of public funding
- Epidemiological or health factors such as AIDS, smoking, and heart disease
- Health service trends, which include the ratio of public to private bed numbers, provision of community services, and changes in care delivery
- Nursing service and labor market trends such as changes to the ratio of nursing staff to average occupied bed, ratio of full-time equivalents to actual numbers, or ratio of registered to enrolled (practical) nurses

The prediction of future trends on these factors is then applied to the numbers to enable calculation of future requirements.

The supply model (see Appendix 2-2) is simpler. It enables forecasting of future supply by taking the current pool of practising nurses

and assessing the turnover or retention of nurses in this pool by calculating the cohort remainder rate. The cohort remainder rate is the percentage of the group of nurses graduating during a given period who remain in the current supply—a measure of retention. The loss to the nursing pool is predicted, and the expected gains from new graduates and immigration are added to arrive at a future supply. A baseline supply projection was calculated on the basis of continuation of current policies, and alternative projections explored the effect of policy changes. The projections can be updated according to new trends.

A review of future predictions of requirement in 1987 confirmed the relevance of the key factors and the assumptions and indicated a projected mismatch between supply and requirements for the early 1990s (see Table 2-1).

Thus present indications lead us to believe that we will be facing a moderate shortage of nurses in the first half of the next decade.

The relevance of the planning model is being questioned in the present climate of rapid change in the New Zealand health service. The underlying assumptions need to be reexamined in the context of these changes. We are currently redeveloping and reviewing our planning model.

INTERNATIONAL INFLUENCES ON NURSING WORKFORCE PLANNING

In New Zealand we, theoretically, are not experiencing a nursing shortage as some nurses are currently having difficulty obtaining positions. However, this unemployment is only in

Table 2-1 Predictions of Future Supply and Demand for Registered Nurses

	1990	1993
Requirements	29,084	30,418
Supply	27,605	27,763
Shortfall	1,321 (4.5%)	2,655 (8.7%)

some geographical areas. A certain percentage of our nursing workforce are immobile because of their family situations so cannot move to take up nursing employment elsewhere if their positions are ended. Predictions of nursing shortages in the future require the development of policies now to alleviate the predicted shortfall.

Our nursing workforce planning could be judged to have succeeded in maintaining an effective workforce. Manipulation of our immigration policy has proved to be an important strategy in the maintenance of effective staffing levels. It is a successful short-term measure with the added advantage that nurses with specific skills and experience can be recruited for specialist clinical areas where needed. Our shortage specialties vary but most commonly include midwives, theatre nurses, nurses experienced in the psychiatric area and in intensive and coronary care. Nurses with forensic psychiatric experience are currently being sought due to the new government policy which increases the provision of national forensic psychiatric services.[3]

A specific current shortage is the shortage of midwives. Nationally the current vacancy level for nurse-midwives is 14 percent, with a further 3.6 percent midwifery positions being filled by nurses without midwifery. We are actively recruiting midwives from overseas at present, and new policies for midwifery education have been developed to address the shortage. Planned legislative change to increase autonomy of midwives will also affect our future requirements and will need to be taken into account in our planning and policy making. Our dependence on overseas midwives is clear: 31.8 percent of all our practicing midwives obtained their qualifications outside New Zealand.

In addition, 10.5 percent of all qualified nurses currently licensed to practice in New Zealand have gained their basic qualifications elsewhere.

A shortage of qualified nurses occurred in 1985. Overall vacancy levels at this time were 10 to 11 percent. (They have since fallen to between 3 and 4 percent). Overseas recruitment was used to address the shortfall. A recruitment campaign was initiated in the United Kingdom with the employment of a British-based liaison person to assist with the recruitment and immigration of British nurses. Restrictions on the entry of overseas nurses to the workforce were also relaxed. Since then numbers of overseas recruits have been carefully monitored by the department (see Figure 2-3).

Last year we faced unemployment of new graduates, so our immigration policy was tightened to prevent entry of all nurses except those with needed specialist experience and skills. It has not been our policy to actively

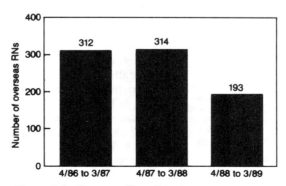

Figure 2-3 Overseas Recruitment.

recruit nurses from countries which are themselves experiencing a shortage, however we accept suitable applications initiated by the prospective immigrant.

Over the past 3 years immigrant nurses have come from a variety of countries, although our major source is the United Kingdom, from where we obtain 63.3 percent of our foreign recruits (see Figure 2-4).

We are affected by international labor market trends, and one factor contributing to our shortage in 1985 was the increased flow of New Zealand nurses to Australia. This could be partly attributed to changes in Australian employment policies for nurses (salary increases) and their transfer of nursing education from hospital to tertiary education institutions, resulting in shortages.

We expect a degree of migration of nurses. The "working holiday" or "overseas experience" is a popular reason for leaving the country. Although the loss to our nursing supply is difficult to assess accurately, in our experience these young nurses can usually be expected to return after a certain period: 2,124 (4.9 percent) of nurses with current practicing certificates are living overseas at the moment. The maintenance of their license to practice seems to indicate an expectation of their return.

The international nursing shortage in countries such as the United States, Great Britain, and Australia while we have an apparent oversupply has resulted in aggressive recruiting campaigns by these countries this year. Many of our new graduates have been employed in Australia. Difficulty in monitoring the level of emigration limits our ability to accurately predict future supply and requirements for nurses. The severe international shortage of nurses raises doubts about our ability to recruit nurses from outside New Zealand in the future, making effective workforce planning an even greater priority over the next decade.

CURRENT ISSUES AFFECTING NURSING WORKFORCE NEEDS

Even though we do not have a nursing shortage, our ability to deliver a high-quality nursing service is challenged by a complex range of factors currently impacting the health service.

Reorganization of the Health Service

As previously mentioned, we have just totally restructured our health care delivery system, a restructuring that was long overdue. The whole style of operations needed to change to meet the demands of a changing society, including the following:

• The need to focus the system more strongly on the needs of consumers, rather than on the concerns of the institutions and providers
• The need to increase the efficiency of the health care delivery service, particularly the hospital system
• The need to restrain government expenditure while improving the quality and quantity of services provided
• The need to improve the management accountability and responsiveness of health service

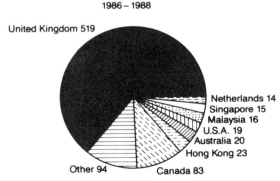

1986 – 1988

United Kingdom 519

Netherlands 14
Singapore 15
Malaysia 16
U.S.A. 19
Australia 20
Hong Kong 23
Canada 83
Other 94

Figure 2-4 Overseas Recruitment by Country of Origin.

• The need to support the primary health care approach and increase the emphasis on prevention and promotion of health rather than the treatment of disease

Strategies employed to address these included the amalgamation of existing health authorities and changing of boundaries to form fourteen area health boards; the replacement of the triumvirate management structure (chief executive, chief nurse, and chief medical officer) with general management; and the provision of much greater autonomy in area health board management than existed in the previous system of largely central government control.

Effective nursing leadership in this new environment requires skills in communication, negotiation, influence, and motivational ability to ensure that nursing workforce needs are met. The changes have several implications for nursing:

• A greater range of opportunities is available for nurses to influence the general health service at all levels.

• Many senior nurses have moved into general management positions. The increasing nursing influence is providing great opportunities for enhancement of the general health service. At the same time it has affected the number of experienced nurse leaders remaining in nursing at a time when nursing needs strong leadership. We must focus our efforts on identifying and developing nurses with leadership potential.

• Strategies need to be developed to ensure that managers have access to sound professional nursing advice when making decisions on nursing utilization and workforce policies which affect nurses.

• The rapid rate of change in health service delivery affects the ability to make valid predictions of future workforce needs.

To increase accountability and meet the needs of their communities, general managers have established a diverse range of management structures within their boards. These management structures with their variety of positions and titles pose challenges for national workforce planning. Previous methods of data collection are no longer so readily applicable, and the regional diversity of employment conditions, roles, and staff utilization make it more difficult to predict nursing needs on a national level.

Strategies

We have developed several strategies to adapt our nursing workforce planning activities to meet the future needs of a restructured, regionally autonomous health service in rapid change.

Development of Regional Workforce Planning Capabilities To cater for the diversity around the country, workforce planning systems must incorporate regional decision making with national coordination. Increasing regional-national interaction would enable identified national workforce needs to be met while promoting regional autonomy and accountability.

The Department of Health is providing a consultancy role in helping boards to develop workforce planning systems. A series of workshops has been held around the country to increase the knowledge and ability of the board personnel in workforce planning and to impart to board personnel the importance of workforce planning in ensuring that their future staffing needs are met. Some boards, however, are not yet prepared to pick up this responsibility.

Dissemination of National Information One method of facilitating the achievement of national goals is to ensure that the decision makers are provided with full information on which to base their policies. Regular publication and broad dissemination of national nursing workforce information will be important to allow for regional decisions made in the national context. Previously we have distributed all our data, but we have become aware that a different presentation is needed to more effectively communicate the information. We plan to change the format of our publication of nursing statistics.

Review of the Nursing Workforce Planning Model   We are currently engaged in an extensive review of the planning model to ensure that it can provide an adequate basis for planning supply and requirements in the current climate of rapid change. All assumptions will be examined for their relevance. New assumptions based on changes in health care delivery (such as increase in day-stay surgery; de-institutionalization of psychiatric and intellectually disabled patients to community-based care; changes in legislation to give more autonomy to midwives; increase in AIDS; and the increasing privatization of the workforce) and current economic factors will be developed, and the projections will be revised in the light of the new assumptions. The use of ''average occupied bed'' as a predictor of nursing requirements is being questioned, and the feasibility of using alternative indicators of nursing workload will be explored. This review is due to be completed mid-1990.

Economic Restraint

The reorganization of the health system, to complicate the situation further, is taking place in a political climate of severe economic restraint. The need for cost containment within the health sector is having major effects on the nursing workforce.

Approximately 80 percent of the government funding allocations to area health boards are spent on staffing, and the nursing services consume 50 percent of this. The sheer numbers of nurses employed make the nursing service budget an obvious target for cost-cutting

in times of fiscal restraint. We are currently seeing hospital restructuring with concurrent cuts in nursing staff levels. Monthly monitoring of nursing staffing levels in the public health sector show an overall 4 percent decrease since December 1988. The effect of this is a national reduction of employment opportunities for nurses, which creates an illusion of oversupply. It is an illusion because, in some cases, the nursing reductions have been made with minimal health service reductions so that the remaining nurses are carrying extra workloads. The challenge is how to ensure patient safety and maintain the quality of nursing care in a time of budget constraint.

Another effect of budget cuts by boards was demonstrated by an unprecedented lack of employment opportunities for new nursing graduates last year. Only 61.7 percent of new graduates had taken up positions with area health boards by March 31, 1989. By June this figure had only risen to 65.5 percent. This is unfortunate at a time when we are predicting future nursing shortages. New graduates are the experienced workforce of the future!

Recent decisions by boards to reduce or discontinue training programs for enrolled nurses (a 1-year hospital-based program) have been largely budget driven rather than needs based. Our planning model recommends national annual intakes of 550. Last year only 308 were trained, and proposed intakes for this year show a further drop to 250. In the event of a shortage of enrolled nurses, boards may choose to employ unqualified staff to meet their staffing needs. This places further strain on registered nurses, who supervise work of enrolled nurses and unqualified staff. It is important to ensure that quality of nursing practice is maintained.

Strategies

Some new strategies for planning nursing staffing may need to be employed to ensure that staffing levels continue to maximise cost-efficiency while maintaining standards of nursing care. National guidelines have been found to be ineffective due to the diversity of nursing use in different areas. Increased emphasis placed on quality assurance programs and hospital accreditation systems suggests that future determination of staffing levels could be based on the agreed standards and criteria for health service delivery.

The need for improving efficiency requires close examinaton of the utilization and mix of staff. It is now more appropriate to study nursing workforce needs in conjunction with those of other health professionals. Increasingly our practice will take a team approach, using the specific competencies which are needed to meet the patient care objectives. The Department of Health is establishing a transdisciplinary approach to workforce planning in the development of a computerized information system designed to store workforce data from a range of health occupations and eventually lead to planning across occupational groups.

Retention

It would be unrealistic not to acknowledge the stress that the current environment of change and need for budgetary constraint is creating for the health workforce. Nurses are expressing anxiety both at a personal level, regarding how the changes will effect their own position, and from a genuine concern about the provision and standard of nursing and health services in New Zealand. An important focus for nursing leadership at present is in uplifting nursing morale. It is important to retain experienced nurses in the health service. Our research has shown[4] that retention in the workforce is by far the most significant determinant of workforce supply. Therefore the effects of increased turnover could be very deterimental for the future supply of nurses.

Demographic Trends

New Zealand is confronting similar population trends to the rest of the world. These will have considerable implications for the nursing workforce. The population is aging (which suggests a greater need for nurses in the future) at the same time as the number of school leavers (our traditional recruits) can be predicted to decline. Current statistics[5] show that the number of secondary school pupils will progressively decrease by around 40,000 between 1989 and 1993 (see Figure 2-5).

The falling school rolls will soon affect numbers of traditional recruits. Recruitment campaigns need to be directed at nontraditional sources such as men and mature students.

Recruitment Difficulties

Our predicted difficulties with recruitment into nursing courses seem to be beginning. We have a planned national intake of 1633 per annum. In 1989, when enrollments had usually closed for the following academic year, enrollments were down by 34.8 percent. Educational institutions responded by extending their enrollment period so, at the time of writing, the final intake numbers remain uncertain. Several causes for this phenomenon can be identified, including reduced popularity of nursing as a career:

• The restructuring of the health service has attracted bad publicity. This is accompanied by a perceived reduction of career prospects.

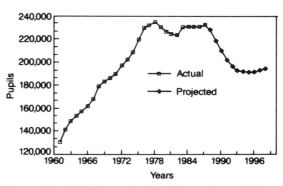

Figure 2-5 Total Secondary Enrollments (Actual 1961–1987, Projected 1988–1998).

• The publicity attracted by the unemployment of last year's new graduates has probably caused anxiety about future employment opportunities.

• The image of nursing is not such as to attract young women (our traditional recruits) into nursing in a climate of much greater variety of career choices and opportunities to move into traditionally male occupations. Research conducted in 1988 showed a disappointingly poor image and popularity of nursing as a career among school pupils.[6]

• Financial support of students in the tertiary education system has been reduced. The government has recently announced a large increase (400 percent) in all student fees for next year. Previously, in New Zealand, the cost of tertiary education to the student has been minimal. The additional costs for nursing students may be putting nursing education out of reach for potential recruits.

Graduates from the intake in 1990 will join the workforce in 1992. This is when our predicted mismatch between supply and requirements for nurses peaks. Several very recent surveys seem to indicate that around 50 percent of second- and third-year students may not continue with their training as a result of proposed increased student fees. In this event, we could experience a severe nursing shortage sooner than anticipated.

Strategies

A strategy employed by the department to increase the level of recruitment is a vigorous campaign to promote nursing. Sponsorship has been provided for activities aimed at marketing nursing and improving its image.

Control of Student Numbers

Since 1980 the Department of Health has established desired national student intake levels in accordance with the workforce plan which planned staged increases in student levels in technical institute courses at the same time as decreasing the levels in hospital-based courses.

The political climate of devolution and accountability which is creating the necessity for new structures and management styles in the health sector has produced similar results in the education sector. Recent political restructuring associated with a climate of economic restraint is challenging the previous relationship between the health and education sectors. Decisions on the nursing intake levels acceptable to both the education service and the health service will need to be reached by mutual agreement.

Area health boards are questioning their role in providing education for the health workforce. They have been making autonomous decisions about enrollments into second-level nursing courses (which are still conducted in hospitals) largely because of need for cost containment.

There are fewer opportunities for clinical experience as health service cuts result in reduction of services. This reduction affects the quality of education and may lead to limitations on the number of student places in the future.

To ensure that we have the number of nurses required for the health service, policies will be needed, developed in collaboration with the boards. Issues relating to control of student intakes will need to be resolved for our workforce planning to be effective.

Strategies

Nursing leaders will need to develop skills in influencing, working collaboratively, and negotiating in order to meet the nursing workforce needs of the future.

We are currently developing a health education policy to address issues of funding for preparation of health professionals. The policy is aimed at ensuring access to the education system for the student numbers required by the health service.

CONCLUSION

Although New Zealand is fortunate in that we are not experiencing a nursing shortage at present, nursing is facing new challenges in planning for its workforce needs for today and in the future. Key issues confronting us have been identified and strategies have been developed for dealing with the issues to ensure that our nursing workforce continues to meet the future health service needs of the next decade.

REFERENCES

1. Department of Health, unpublished statistics.
2. Department of Education, *Nursing education in New Zealand*, 1972, p. 22.
3. Mason, K.H. et al, *Psychiatric Report—Report of the committee of inquiry into procedures used in certain psychiatric hospitals in relation to admission, discharge or release on leave of certain classes of patients* (Department of Health: Wellington, 1988).
4. Nursing Manpower Planning Committee, *Nurse workforce planning* (Department of Health: Wellington, 1985).
5. Department of Education statistics, 1988.
6. National Action Group, *To nurse?! Attitudes towards nursing as a career* (Wellington, National Action Group Publication No. 3, 1989).

Nursing Workforce Planning Model: Requirements

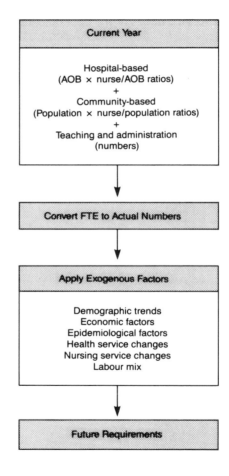

Nursing Workforce Planning Model: Supply

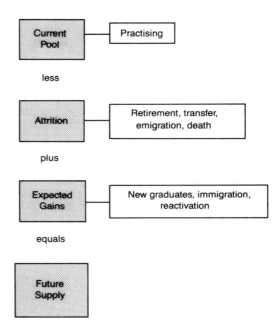

Chapter 3

Manpower Needs: Womanpower Demands

Christine Hancock

INTRODUCTION

"Shortages" of nursing staff have been a recurring problem in the United Kingdom, as elsewhere, over the last 50 years. As the problem has recurred, so have the proposals for innovative and radical solutions. Sometimes these proposals have been considered responses, based on research and evaluation, but on other occasions both proposals and proposers have displayed a fundamental ignorance of nurses and nursing.

This chapter outlines the current state of nursing in the United Kingdom and has two guiding themes. First, to devise solutions you

must define the problems. Second, any proposed solutions must recognize that over 90 percent of nurses in the United Kingdom are female. A shortage of "manpower" may be the problem; womanpower will have to provide the solution.

DEFINING THE PROBLEM

There are over 400,000 nursing staff employed in the United Kingdom. Their numbers have increased markedly over the last 40 years (see Figure 3-1). Despite this increase, there are

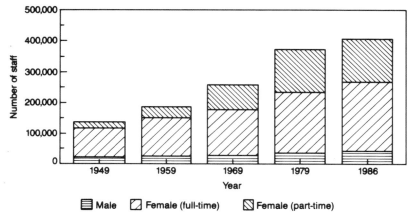

Figure 3-1 Nursing Staff, England, 1949–1986 (*Source: Health and Personal Social Services Statistics Annual, HMSO*).

widespread concerns about nursing shortages in the United Kingdom. The classic definition of *shortages,* in staffing terms, is a situation where the demand for staff exceeds the supply. A shortage may occur when demand increases, outstripping the capability of the system to respond with sufficient numbers of staff or when the supply of available staff reduces but demand for their services does not. The United Kingdom is currently experiencing the combined effect of both phenomena, primarily as a result of demographic changes but also because of developments in health care provision and policy.

The supply of school leavers, the traditional source of new recruits to nursing, is reducing markedly as a result of demographic change. Between 1983 and 1993 an overall 31 percent decline in the annual number of school leavers is projected. There is some evidence that the reduction may not be as marked in the social and qualification levels, which nursing traditionally recruits from, but clearly the potential pool of new young recruits will be drying up when other employers are devoting increasing resources to maintaining or expanding their "market share" of school leavers.

At the other end of the age spectrum, demographic projections indicate that the elderly

will increase in significance, both in numerical terms and as a proportion of the total population. The increasing demands which will be made on the health service by the growing numbers of elderly will be compounded by an associated projected increase in the number of patients suffering from dementia.

Demographic change can all too easily exert a debilitating, almost hypnotic effect on the willpower of those responsible for forward planning in the health service. The unstoppable certainty of demographic projections may cause difficulties in matching supply and demand, but at least their predictability provides time for organizations to respond to and plan for these changes. The phrase "demographic time bomb," often used in the United Kingdom to describe the labor market impact of the reduction in school leavers, is singularly inappropriate. The time bomb cannot be defused—but neither is it ticking away, ready to create instant, explosive chaos. The reality is that the demographic change has been predictable, and predicted, for many years, and will take a further 5 or 6 years to "bottom out."

Another demographic trend tends to get overlooked in the doom and gloom scenarios. Although there are likely to be 1 million fewer 18 to 25 year olds in the labor force in the

1990s, 2½ million *more* 25 to 55 year olds are projected. Nine out of every ten new additions to the UK labor force in the 1990s are projected to be women. The participation rate of women in employment is predicted to increase, while male participation declines.

So, in beginning to define the underlying problem—demographic change—we can begin to perceive potential solutions. Demography is, of course, not the only factor affecting supply and demand which is changing, or will change over the next decade. Health care provision is itself changing, as new procedures, new technology, and new drugs are introduced. Their impact is often to increase demand for nursing staff. As the frontiers of medicine move forward, many patients, who 10 or 20 years ago would have been beyond treatment, are now being cared for, often in a high-dependency status. An increasingly old population is being kept alive for longer. The projected increase in the number of patients with dementia has already been noted; another issue which the health service is having to face is the growth in the number of patients with AIDS, and the related impact on the demand for nursing staff.

Finally, changes in health policy will continue to affect the demand for nursing staff.

One major factor increasing demand is the long-term trend in the reduction of length of stay of patients in hospital (Figure 3-2). "Patient throughput" has increased significantly over the years, as average length of stay declines (see Figures 3-2 and 3-3). This trend may make sense in terms of best accommodating an ever-increasing demand for health services, but two unintended side effects have resulted. First, increased throughput and shorter stays places additional burdens on nursing staff, who have to provide care to more patients, at an increasing average dependency state, in a shorter time. The result is, as one survey of nurses showed (Figure 3-3), that frustration, stress, and demoralization can increase as nurses can no longer provide the level of care they know they can provide and have been trained to provide. A second side effect is that higher patient turnover and shorter stay in hospital have led to much higher readmission rates—the quicker the patient is discharged, the more likely he or she will have to be readmitted (Figure 3-4). This is clearly a false economy, but the ensuing double counting assists government ministers in claiming each year that the health service is "treating a greater number of patients than ever before." The fact that they are also read-

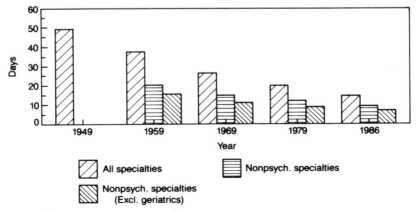

Figure 3-2 Average Length of Patient Stay, England, 1949–1986 (*Source: Health and Personal Social Services Statistics Annual, HMSO*).

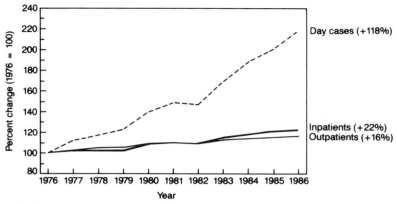

Figure 3-3   Change in Hospital Activity, England, 1976–1986 (Change in Nursing Staff = 16%)
(*Source: Health and Personal Social Services Statistics Annual, HMSO*).

mitting more every year is less widely publicized.

Thus we have begun to define the problems facing UK nursing over the next decade, in relation to the supply of, and demand for, staff. Forecasting future supply and demand is always an inexact science, but all the indicators clearly point to the potential for a greater mismatch between supply and demand—and hence greater likelihood of "shortages." Next we will examine the current extent of nursing shortages in the United Kingdom and we will outline the available methodologies for forecasting demand.

MEASURING THE PROBLEM

Defining the "shortage" is problematical. Measuring, or putting some quantitative label to the extent of mismatch between supply and demand is even more difficult. However, by drawing together a number of different indicators, the nature and extent of the problem can be measured. Evidence of shortages can be

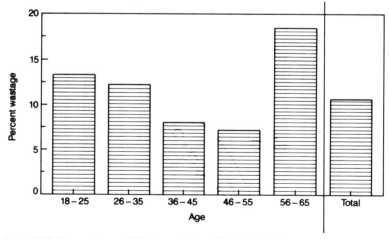

Figure 3-4   NHS Nurse Annual Wastage Rates, 1986–1987 (*Source: Institute of Manpower Studies/RCN*).

discerned from vacancy rates, turnover/wastage rates, and increased waiting lists and/or ward closures as a result of staff shortages. It should be stressed however, that a detailed analysis of staffing levels and activity rates at national level is precluded by an absence of systematically and regularly collected data.

Vacancy Rates

An annual "snapshot" survey of vacancy rates of nursing staff is undertaken for the Review Body, the independent board which determines nurses' pay. The information from this survey provides an indication over time of trends in vacancy rates for various specialties of nursing staff. Year on year variations in the sample base prevent detailed analysis, but the overall trend in vacancies has been upward, over the period since surveying began in 1985. The definition of vacancy used in the survey is "posts unfilled for 3 months at the time of survey," a measure of vacancy rates which effectively excludes transitioned vacancies. The overall 3-month vacancy rate in March 1989 was 3.2 percent, with markedly higher rates in some specialties, such as intensive care and psychiatric nursing (see Figure 3-5).

As an indicator of trends in shortages and variations between specialties, the annual monitoring of vacancy rates is relevant. How-

ever, the survey cannot be taken as a measure of the magnitude of shortages, because hard-to-fill or impossible-to-fill posts may not be funded, and other posts may be filled by staff underqualified for the responsibilities of postholder.

Furthermore—and crucial—the number of nursing posts is constrained by the extent of available funding. Vacancy rates merely measure the shortfall between staff in post and funded posts, they do not provide any indication of the adequacy of available funding or available posts to meet demand for nursing staff.

Turnover and Wastage

In assessing the level of job mobility of UK nurses, a distinction can be made between *turnover,* which is an indicator of the rate of job moves, and *wastage,* which is a measure of the extent of loss, to the health service, of nursing staff.

Accurate measurement of turnover and wastage of UK nurses has been difficult because of the lack of comprehensive data—many health authorities only assess turnover, which does not allow an assessment of wastage from the stock of nurses working in the health service. However, recent research commissioned by the Royal College of Nurs-

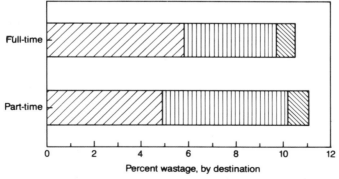

Figure 3-5 NHS Nurse Wastage, by Destination, 1986–1987 *(Source: Institute of Manpower Studies/RCN).*

ing (RCN), and undertaken by the independent Institute of Manpower Studies, has provided detailed data which allow for an assessment of turnover rates and wastages rates, at regional and national level. Crucially, the data also allow for an examination of the underlying causes for turnover and wastage and a quantification of the "destination" of nurses who have moved jobs.

The study found that the annual wastage rate—the proportion of nurses leaving the National Health Service (NHS)—was 10.9 percent for female nurses, and 7.5 percent for male nurses. Younger nurses were more likely to leave the NHS, but wastage rates of part-time did not differ markedly from full-time nurses. Many of the nurses, particularly those that were younger and female, were not moving to other jobs but were taking a break in their career (Figures 3-4 and 3-5). Turnover rates were much higher, particularly among younger staff nurses, who were moving jobs and locations as they broadened their experience and developed their career.

An overall wastage rate of approximately 10 percent suggests that about 30,000 nurses leave the NHS every year. As noted above, many were not moving to other jobs but were taking a career break. The three most cited reasons for leaving the NHS were "stress", "bad atmosphere," and "workload." These factors raise an important issue relating to nursing shortages—the potential for an unfortunate interrelationship between staff shortages and low morale: As shortages increase, so do workloads and stress; more nurses become demoralized and leave; and the shortage problem becomes more pronounced.

Waiting Lists, Ward Closures

Waiting lists, which detail the number of patients waiting for treatments, can be used as a broad indication of a mismatch between demand for the health service and the health services capabilities immediately to meet that demand. Recent data suggest that waiting lists are increasing despite strenuous efforts by government to effect a reduction. In March 1989, 704, 700 people in England were waiting for in-patient treatment, the highest figure for 6 years, and 3.8 percent higher than the previous year. A further 172,100 were waiting for treatment as day cases, 14.7 percent higher than in 1988.

Recent reports also indicate that funding and staffing difficulties are forcing hospitals to cut back on bed provision: Only a few weeks ago it was announced that St. Bartholomews, the famous London teaching hospital, would have to close 75 beds and reduce operating sessions because of lack of funding. Waiting lists and bed closures are not necessarily a direct indicator of nursing shortages. They are, however, a clear sign that demand for health service provision is outstripping the available funds and resources, and in specific local cases ward closures or suspension of services have occurred directly as a result of a lack of appropriately qualified nursing staff.

This brief overview of the available data has demonstrated a fundamental point. First, there are indications of a nursing shortage, but the lack of comprehensive national data prevents an accurate assessment of the extent of these shortages. The quasi-autonomous nature of the 200+ employing authorities in the United Kingdom makes obtaining standardized detailed data with which to establish an accurate national picture very difficult.

This devolution of employment responsibilities also means that there is no "national" plan for balancing supply and demand. Many authorities will independently make an assessment of their own supply-demand balance, by using one of a number of methodologies, e.g., weighted or unweighted population-staff ratios or staff-bed ratios, or staff-patient ratios (with or without some attempt to assess dependency levels, and with or without an element of "professional judgment'' being built into the procedure). No single methodology is generally accepted or used in all employing authorities. This ''bottom-up'' approach to assessing staffing levels also contributes to the lack of detail at national level.

SOLVING THE PROBLEM

Having defined and ''measured'' the shortages, to the extent that available data makes such analysis possible, potential solutions to the shortages will be examined in this final section. Four possible solutions are proposed:

- Improve recruitment from ''traditional'' sources
- Increase substitution (i.e, recruit from nontraditional sources, including overseas)
- Enhance utilization of staff
- Improve retention of staff

It is not intended to go into detail as to the actual and potential merits of the myriad policy options which could be utilized to solve the shortages. Many will be familiar to nurses in the United Kingdom and in other countries; indeed some have been recently highlighted in two reports on nursing shortages in the United States. In highlighting the main solutions, the guiding principle should be, as noted in the introduction, that more than nine out of every ten nurses are female. Only policies which take due account of this rather obvious, but sometimes overlooked, factor should be considered or are likely to succeed.

Improve Recruitment from ''Traditional'' Sources

Female school leavers are the main source of recruits to nursing in the United Kingdom. As discussed earlier, the size of this potential pool of recruits will decline markedly over the next few years—a factor which also affects other European and North American coun-

tries to a greater or lesser extent. To compete in a ''sellers market'' for labor, nursing will have to be perceived as an attractive and rewarding career. Recent developments in the system of nurse education in the United Kingdom, with the establishment of college-based, supernumerary status for nursing students, should help achieve this objective, but constant review of starting salaries and benefits in comparable professions will also be required. Promoting a positive image of nursing is also a priority, and the UK government is currently funding a national advertising campaign to heighten awareness of nursing as a career. Of course, the reality of nursing will have to match up to the marketed image.

Increase Substitution

There is much potential in the United Kingdom for nursing to concentrate greater efforts on recruiting from nontraditional sources of recruits. Ethnic minorities are currently underrepresented in the profession, particularly in promoted posts. As progress is made toward establishing equal opportunities in the United Kingdom, and in the health service, it is to be hoped that more recruits from Asian and black backgrounds are encouraged to enter nursing. Mature entrants to training drawn from the increasing pool of 25 to 55 year olds present another potential source, but the needs for training and childcare facilities will have to be recognized and accommodated. Another source, currently underrepresented in nursing, are men. Only 7 percent of the NHS nursing workforce is male (although they do occupy a disproportionately large percentage of promoted posts). Whether increasing numbers of men can be recruited to a female-dominated profession where salaries are lower than in most male-dominated professions is debatable.

One other option is for the United Kingdom to expand its recruitment from overseas.

There have been recent reports of health authorities mounting recruitment drives in the Caribbean, Eire, and mainland Europe (particularly Spain), but in terms of overall numbers, flows of nurses to and from the United Kingdom are comparatively small. In 1986-1987 a total of 5216 verifications were issued to UK nurses wishing to practice abroad (Australia being the main destination) and a further 308 to nurses wishing to practice elsewhere in the European Economic Community (EEC). There were 1978 admissions to the UK register from nurses from non-EEC countries and a further 599 from EEC countries. In overall terms, the United Kingdom was therefore a net 'loser' (outflow approximately 5500, inflow approximately 2500), but neither flow was large in comparison to the overall stock of U.K. nurses.

Although the RCN favors international mobility of individual nurses in the pursuit of career development and the exchange of ideas, it would not wish to see any country meet its requirements for nursing staff by recruiting from other countries at a level which damaged health care provision in these other countries. Exploitation of the nursing resources of one country by other "richer" or more "developed" countries is unacceptable.

Enhance Utilization of Staff

Improvements in the effectiveness of the deployment of available staff is the third area of potential solution. Such action does not directly address the issues underlying the shortages, but it does ameliorate the effect on health-care provision. Ensuring the availability of appropriate administrative and domestic support staff and establishing the appropriate skill mix of nursing staff for different patient numbers and dependency levels (including retraining and redeploying where appropriate)

should be an ever-present tenet of good management.

Improve Retention of Staff

The need to take good care of nursing staff already employed in the organization should be a fundamental part of any strategy to combat shortages. The RCN-commissioned IMS report, referred to earlier, listed the following agenda for action:

1 Improve staffing levels in relation to workloads (e.g., by increasing establishments or, more likely, given present funding and recruitment problems, by ensuring that daily fluctuations in the match of staff to workloads do not produce overload on some days, or by decreasing overall workload levels)
2 Provide support and occupational health counseling services for staff to help them cope with workload-related stress
3 Improve pay and conditions (some progress has been made here with the establishment of a clinical career salary structure)
4 Initiate "stay-in-touch" retainer schemes during career breaks
5 Provide part-time and flexible hours
6 Provide career opportunities for part-timers
7 Provide childcare facilities

Clearly the style of management adopted by the health service in its approach to retaining nursing staff has to be founded on a recognition that nurses are career-oriented professionals—be they full-time or part-time, male or female, black or white. The primacy of a "male model" of unbroken full-time service as the prerequisite for career development and promotion in a female-dominated profession has always appeared illogical; with increasing shortages of staff this illogicity is no longer sustainable. Effective "manpower" planning may provide the key to solving nursing shortages, but it will be womanpower that unlocks the solutions.

REFERENCES

Department of Employment Gazette, April 1989.

Health and Personal Social Services, *Annual Abstract of Statistics,* HMSO.

Henderson J, Goldacre M, Graveney M, Simmons M, "Use of medical record linkage to study readmission rates." *British Medical Journal* September 16, 1989.

Office of Manpower Economics, United Kingdom, 1989.

United Kingdom Central Council for Nursing Midwifery and Health Visiting, *Annual Report.*

Waite R, Buchan J, Thomas J, "Nurses in and out of work: A report for the RCN." Institute of Manpower Studies, 1987.

Waite R, Hutt R, "Attitudes, jobs and mobility of qualified nurse: A report for the RCN." Institute of Manpower Studies, 1987.

"What to do about the Nursing Shortage," Commonwealth Fund, 1989; The Secretary of Health's Commission on Nursing. *Final Report,* 1988.

The Greek Nursing Workforce: Present Needs and Future Predictions

Dimitri Monos
John Yfantopoulos

There seems to be an almost inescapable inclination on the part of the people living toward the end of a century to project to the next many of their collective hopes and dreams.

Since historical evidence has provided no support for the justification of this inclination, humankind's collective hopes might stand a better chance if they were based on rational planning rather than wishful thinking.

One such goal for the twenty-first century is the improvement of health care, which, among other problems, is facing a worldwide nursing shortage.[1] However, the nursing workforce around the world has not in all cases decreased in proportion to the population. In several developed countries, in fact, the ratio of nurses to population has doubled several times during the last 10 to 20 years (Table 4-1).

However, the nursing shortage, as a consequence of public demand, is a reality. This demand is possibly understandable in view of the improvement in the quality of other aspects of communal life.

Chapter 4 examines the nursing shortage in Greece and nursing's future trends and pro-

Table 4-1   Number of Persons per Nurse

Countries	1960	1980
Germany	485	310
Belgium	—	133
France	—	—
Luxembourg	—	—
Netherlands	—	—
Denmark	—	143
United Kingdom	—	129
Spain	1,204	298
Greece	—	416
Italy	1,007	266
Portugal	1,458	447
United States	343	196
Japan	382	—
Sweden	324	150

Source: Organization of Economic Cooperation and Development (OECD), Paris, 1988.

vides suggestions which will possibly ameliorate the shortage. Greece is compared to the three other Mediterranean *European Economic Community* (EEC) countries (Portugal, Spain, and Italy), which share with Greece certain common cultural, political, and sociological similarities. In addition, this cluster of Mediterranean countries is compared to the rest of the EEC members as well as Japan, Sweden, and the United States, since these three are used as health-care models by many other developed countries.

The observations and commentaries presented here are not based on objective research, since nursing research in Greece has yet to be developed for the following reasons.

The first university nursing department was founded as a branch of the School of Medicine of the University of Athens in 1980, achieved an independent status within the School of Health Sciences in 1983, and graduated its first class in 1985. Its original core faculty of seven could not possibly concentrate on research, as they were overwhelmed by basic problems such as the total absence of office and classroom space, lack of secretarial help, lack of textbooks for a university-level science, and, at times, the open hostility on the

part of a considerable number of medical faculty. With the hiring of some younger research-oriented faculty members, however, a corpus of research ought to be developing in the next several years.

For these reasons, the authors have used their own and other colleagues' observations and experiences as medical and nursing professionals, hospital administrators and government health advisors to create commentaries presented here.

WORLDWIDE NURSING SHORTAGE

There is a shortage of nursing personnel in most Western European countries (Table 4-1). In Greece, 416 inhabitants compete for the services of one nurse. In Italy the nursing personnel have developed at a much faster rate, and there this ratio is much smaller—250 inhabitants per nurse; in Spain the ratio is 300: 1, and in Portugal 450: 1. In southern Europe, then, Greece and Portugal show severe shortages of nursing personnel.

The rest of the European countries present a better indicator of nursing personnel. The United States and Sweden show an even better picture, probably due to a long-standing tradition in the organization of health-care services.

The nursing shortage in Greece is even more severe, in terms of qualified nursing personnel. In this country, there is a distinction between the nonqualified practical nurses, the graduates of one- and two-year programs housed within hospitals, and the qualified graduates of three-year programs from technical institutes (T.E.I.). There are also the recent degree holders of the four-year program of the University of Athens, but since the first class graduated in 1985, these are too few to be included in this comparative analysis.

There has been a considerable expansion in the Greek nursing workforce during the last few years (Figure 4-1). This expansion results,

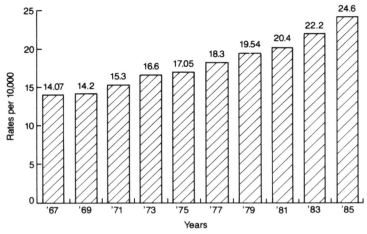

Figure 4-1   Nursing Evolution.

however, largely from an increase in the number of nonqualified nurses. In terms of qualified nursing personnel, the evolutionary changes are very small (Figure 4-2).

It is to be noted that during the same period that the Greek nursing workforce has increased, the population of the country has remained almost constant. Greece, then, resembles some developed countries, such as the United States, where an increase has been followed by a greater demand for nursing personnel.

Two major factors may explain this new demand. During the last 20 years, a very rapid urbanization has taken place in Greece, a consequence of which is the reorientation of the population from a traditional folk medicine to a more professional system of health care. In addition, the unhealthy conditions associated with urban living have increased considerably the incidence of hospitalization and the consequent need for more nursing personnel. Athens, for instance, which contains almost one-third of the Greek population, is also one

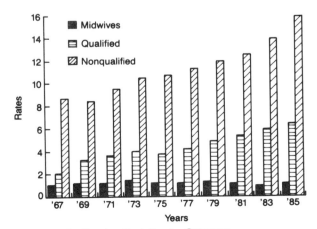

Figure 4-2   Nursing Evolution by Category.

of Europe's most polluted cities. The levels of pollution frequently surpass the dangerous limits, and hundreds of people require medical care for respiratory, heart, and other complaints.

THE QUANTITATIVE ASSESSMENT OF THE NURSING SHORTAGE

To assess the nursing shortage we have focused on the expenditure and the utilization aspects of the health-care system, vis-à-vis the nursing workforce needs of the present and the future.

Empirical evidence indicates that, in terms of the evolution of health-care system, there is a time-lag of approximately 5 to 10 years between the Mediterranean and the other EEC countries.[2] This lag is due to political as well as economic reasons.

The existence, for years, of nondemocratic governments (Spain, Portugal, Greece), are associated with restrained social policies. The reestablishment, however, of democracies in these countries has brought about a new era of social policies, including an increase of health and nursing services. In addition, the reestablishment of democracies precipitated an economic development which brought an increase in the GDP (gross domestic product), as well as substantial improvements in the distribution of income. Empirical evidence reveals that, in all these countries, the income-inequality measures have been substantially reduced. The proportion of poverty, in comparison to Northern European countries (except Ireland), however, still remains high.[3] Finally, to satisfy the accumulated social needs and to combat previous economic and social stagnation, the expenditures of these countries were increased substantially, followed by increased coverage for primary, secondary, and tertiary health care.

An established method of drawing meaningful economic comparisons is the use of purchasing power parity rates. This indicator is equivalent to what is known in the Greek economic language as "the housewife's shopping cart," and this indicator assesses the amount the average person has to spend on health.

Economic indicators show that the Southern European EEC members spend on health much less per capita than do the Northern European countries. Greece spends 256 per capita per year on health and exceeds slightly only Portugal, which spends 248 (Table 4-2).

Specifically, the wealthier European countries—Germany, Belgium, Denmark, and the Netherlands—spend approximately 8.2 to 9.3 percent of their GDP on health-care activities. The percentage that the Southern European countries spend on health is much smaller. Greece has the lowest expenditure (4.4 percent) of all the European and non-European countries compared.

With regard to the form of health service—whether it is private or public—with the exception of Greece, the proportion of public expenditures (Table 4-2, column 3) is quite high, an evidence of the dominance of the public health system in the majority of the European countries. In Southern Europe approximately 80 percent of the health-care activities are carried out by the public sector, which has, of course, many implications for the quality and the provisional aspects of the health-care system.

For the analysis of the performance aspect of the health-care systems, hospital admission rate, average length of stay, and number of persons per physician have been used as indicators of health-care utilization (Table 4-3).

With regard to hospital admission rate, and in contrast to the northern EEC countries, considerably fewer people in the south of Europe are admitted to the hospitals (Table 4-3). The Greek rate (11.9 percent) is equal to the lowest in Northern Europe, found in the Netherlands. And this low Greek rate is probably inflated: The recently (1983) introduced

Table 4-2   Public Expenditure on Health

Countries	Per capita expenditure on medical care (at current GDP purchasing power parity rates), 1982	Percentage of total expenditure on health in GDP, 1982	Percentage of public expenditure on health in GDP-1982	Total expenditure on health in constant prices, 1975–1982	Public expenditure on health in constant prices, 1975–1982
Germany	883	8.2	6.6	0.8	0.7
Belgium	636	6.2	5.8	2.3	2.8
France	996	9.3	6.6	1.2	2.5
Luxembourg	719	6.5	7.4	—	—
Netherlands	851	8.7	6.9	0.7	1.1
Denmark	736	6.8	5.9	1.8	1.4
United Kingdom	539	5.9	5.2	1.2	0.9
Ireland	532	8.2	7.7	1.0	1.5
Spain	417	6.3	4.6	—	—
Greece	256	4.4	3.4	2.1	3.6
Italy	673	7.2	6.1	0.8	0.7
Portugal	248	5.7	4.0	—	—
United States	1.388	10.6	4.5	1.4	
Japan	673	6.6	4.8	1.4	
Sweden	1.239	9.7	8.9	3.9	

Source: Organization of Economic Cooperation and Development (OECD), Paris, 1988.

Table 4-3   Indicator of Health-Care Utilization

Countries	Percentage of inpatient care	Hospital admission rate	Average length of stay	Number of persons per hospital bed	Number of persons per physician
Germany	3.4	18.1	18.7	90	422
Belgium	2.8	13.9	13.5	106	384
France	3.1	12.1	14.1	90	480
Luxembourg	3.8	17.8	21.0	76	605
Netherlands	4.0	11.9	34.1	83	497
Denmark	2.2	18.7	11.9	130	416
United Kingdom	2.4	12.7	18.6	124	775
Ireland	1.6	17.6	9.0	103	845
Spain	1.3	9.2	14.6	185	498
Greece	1.6	11.9	13.0	162	394
Italy	2.2	15.6	12.4	127	798
Portugal	1.4	9.6	14.4	195	454
United States	1.7	17.0	9.0	124	498
Japan	3.6	6.4	56.1	84	738
Sweden	4.8	18.9	22.9	71	427

Source: Organization of Economic Cooperation and Development (OECD), Paris, 1988.

National Health Care system established a number of local health-care centers in the various parts of the country which are permanently underused, as the Greek patient prefers to seek medical help in the larger urban centers. As a result, to justify the existence of these centers, the local staff keep in them patients for minor ailments and for longer treatment periods than are actually needed.

Not only are fewer Southern Europeans admitted to hospitals, but their average hospital stay is considerably shorter than what is found in the north of Europe. This could be mistakenly taken as an indicator of more health and greater health-care efficiency in Southern Europe.

However, a look at the number of persons per hospital bed (Table 4-3, column 4) clearly shows a severe shortage of beds in the Mediterranean EEC countries as compared to the north of Europe and to the other three non-European countries. Therefore, a reasonable conclusion is that the shortage of beds in Southern Europe, on one hand discourages hospital admission and on the other encourages early dismissal from the hospital. This conclusion is supported by the evidence provided by the picture of the average public Greek hospital, where cots placed in the corridors to accomodate the great number of patients is part of the daily routine.

The workforce issue of health-care utilization indicators is analyzed in terms of number of persons corresponding to one physician and/or one nurse. Greece, with 1 physician per 394 persons, presents an oversupply of medical doctors. This ratio is the highest among all the European and non-European countries compared, with the exception of Belgium, whose ratio is 1 physician per 384 persons.

In Greece, this oversupply of physicians goes hand in hand with an undersupply of nursing personnel, which, with the exception of Portugal, is also the largest among the countries compared.

One of the problems of an oversupply of physicians is their underemployment, if not unemployment, at times. To a degree, this problem has been averted in Greece—in a number of hospitals and other health-care establishments much activity which could be carried out by scientifically trained nursing personnel is actually being carried out by physicians. It is not accidental, then, that Greece did not introduce nursing into its university curriculum until 1980, and then it received much opposition from the medical establishment and the medical faculty. The oversupply of physicians, then, can be considered as one of the obstacles to both the quantitative and qualitative evolution of the nursing profession in Greece.

In summary, and in terms of the health-care untilization indicators in Europe, Greece follows the same pattern of evolution as do the rest of the Southern European countries. Greece most resembles Portugal, Spain exhibiting a somewhat more progressive picture. The Italian model resembles more that of the Northern European countries, which show higher per-capita expenditures for health, higher percentages of total and public expenditures on health, and higher supply of hospital beds.

FORECASTING GREEK NURSING WORKFORCE EVOLUTION

Under public law 1397, the National Health System was established in Greece in 1983. A committee formed to identify nursing workforce needs concluded that the desired goal was a 300 percent increase of the qualified nurses in the country. If these nurses were to materialize overnight, the ratio of persons per nurse would be diminished from 416: 1 to 188: 1 (or from 24 to 53 nurses per 10,000 inhabitants), which would be the smallest ratio in the Mediterranean EEC countries.

However, at the rate at which the nursing personnel is increasing at present, the desired nursing workforce goal could not be reached for 35 years. To make this forecast, data have been gathered covering the period 1967 to 1985 (Figure 4-1). During this period the total (qualified, practical nurses, and midwives) nursing personnel was increased from 14.7 to 24.6 per 10,000 inhabitants.

To forecast the nursing workforce from 1985 to the year 2025, the following linear regression analysis has been used: $Y = 10.1077 + 0.738t$, where the coefficient of determination is $R^2 = 0.733$. Y represents nursing personnel per 10,000 inhabitants and t stands for time.

As the formula interprets 73 percent of the variation of the dependent variable, it is a good indicator of the quantitative evolution of the nursing workforce.

Using this analysis, then, it is determined that by the year 1990, about 27.10 nurses will correspond to 10,000 inhabitants; in 1995, the number goes up to 30.77, in the year 2000 to 35.21, in 2010 to 42.60, and it will not be before the year 2025 that the desired ratio of 54 nurses per 10,000 people will be reached.

Note that this predictive model is based on the existing evolutionary patterns and has not taken into account any other forms of intervention such as new technologies which might reduce the quantity of required nursing personnel. Without such helpful interventions, however, Greece needs to develop very rapidly strategies to increase its nursing workforce.

THE GEOGRAPHY OF THE NURSING SHORTAGE

As serious as the nursing shortage is in Greece, the regional distribution of nursing workforce gives an even greater reason for concern. Greece resembles many other countries where the medical services have been disproportionally concentrated in the large urban areas. Athens, for instance, which houses almost 30 percent of the country's population, has 49 percent of the country's hospital beds, 52 percent of the nursing workforce, and 60 percent of the physicians (Table 4-4).

In terms of qualified nursing personnel, the picture is even grimmer, as 75 percent of them are concentrated in Athens, and the rest of them (25 percent) offer their services to 70 percent of the population.

This shortage of qualified nursing personnel at the regional level undermines seriously the quality of services. It also creates problems to nursing planning activities related to social

Table 4-4 Hospitals, Beds, Doctors, and Nursing Personnel in Greece by Geographic Region, 1987

	Hospitals		Beds		Doctors		Nursing		Nurses per Bed	Nurses per Doctor
	Number	Percent	Number	Percent	Number	Percent	Number	Percent		
Athens	124	27.3	25,471	49.2	9,131	60.0	14,270	51.9	0.56	1.56
Central Greece	39	8.5	2,054	3.9	349	2.3	861	3.1	0.42	2.46
Peloponnesus	59	13.0	3,133	6.0	736	4.8	1,690	6.1	0.54	2.30
Ionian Islands	12	2.6	964	1.8	131	0.9	400	1.4	0.42	3.05
Epirus	13	2.8	844	1.6	288	1.9	629	2.2	0.75	2.18
Thessaly	45	9.9	2,386	4.6	434	2.8	1,095	4.0	0.46	2.52
Macedonia	93	20.5	11,303	21.8	3,145	20.7	5,770	21.0	0.51	1.83
Thrace	11	2.4	780	1.5	278	1.8	669	2.4	0.86	2.40
Aegean Islands	22	4.8	2,528	4.9	227	1.5	945	3.4	0.37	4.16
Crete	36	7.9	2,282	4.4	486	3.2	1,125	4.1	0.49	2.32
Total	454	100.0	51,745	100.0	15,205	100.0	27,454	100.0	0.53	1.81

Source: National Statistical Service of Greece, "Social Welfare and Health Statistics," 1989

medicine and primary health care which require qualified, expert nursing personnel. The gulf between Athens and the rest of the country has increased dramatically since 1977 and will probably continue to increase in the same fashion, since most qualified nurses are educated in Athens and many choose to remain there.

IMPORTED NURSING PERSONNEL

Greece does not export nurses, as it has a serious nursing shortage. On the contrary, the country is an importer of nursing personnel and, particularly, at the qualified and the specialized level.

Concerning the regulating of the employment of foreign nursing personnel, Greece complies with the 1951 Treaty of Rome whose aim was to increase competition of goods and services through the free movement of personnel and services across the borders.

But the mutual recognition of courses and standards of personnel did not occur until 1967, when the first recognition of mutual qualifications of medical personnel was agreed upon. The first regulation which enhanced the free movement of nursing personnel was signed in Brussels in 1977. At the beginning, this movement was aimed at the general nursing personnel, but later it was expanded to include the qualified nurses as well. As there are no national data gathered by a governmental agency, the present analysis was accomplished by resorting to a sampling procedure which discovered in some health care institutions in Athens—such as the Red Cross Hospital—as well as in hospitals in other areas a small number of foreign nurses from the Netherlands, England, and other European countries. These nurses are well trained and are mainly used in qualified activities, such as intensive care units.

Greece, so far, has such a tremendous shortage of nursing personnel, that the presence of foreign nursing personnel has not created a problem. On the contrary, the high training of these nurses has facilitated the operation and even raised the standards of nursing care in some Greek hospitals.

The imported highly trained nurses constitute only a minute part of the great need for qualified nurses in Greece. A coherent plan, therefore, is soon needed, including financial and other incentives, which will produce more qualified nurses and encourage a good number of them to move to various regions of the country.

SUGGESTIONS FOR SOLVING NURSING WORKFORCE PROBLEMS

As has been discussed, three main nursing workforce problems exist in Greece—a general severe nursing shortage, an even more severe shortage of qualified nurses, and a highly uneven distribution of general and qualified nursing personnel around the country.

So far, there is no national plan to deal with these problems. The agency which has undertaken the responsibility of balancing supply and demand for nursing personnel is the Ministry of Health and Welfare Services. Unfortunately, in this Ministry there is not even an office or directory for nursing personnel; no type of planning, let alone scientific planning, is being carried out to balance the present supply and demand or to forecast future needs.

The first proposal, therefore, is that this responsibility is assumed by the so-called KESY (the central health council), whose primary goal ought to be the creation of a nursing study committee which will undertake the scientific and planning activities of balancing supply and demand. The first two tasks that this committee will have to work on are the retention of existing and creation of new nursing personnel. The solution of the problem of retention is a difficult but a primary one, as it is directly related to attracting young persons into the profession in the future.

Greece is a country of dramatic social, organizational, and bureaucratic contrasts. Many government employees do very little, as they were hired not because there was work to be done but rather because there were political debts to be paid off to political constituents by elected deputies and new ministers. However, there are professional people of vital importance, such as nurses, who are severely overworked and terribly underpaid. In addition, nurses in Greece enjoy a very low social status.

An additional problem concerning the retention of nursing personnel is a law which had made it attractive for married nurses, for years, to leave the profession and receive retirement benefits after only 15 years of work. This law has been rescinded for those who began work in the present decade, but thousands who began employment while the law was in force will be taking advantage of its benefits during the next several years.

To achieve the retention, therefore, of the nursing personnel, Greece needs to create economic, social, and educational incentives, such as tertiary, university, and other educational opportunities. At the present, the country has, possibly unintentionally, created an excellent opportunity to accomplish this goal.

Due to the peculiarities of the Greek university entrance examination system, and after the creation of the department of nursing, the students who, as a result of extremely competitive examinations, barely fail to gain entrance into the department of medicine, can enroll in the school of nursing.

Consequently, at present, the department of nursing of the School of Health Sciences of the University of Athens receives approximately eighty students of both sexes of very high academic potential every year. Unfortunately, fewer than two-thirds of them conclude their studies there. The others repeat their effort to gain entrance into the department of medicine.

But even if all of these students graduated from the department of nursing, they would comprise only a faint answer to the quantitative nursing personnel needs of the country. Consequently, the answer to the shortage of nursing workforce in Greece depends on the following:

1 Economic, educational, and social incentives to retain the existing nursing workforce and attract considerable numbers of young people into the profession
2 The opening of nursing departments in all the Greek universities
3 The elevation to the university level of the Greek three-year technical institutes, whose nursing departments graduate the greatest number of nurses

Those three goals could gradually alleviate the shortage of well-trained qualified nurses. The great need for specialized nursing personnel, such as psychiatric and intensive-care nurses, will have to be satisfied by the programs which will be developed in the aforementioned new university nursing departments.

The redistribution of nursing personnel according to each region's needs has, at least theoretically, already been addressed. KESY is planning to adopt a system similar to the one existing in England, dividing the country into health regions. So far there have been specified thirteen such regions.

The plan is that each region obtains tertiary hospital, university hospital, and eventually, secondary and tertiary care. In this way, the educational and training needs of nurses are expected to be met at the regional level, avoiding the lure of the large urban centers.

NURSING LEADERSHIP

The serious nursing workforce problems facing Greece obviously require competent leadership at the hospital, the university, the regional, and the national planning level.

The nursing school of the University of Athens, as the first and the leading such school of Greece, is well aware of the responsibility it carries, in this respect.

Some of the first university nursing students were graduates of three-year programs who had several years of working experience. By providing them with extended leaves-of-absence with full salary, the hospitals they were working for encouraged them to finish their university degrees. Upon graduation, these nurses were placed as assistants to the nursing director's office. Soon afterward, some of them assumed the nursing director's offices at some of Greece's larger hospitals, including the university hospital of the University of Athens. These new nursing directors are expected to play an important role in reshaping the image of the Greek nurse, modifying the interpersonal and working relationships with the physicians and improving the nursing administration activities.

At the university level, the Faculty of Nursing of the University of Athens offers the doctorate in nursing, which, using the standard European model, is solely based on the preparation and defense of a dissertation. A more comprehensive program modeled after the U.S. Ph.D. is still in the planning stage.

The department of nursing is producing a considerable number of doctorates at an impressive pace. Some of the school's faculty are concerned that the impressive quantity may be obtained at the expense of quality. The opposite view is that the urgent need for nursing Ph.Ds (the Ph.D. is a prerequisite for teaching in a Greek university) to fill the positions in the nursing departments of other Greek universities calls for some sacrifices in quality, at least for the time being. In any event, these nurses who already have or will soon obtain their doctorates will, undoubtedly, play a leading role in the development of the new university nursing departments.

Some of the first Ph.D. graduates wrote dissertations dealing with hospital management and administration, workforce issues, and nursing education. These graduates, therefore, are the obvious people to assume leading roles and positions within the nursing establishment. One of the most important of these roles is undoubtedly membership in KESY's study committee, which will undertake the scientific and planning activities of balancing the supply and demand of the country's nursing workforce. This chapter has proposed that the creation of this committee is of urgent importance, as it constitutes the major factors for the improvement of health care in Greece in the twenty-first century.

REFERENCES

1 World Health Organization (1985). *Health Manpower Requirements for the Achievement of Health for All by the Year 2000 through Primary Health Care*, WHO Technical Report, Series 717. Geneva.
2 Yfantopoulos J. (1988). *Health Planning in Greece, Some Economic and Social Aspects*. National Centre of Social Research. Athens.
3 O'Higgins, M., and Jenkins S. (1984). "Poverty in Europe." Paper presented in the European Conference on Poverty. University of Leyden, Holland.

Chapter 5

Health Manpower in Korea: Demands, Supply, and Education

Mo-Im Kim

INTRODUCTION

There is a growing awareness that health is not only a basic human right but also an important objective of social development for a nation, a prerequisite for socioeconomic progress. This awareness is noted not only among policy makers and administrators but among the public as a whole. Surveys conducted jointly in 1984 and 1985 by Korean television and a daily newspaper disclosed health as one of the most important goals among the items listed. High-ranking policy makers should now ask themselves if this country can achieve national pro-

gress without health management rather than ask whether we have the resources to manage health. Today our living standards are such that we can appreciate the meaning of the adage, "a healthy person has hope, and he who has hope has everything."

Research findings indicate a positive correlation between a public's demands for health services and its socioeconomic and educational standards. We should anticipate that popular expectations for health services will continue to rise, and the availability of personnel to meet this certain challenge is a major health issue.

The meaning of human resources can vary significantly depending on the terms we choose. The World Health Organization (WHO) has defined health professional to include everyone from a community health worker to a cardiac surgeon, that is, anyone who can perform duties efficiently within a health system. Mejia and Fulop define human resources in public health as including: (1) health workers already involved in the field of public health; (2) potential health workers, i.e., persons with experience or training in a specific area of public health; and (3) future health workers currently receiving education or training to work in the field of public health.

These are broad definitions, but each encompasses widely different types of workers. Timothy D. Baker (1968) does not define as health workers individuals such as drivers and administrative workers who have not received any special training even though they work for medical and public health institutions.

The concept of a health work force used here is taken from medical law in Korea:

1 Medical doctors, doctors of Oriental medicine, dentists, midwives, and nurses as stipulated in the Medical Law, Article 2; nurses' aides as prescribed in Article 58 thereof; paramedical personnel such as chiropractors, acupuncturists, and "moxacauterists" as defined in Article 60; and physiotherapists as defined in Article 61.
2 Pharmacists as prescribed in the Pharmaceutical Affairs Law, Article 2.
3 Clinical pathologists, radiologists, physical therapists, occupational therapists, dental technicians, dental hygienists, and medical clerks as defined in the Medical Law, Article 2.

THE PRESENT STATUS OF HEALTH PROFESSIONALS IN KOREA

The status of the health work force in Korea will be examined in terms of the following: (1)

categories of health personnel and educational requirements, (2) the population as it relates to health personnel, (3) composition of the health work force, (4) employment and registration, (5) employment by health facilities, and (6) urban and rural distribution.

Categorizing Health Personnel and Educational Requirements

The qualifications of health personnel are strictly regulated by law because their activities have a direct impact on people's lives. Only qualified and licensed/certified persons can engage in health work (see Table 5-1).

The qualifying standards and duration of education required for licensure of health professionals vary depending on the degree of expertise required for each role in health work. The licensing for medical doctors, doctors of Oriental medicine, dentists, midwives, and nurses is described in the Medical Law, and pharmacists' licensing procedures are defined in the Pharmaceutical Affairs Law. All licensing procedures are subject to approval by the minister of Health and Social Affairs. All candidates must pass a national licensing examination. To be eligible for such tests, a candidate must finish high school, pass the national college entrance examination, and successfully complete 3 to 6 years of professional education.

The certifying of paramedical personnel is subject to approval by the mayor or governor of a province upon (1) passage of qualifying certification tests supervised by the head of a local government, and (2) completion of a specified training program.

The paramedical personnel stipulated by the Medical Technician Law include clinical technicians, radiologists, physical therapists, occupational therapists, dental technicians, dental hygienists, and medical clerks. Eligibility for certifying examinations for these positions requires a high school diploma plus a 1- to 2-year junior college degree and success in examinations required by law.

Table 5-1 Categories of Health Personnel and Education Requirement in Korea

Type of law	Categories	Education requirement	Eligibility test for college	Length of education training	License or certificate	Government authority involved
Medical law Article 2	Medical doctor	High school	Yes	6 years	License	Minister of Public Health & Social Affairs (PHSA)
	Oriental doctor	High school	Yes	6 years	License	PHSA
	Dentist	High school	Yes	6 years	License	PHSA
	Midwife	Nurse/Lic.	Yes	1 year	License	PHSA
	Nurse	High school	Yes	3 to 4 years	License	PHSA
	Clinical technician	High school	No	2 years	Certificate	PHSA
	Radiologist technician	High school	No	2 years	Certificate	PHSA
	Physical therapist	High school	No	2 years	Certificate	PHSA
	Occupational therapist	High school	No	2 years	Certificate	PHSA
	Dental technician	High school	No	2 years	Certificate	PHSA
	Dental hygienist	High school	No	2 years	Certificate	PHSA
	Medical clerk	High school	No	2 years	Certificate	PHSA
Medical law Article 58	Nurses aides	Middle school till 1984; high school since 1985	No	9 months	Certificate	Mayor/governor
Medical law Article 60	Chiropractor	None	No		Certificate	
	Acupuncturist	None	No	1 year	Certificate	
	Moxacauterist	None	No		Certificate	
Medical law Article 61	Physiotherapist	None	No		Certificate	
Pharmaceutical law	Pharmacist	High school	Yes	2 years	License	PHSA

Source: Ministry of Justice, B vol. 22, no. 23, 1985

One of the problems with our paramedical personnel is that training has been taking place in facilities outside the formal education system. Given the quality of this training, one is skeptical about whether such health workers can perform their duties properly. (Korea is just entering the age of information with its recent socioeconomic progress. In 1985 the nation was able to stipulate the completion of high school as part of eligibility for the training of nurses' aides.)

Population and the Health Work Force

One index used to depict the health care status of a country is the ratio of health work force to the population. As of 1975, the ratio of pharmacists and nurses' aides in Korea was high compared to other developing countries, but the relative numbers of doctors, dentists, nurses, midwives, and medical technicians was low.

In 1984 Korea's ratio of doctors, dentists, and nurses (including midwives) per 100,000 population as compared to Japanese workers in these categories was approximately 1:3, 1:3, and 1:8 respectively (see Table 5-2).

These figures suggest that the number of doctors and dentists in Korea is less than that of Japan and the averages of other developing countries, and the number of nurses and medical technicians is even smaller. The number of pharmacists and nurses' aides far exceeds that of other developing nations. Obviously there are problems in the supply side of our health work force.

At the end of 1984, the total number of health workers as defined by current medical laws and regulations was 117,142—a mere 0.78 percent of the nation's economically active population. When compared with the statistics of developed countries in Table 5-3, our situation is equivalent to that of Hungary in the 1950s. Of course the interpretation of comparative data on a global scale requires a great deal of caution as the definitions of socioeconomic growth and health personnel differ from country to country, but the data presented here indicate that the overall ratio of our health workers to the population is comparatively low. Korea is an underdeveloped nation when it comes to health services; the efforts by the government have been insufficient.

Table 5–2   Selected Health Personnel Density per 100,000 Population by Country

Health personnel	Korea (1984)	Developing country (1975)	Developed country (1975)	Japan (1984)
Doctor	51.8	28	87	144.3
Doctor of oriental medicine	(7.0)	—	—	—
Dentist	10.0	5	17	51.0
Nurse-midwife	64.5	29	153	528.5
Health care nurse	N/A	N/A	N/A	7.3
Midwife	N/A	N/A	N/A	20.3
Nurse	N/A	N/A	N/A	490.9
Nurse's aid	87.2	32	63	N/A
Medical engineer	21.7	13	96	N/A
Dental technician	N/A	N/A	N/A	24.4
Dental hygienist	N/A	N/A	N/A	24.3
Pharmacist	45.6	9	23	62.1

Source: "A Study on Long-term Demand and Supply of Health Professionals," KIPH, 1986; Bul Dang Ha Doan, "Statistical Analysis of the World Health Manpower Situation Circa 1975," *World Health Statistics Quarterly,* WHO, vol. 33, no. 2, 1980; Ministry of Health, Japan, *Reports on the Status of Doctors Dentists and Pharmacists, in Japan,* (N/A) Data not available, 1986

Table 5–3 Percent Distribution of Health Personnel among Economically Active Population of Six European Countries by Year

Country	1950	1960	1970	Remarks
Korea		0.16	0.58	0.78 in 1984
Austria	1.5	1.8	2.3	
West Germany	1.5	1.6	2.1	
Hungary	0.7	1.5	2.1	
Sweden	2.0	3.4	6.0	
Switzerland	1.7	2.1	2.5	
United Kingdom	1.8	2.0	2.4	
Average	1.5	1.8	2.3	

Sources: Figures for Austria from C. P. Hogan, "Health Sector Growth and Changes in the Blend of Health Groups in Seven Countries over Two Decades," *World Health Statistics Quarterly,* WHO, vol. 32, no. 2, 1979; figures for Korea 1984 are from "A Study on Long-term Demand and Supply of Health Professionals," KIPH, 1986; Korean figures for 1960 and 1970 from Economic Planning Board, Census of 1960 and 1970.

Composition of the Health Work Force

Another index of the status of health care is the proportion of different categories of health professionals. Table 5-4 indicates that (1) the ratio of dentists in Korea is low compared to developing countries, (2) the ratio of nurses and midwives is low compared to developed countries, and (3) the ratio of nurses' aides and pharmacists is high as compared to both developed and developing countries. The ratio of medical technicians is low for both comparisons.

Data in Table 5-5 indicate that in Japan nurses comprised 67 percent of the cumulative total for the four representative health professionals, whereas in Korea they comprised only 36 percent.

In Korea, the excessive number of nurses' aides may be characterized as a case of "overemployment," whereas the number of pharmacists and doctors relative to nurses is so great that many are underemployed, a situation that inflates the cost of medical care nationally.

WHO has proclaimed that "prevention is better than care and a lot cheaper," contending that developing nations are jeopardizing the health of millions of their people by allocating 80 percent of their public health budget to preparing doctors. Put bluntly, educating

Table 5–4 Percent Distribution of Selected Health Positions by Country

Health position	Korea (1984)	Developing Country (1975)	Developed Country (1975)
Doctor	17.9	24.1	19.8
Doctor of oriental medicine	(2.4)		
Dentist	3.5	4.3	3.9
Nurse-midwife	22.7	25.0	34.8
Nurse's aid	30.2	27.6	14.4
Medical technician	7.5	11.2	21.9
Pharmacist	15.8	7.8	5.2
Total	100.0	100.0	100.0

Source: Korean Population and Public Health Research Institute, "A Study on Long-term Demand and Supply of Health Professionals," April 1986.

Table 5–5 Health Professionals in Korea and Japan, 1984

Health professionals	Korea	Japan
Doctors (doctors of oriental medicine included)	32.71%	18.36%
Dentists	5.55	6.48
Nurses (midwives included)	36.39	67.26
Pharmacists	25.35	7.90
Total	100.00	100.00

Sources: Korean data from *Survey on Professional Health Manpower* conducted by KIPH in 1984. Japanese data from *Reports on the Status of Doctors, Dentists, and Pharmacists,* Ministry of Health, 1986.

doctors is a drain on financial resources. The WHO report indicates that we need to change the structure of our professional health work force in keeping with socioeconomic advancement and attendant on the demands of the public for quality health care.

Employment and Registration

As Table 5-6 displays, on December 31, 1984, the total number of licensed/certified health workers in Korea was 217,445. In the same year, only 117,142 of these (54 percent) were actively employed. No organization has reliable statistics on emigrants, and the official employment rate simply accumulates all persons who have been registered. The paucity of reliable data is a problem when such data become the basis for government policies.

Song's calculation suggests that the 1984 figures on registered doctors included 16.4 percent who had left the country and 9.6 percent who were deceased. Hence the actual employment rate for medical doctors would be about 75.1 percent. Kim (1983) estimated that, as of 1983, 27.9 percent of the registered nurses were employed or had emigrated overseas and 18.3 percent were retired. Thus the real employment rates for nurses in 1984 would have been much higher than that shown in Table 5-6.

Although data are not available, it is safe to expect that a higher employment rate would similarly apply to doctors, doctors of oriental medicine, dentists, pharmacists, and midwives who engage in private practice.

Among the registered professionals, slightly over 50 percent actually contribute to health care for people in Korea. These data give administrators and educators of public health a lot to think about.

Employment by Health Facilities

Among the health professionals stipulated in the Medical Law, the following percentages

Table 5–6 Number and Percent Distribution of Selected Health Positions and Employment Status

Health position	Total registered	Employed	Not employed*
Doctors	28,015	21,033 (75.1%)	6,982 (24.9%)
Doctors of oriental medicine	3,591	2,828 (78.8)	763 (21.2)
Dentists	4,972	4,051 (81.5)	921 (18.5)
Nurses	54,081	24,624 (45.5)	29,457 (54.5)
Midwives	5,991	1,920 (22.0)	4,071 (68.0)
Pharmacists	28,531	18,497 (64.8)	10,034 (35.2)
Nurse's aids	92,264	35,377 (38.7)	56,587 (61.3)
Medical technicians	7,501	8,812 (50.4)	8,689 (49.6)
Total	217,445	117,142 (53.9)	100,303 (46.1)

* Includes deceased and retired.

Sources: Data from Ministry of Health and Social Affairs, *White Paper,* 1985, and *Census on Health Manpower* conducted by KIPH for 1984.

work in hospitals and doctor's private clinics: doctors, 86 percent; doctors of oriental medicine, 98 percent; nurses, 68 percent; midwives, 40 percent; and nurses' aides, 91 percent. Of pharmacists described by the Pharmaceutical Affairs Law, 7 percent work in hospitals and clinics, and 91 percent have their own pharmacies or work in other areas (see Table 5-7). Seventy-six percent of medical technicians work in hospitals and doctor's clinics. Only 5 percent of the 117,142 health professionals work in various health centers,

and 9 percent are employed by administrative, training, or research institutes. A preponderance of 85 percent of Korea's health professionals are engaged in curative services.

Urban and Rural Distribution

Table 5-8 looks at the geographic distribution of health professionals; it shows that they are concentrated in urban areas. In 1975, 48 percent of the population was rural, and 52 percent was urban. In 1980, 43 pecent was rural and 57 percent urban. By 1983, only 37 per-

Table 5-7   Number and Percent Distribution of Selected Health Professionals Employed, by Health Facility, 1984

Institution	Doctor Number	Doctor Percent	Doctor of oriental medicine Number	Doctor of oriental medicine Percent	Dentist Number	Dentist Percent	Pharmacist Number	Pharmacist Percent
Hospital	10,095	48.0	145	5.1	682	16.8		
							1,317	7.1
Clinic	8,032	38.2	2,634	93.1	2,789	68.9		
Subtotal		86.2		98.2		85.7		7.1
Health center (branches incl.)	1,245	5.9			399	9.8	70	0.4
Administrative works	75	0.4					121	0.6
Subtotal		6.3				9.8		1.0
Training, research and others	1,435	7.5	49	1.8	181	4.5	231	1.3
							16,758	90.6
Subtotal		7.5		1.8		4.5		91.9
Total	21,033	100.0	2,828	100.0	4,051	100.0	18,497	100.0

Institution	Nurse Number	Nurse Percent	Midwife Number	Midwife Percent	Nurse's aid Number	Nurse's aid Percent	Medical technician Number	Medical technician Percent
Hospital	15,995	65.0	686	35.7	12,832	36.3	4,911	56.7
Clinic	623	2.5	85	4.4	19,196	54.3	1,770	20.1
Subtotal		67.5		40.1		90.6		75.8
Health Center (branches incl.)	2,864	11.6	402	20.9	3,349	9.4	585	6.6
Administrative works	361	1.5	85	4.4			275	3.1
Subtotal		13.1		25.3		9.4		9.7
Training, research	3,829	15.5	159	8.3			868	9.9
and others	952	3.9	503	26.3			403	4.6
Subtotal		19.4		34.6				14.5
Total	24,624	100.0	1,920	100.0	35,377	100.0	8,812	100.0

Sources: Data from *Census on Health Manpower,* conducted by KIPH for 1984, and Ministry of Health and Social Affairs, *Statistical Yearbook, 1985.*

Table 5–8   Distribution of Population and Health Workers by Urban and Rural
            Areas, 1980 and 1983

	1980		1983	
	Urban	Rural	Urban	Rural
Population	57.3%	42.7%	62.9%	37.1%
Distribution of health workers				
Doctor	89.3	10.8	87.1	12.9
Dentist	92.4	7.6	91.2	8.8
Doctor of Oriental Medicine	86.3	13.7	85.9	14.1
Nurse	85.5	14.5	85.1	14.9
Midwife	79.6	20.4	85.7	14.3
Pharmacist	N/A	N/A	88.0	12.0

N/A = Data not available
Source: Ministry of Health and Social Affairs, Statistical Yearbook, 1981 and 1984.

cent was rural and 63 percent urban. In 1980, more than 80 percent of all health professionals provided services for the urban people, who represented only 57 percent of the population. In 1983, more than 85 percent of all health professionals provided services for the urban people, who represented only 63 percent of the population. These figures indicate there has been no improvement in the maldistribution of health professionals between urban and rural communities.

DEMAND FOR HEALTH PROFESSIONALS

Several methods are used to estimate human resource requirements for health professionals. T. L. Hall identifies the following bases for this calculation: (1) health needs, (2) service targets, (3) health demand (economic), and (4) work-force-to-population ratios (Hall & Mejia, 1978).

Today public awareness of and expectations for health care are visibly heightened. Since the government has expressed its intent to set up policies aimed at providing people with equal health care, demand will continue to increase.

The fourth Five-Year Economic and Social Development Plan, in a notable change, incorporated primary health care into a national

policy. Previously, work force planning for health professionals had been old-fashioned, with a focus on the demand and supply of medical doctors only. Conventional health planners were preoccupied with the traditional notion of medical doctors as the answer to increasing demands for health care.

This was the situation until 1984, when the Korea Population and Public Health Institute (KP&PHI), by request of the Ministry of Health & Social Affairs, made a study of long-term demand and supply for health professionals, including nurses and pharmacists as well as medical doctors. The concept of health professionals is rather new, and the history of pertinent research is short. Data available for the study of demand and supply of health professionals are scanty.

It is generally believed that the planning of health professionals should consider not only the necessary numbers but also the types and mix of professionals. Furthermore, work places in which trained people can utilize what they have learned should be taken into account.

Long-term health work force findings by the Korea Population & Public Health Research Institute, supposedly fed into the sixth Five-Year Economic and Social Development Plan, along with other recent studies, were used to forecast for the year 2004. Based on information such as population forecasts, economic growth rate, and medical insurance coverage, the estimate for the year 2004 is that the Korean population will increase to 50,994,000 (up 1.26 times as compared to 1984) with per capita income expected to be around $6000. It is anticipated that medical insurance will be applied nationwide by that time. Table 5-9 illustrates the estimate for the demand for health professionals, assuming there are no major difficulties in people's buying power. In summary, by the year 2004, Korea will need 45,600 to 58,900 medical doctors, 76,000 to 100,500 nurses, and 18,200 to 28,200 pharmacists, or 139,000 to 188,600 professionals from these three categories. To meet this goal will require more doctors and nurses.

No single estimating procedure is ideal, but the assumptions behind each method must be kept in mind. Some questions to be raised in applying these techniques include:

1 In existing research, the target of medical treatment is the basis for estimating demand for doctors, nurses, and pharmacists. Even in the case of public health centers, demands are estimated on the basis of frequency of visits that people pay to doctors for the purpose of cure. Estimates based on such assumptions cannot be expected to reflect all the needs of comprehensive health care including health maintenance and enhancement, disease prevention, early detection and cure of diseases, and rehabilitation.

2 The increase in number of health professionals desired for the year 2004 reflects the natural increase in population but doesn't reflect much more than maintenance of the present situation. Thus the problems related to the present delivery modalities cannot be modified or improved within this model.

If we want predictions that reflect promise of improvement, we must identify the valid premises and estimate what work force would be capable of managing health care in a solid, dynamic delivery system. The situation is reflected in a passage from Shakespeare's tragedy, *Macbeth:* Macbeth urged the three witches on that bleak Scottish heath: "If you can look into the seeds of time and see which one will grow and which will not, speak then to me." Would that we had the seeds that would grow to fulfill the goal of adequate health care for people. Projections of demand for health professionals in the future must not simply continue the present situation but must reflect changes in health demand.

T. L. Hall admits that factors affecting demand are extensive and diverse, but he offers the following eight items for responsible work force planning:

1 Demograhic factors (e.g., size, distribution, density, rate of increase, age)
2 Economic factors (e.g., buying power)
3 Social and cultural factors (e.g., educational level, awareness of health, level of knowledge about available health resources)
4 Health condition, health demand, disease
5 Accessibility (travel time and waiting time for available medical resources)
6 Available resources (e.g., facilities, health professionals)
7 Capability to generate resources (e.g., facilities, human resources)
8 Health management technology

R. J. Carlson points out the significant trends in contemporary U.S. society that will affect health care in the 21st century:

1 Shift in population structure, that is, an aging population
2 Public endeavor to enhance health (prevention rather than cure)
3 Application of new technology such as the computer and telecommunications
4 Enhancement of people's ability to manage their own health, that is, improvement in knowledge about health as we move into an "information society"

Table 5–9   Estimation of Demand for Doctors, Nurses, and Pharmacists for 2004

Estimates for demands		Basis of estimation
Doctor	Direct service	Demand of medical services is based on the frequency of visits to doctor and the period of hospitalization per person per year, and from previous statistics and professional opinion.
	Hospital: 24,000	Bed ratio per doctor (6.8) is estimated on the ground of previous statistics and expert opinion.
	Physician's office	Number of doctors needed by 2004 was presumed on the basis that 9 outpatient visits, save the cases seen by hospital doctors and cases seen by doctors working at public health centers or subcenters, should be dealt with in the doctor's office.
	Health center and subcenters: 3600	Assumed that 4 doctors in each public health center and 2 doctors in each public health subcenter are required to meet the demand for outpatient examination and treatment
	Indirect service Education: 2500	To fill up the shortage in personnel supply on the premise of no change in the number of existing medical schools or students.
	Administration and research: 500 Subtotal: 45,600 to 58,900	The number in 1984 indicates below 100 in 1984; continuous increase in demand is expected.
Nurse	Direct service Hospital: Physician's office: 10,000	A nurse-to-patient ratio of 1:25 or 1:3.93 prescribed by medical service laws which assume 90 percent bed occupancy. Physician's offices (9.985) are estimated based on the increasing trends from 1978 to 1984. One nurse per each physician's office is presumed.
	Health centers (rural and urban) and subcenters: 6200	Assuming that 1 public health nurse is required for 5000 people.
	Primary health care posts—public: 2000	The present condition to be maintained.
	Mother-child health center: 400	The present condition to be maintained.
	School health: 141,200	School Public Health Laws (Article 6): a nurse-teacher in each grade at elementary, middle, and high school.
	Occupational health: 5,800 Indirect service	Based on current Industrial Safety & Health Law (Article 16)
	Education College: 246 Junior college: 864 Subtotal: 76,000 to 101,500	To secure by 2004 the number of professors at least required by Ministry of Education.
Pharmacist	Direct service	Minimum-maximum demand was estimated on the basis of assumed frequency of visits (range from 10 to 600) by each person to a doctor.
	Hospital and physician's office: 733 to 1,223	Same as above.
	Pharmacy: 12,600 to 21,100	Same as above.
	Education, pharmaceutical company, others: 3500 to 3600 Subtotal: 18,200 to 28,200	Education to be maintained at the present level. Pharmaceutical companies: 50 to 100% increase is expected.
Total	139,000 to 188,600	

* The number of patients taken care of by each nurse in 1984 (research by Korea Population and Public Health Institute).
** Korean Education Development Institute. The 6th data provided by Office of Planning and Management, 1985
Sources: Korean Population and Public Health Research Institute, "A Study on Long-term Demand and Supply of Health Professionals," 1986.

5 Positive efforts between government and the private sector to coordinate increased medical costs

These five trends are not unique to U.S. society; they also apply to Korean society to a lesser extent.

Since medical costs have increased faster than the pace of inflation—causing an excessive burden on the federal budget—the U.S. government commissioned a public health economic research team at Michigan School of Public Health to analyze total, nationwide medical costs. The aim of this study is to use the federal public health budget efficiently. According to the report by the researchers, the U.S. federal budget for public health increased 65.3 percent from 1979 to 1983. In the same period, hospital budgets increased 77.3 percent. The U.S. gross national product (GNP) increased only 36.7 percent over the same period.

Approximately 60 percent of the total medical cost was for hospital coverage. What was astounding was that most of it was used for only 2 percent of the whole U.S. population. More than 60 percent of the money allocated for direct care was spent to treat conditions such as (1) vascular disease, (2) cancer, (3) injury and intoxication, and (4) upper respiratory disease. A great deal of money was spent on conditions that were preventable, e.g., 39 to 77 percent of cardiac and neural cases, 25 to 79 percent of cancer victims, and about 39 percent of accident-related deaths. These statistics are eloquent proof of inefficiency in the current medical system.

In 1983, the U.S. government put into effect a new payment system using Diagnostic Related Groups (DRGs). The system aimed at reducing the strain on the federal budget due to rising medical costs. Prior to the DRG system, U.S. hospitals were burdened with an economic dilemma: Following the government's health policy stressing accessibility to medical service, facilities had expanded, and bed occupancy fell below 70 percent.

To ameliorate the economic dilemma, U.S. hospitals now try to (1) attract the most lucrative types of services; (2) offer hotel-quality services; (3) replace high-cost personnel with less expensive human resources; and (4) take many conventional hospital services outside of the hospital, including ambulatory care centers or walk-in clinics, birthing centers, nursing homes or home health units, and independent emergency care centers.

In line with social changes in the United States, hospital work forces are undergoing changes. Teams of highly specialized professionals manage special diseases or complications caused by multiple diseases. In a new trend, about 80 percent of the diseases that once were treated in hospitals are now being treated in outpatient facilities where a few doctors serve as super-specialists, and nurse practitioners and physician's assistants are largely responsible for patient care.

What is happening in U.S. hospitals could very well become a reality in Korean hospitals in the 2000s. Recent data compiled by the Korean Hospital Association (KHA) indicate that, from April of 1985 to the end of 1986, a total of 24 medium- and small-sized hospitals either closed or were downgraded to physician's offices. Some hospitals are crying for realistic adjustments of the low medical insurance premium rate which, they argue, makes hospital financial management difficult. Hospitals also are asking for tax incentives and financial assistance. Equally strong critics are demanding more professional hospital management, avoidance of unnecessary competition among hospitals, and reduction of operational costs.

National health insurance coverage (effective in July 1989) was designed to spur intensified government and social intervention to curb the skyrocketing medical cost. Some Korean hospitals already show signs of the problems now plaguing U.S. hospitals.

Doctors, nurses, and pharmacists will have new functions and new roles to play in the twenty-first century. It is essential that the new functions and roles be incorporated into the assumptions and calculations used to forecast demand for health professionals for the twenty-first century, especially if we are to reach the goal of health for all through primary health care.

The development of Western-style health care is generally classified in three historical eras:

1 The period from the late nineteenth century to World War II represents "the individual care era," when policy was to take care of as many patients seeking doctors as possible under what was then a single-tier system.
2 World War II was a period marked by an interest in extending population coverage, social factors, and preventive medicine. By this time health care had evolved into a two-tier system under which doctors and nurses became the axis of public health. Interest in population health coverage was great, but the size of the population actually enjoying health management was very small. This period is called the "community care era."
3 At its 1977 convention, WHO declared the contemporary period an era of "health for all" (the population care era), calling for a three-tier system to deliver primary health care.

Experts in public health, including policy makers and even health and medical professionals, generally believe that the current system, using the medical model, would have been more suitable for the individual care era rather than for the community care era or the population care era that has just begun.

R. J. Carlson predicts that diseases in the twenty-first century will be quite different

from those which we see today. As he envisions it, the early part of this century began as an "era of acute disease," but we are now in an "era of chronic disease." The twenty-first century will be an "era of frailty of the organism" stemming from an aging population, a period in which specific diseases will not matter as much as they used to.

According to Carlson, major health concerns in the future are expected to shift from acute diseases to known causes to chronic diseases of unknown causes and eventually to organic frailty and organ malfunctions. The medical model is most applicable to the treatment of diseases whose causes are known and that require hospitalization. The medical model is not equally satisfactory in managing chronic diseases—let alone health concerns of the future society.

To bring about fundamental changes within our existing health care system, health professionals must see the social trends and changes taking place around them and develop the right kind of system, personnel, and facilities to meet the changing health needs of the society. The important question, says Carlson, is who will bring about such changes? If health professionals don't, the insurance companies and governments will take charge. Were this to happen, the consequences could be disadvantageous to the society and to all health professionals.

SUPPLY OF HEALTH PROFESSIONALS

It is important to look at the supply side for health professionals in Korea and to consider a course of action to provide human resources for the future health needs. The educational (or training) institutions are charged with supplying health professionals and projections of the supply side for future human resource needs by looking at the number of educational (or training) institutions and their graduation quotas. As indicated in Table 5-10, there are at

Table 5-10 Number of Graduation Quorum of Schools of Health Professionals and Success Rate of National Licensure Examination

	Doctor	Dentist	Oriental doctor	Nurse-midwife	Nurse	Clinical technician	Pharmicist	Nurse's aid	Total
Number of institutions	26	10	5	53	60	65(261)*	20	(37)*	186(351)*
Graduation quorum	1940	580	260	802	4680	6,620(853)*	1220	7740	23,842
Success rate of national licensure examination	95.9%	99.4%	98.9%		98.8%	41.9%	92.0%		

* Numbers in parentheses refer to those trained in state institutions (not informal education system).
Source: Korea Population & Public Health Research Center, ''Long-term Health Medical Professional Plan Workshop Report,'' 1985.

present 186 institutes from which 23,842 health workers are produced each year. About 5,000 new nurses are graduated from 60 nursing schools annually.

We have both formal and informal institutions for the basic education of health professionals. Doctors, dentists, oriental doctors, nurses, and pharmacists receive their training through the formal system, but only 14 percent of medical technicians are trained in formal institutions. However, the apprenticeship agencies for medical technicians represent 80 percent of all the training institutions. According to 1984 statistics, the ratio of successful applicants for six different certificates were: 28 percent, clinical technicians; 20 percent, radiology technicians; 47 percent, physical therapists; 91 percent, occupational therapists; 66 percent, dental technicians; and 75 percent, dental hygienists. These figures indicate that about 40 percent of the total 6155 applicants successfully obtain their certificates.

Table 5-11 estimates the supply of doctors, nurses, and pharmacists by the year 2004. It is easy to see that a state of enormous imbalance is going to exist between supply and demand.

Unlike ballpoint pens, surplus health professionals cannot be stored and released when needed to control prices. Those who go into private practice create demand for their own employment. Having surplus personnel requires huge investments in the form of re-

education. (Even those who are active professionally need additional training each year so they don't get rusty.) Thus overproduction contributes to the increase in medical fees, bringing great financial losses to the national economy. What we need is a radical change in policies to supply health professionals in the right numbers and of the right mix.

REORIENTATION OF EDUCATION OF HEALTH PROFESSIONALS

Dr. Haefdan Mahler, WHO general secretary, observed that, "If the doctors who graduated from medical schools in the developing nations were to be tested on primary health care, a majority of them would fail. And yet there will be nearly 200,000 new doctors in Latin America within the next six years." He said that this figure is higher than necessary for the health needs of people; what Latin America needs is not 200,000 new doctors but 1 million primary health workers.

Korea is in the same boat. If Korean doctors and nurses (except community health nurse practitioners) were to take a test on primary health care, most would fail. Korea's education for health professionals is partial to cure, failing to provide adequate training for response to the different health needs of the people.

One might make an educated guess that the majority of people who finish the master's or higher-level education in public health or health-related fields are not providing stimulus for change in the content of curricula for professionals. What we must do is teach all health professionals, whether in basic or specialized training, the concept and philosophy of public health care and health for all. We must enable professionals to acquire the knowledge and experience necessary to make these concepts and this philosophy a reality.

Public health care cannot succeed without the help of hospitals. With this in mind, we

Table 5-11   Estimates for Supply, Employment, and Demand for Health Professionals for 2004

	Supply	Demand
Doctor	68,205	45,600– 58,900
Nurse	160,011	76,200–101,500
Pharmacist	43,440	18,200– 28,200
Total	271,656	139,800 88,600

Source: Korea Population & Public Health Research Institute, "A Study of Long-term Supply and Demand Plans for Health and Medical Professionals."

should redefine the functions and roles of hospitals, doctors, public health institutions, and people working in such institutions as well. Then we should offer proper education to make public health care and the goal of health for all work. This education is as important as the knowledge of diseases and health problems. This kind of education would humanize today's hospitals, which have become "disease palaces" or repair shops, as Dr. Nakajima bluntly described them. This education also would make health professionals regard their patients as whole human beings.

Public health care and health for all call for a new system of health care, one that can be delivered by teams of competent health professionals working together. According to Fulop, a health team is: "A group of persons who share a common health goal and common objectives, determined by community needs, towards the achievement of which each member of the team contributes, in a coordinated manner in accordance with his/her competence and skills and respecting the function of others."

To learn how to carry out team activities effectively, we must employ the multiprofessional education (MPE) method. *Multiprofessional education* is defined by Areskog as follows: "In the training of a group of health students and/or health workers of different educational backgrounds, they learn together so as to be able to collaborate efficiently in the health system in promotive, preventive, curative, rehabilitative and other health-related activities."

It is important to have increased instruction in a group or team setting; it is suggested by Yy sohlid that if health workers of different background and levels learn together, they will be better able to work together effectively as part of a health team.

To make MPE work, the professors of medical and nursing schools could, through joint appointments, participate in the education of both schools, or students could learn the sub-jects common to all health professionals together with the students who will specialize in other fields. At the least, there should be an opportunity for each professional to learn in each university what function and role each other member of a team has in the health care system and to find out what to expect from one another. Accomplishment begins with knowledge, but knowledge alone does not lead to accomplishment. What we need is motivation and resolution, two important prerequisites concerning which A. Low said, "As long as we rest on the security of our certainty, nothing new can come to us."

BIBLIOGRAPHY

Alexeev, V. (ed.), Report of the Second WHO interregional consultation on Strengthening Health Manpower Management, Tashkent, USSR, April 1985 (Geneva: W.H.O., 1985).

Andreano, R., Economic Consequence of Alternative Manpower Strategies, unpublished paper, 1985.

Baker, T. D., Health Manpower Planning: A Seminar for the University of Hawaii School of Public Health, 1968.

Deiman, P., Guide to Staff Nursing Needs, unpublished paper, 1984.

Economic Planning Board, *Korea Statistics Yearbook, No. 13, 1966, Korea Statistics Yearbook, No. 18, 1971.*

Hall, T. L., and Mejia, A. (eds.), Health Manpower Planning— Principles, Methods, Issues, Geneva: W.H.O., 1978.

Japanese Department of Public Welfare, Trend of People's Hygiene, Sohwa 61 (1986).

Japanese Nursing Association, Statistics Data on Nursing, Sohwa 60 (1985).

Jeffers, J. R., Economic Issues: Korea Health Planning and Policy Formulation, Seoul: Korea Development Institute, 1976.

Kim, Mo-Im, "Aspiration," KNA Nursing, Vol. 22, No. 3, July 8, 1983, pp. 22–29.

Kwon, Sun-Won, "Research on Medical Fees in Korea: Estimation & Analysis,: Sociomedical Science Research Center, Hallim University, 1986.

Mejia, A., World Trends in Health Manpower Development, Workshop on Health Manpower Development, 1985.

Ministry of Education, Education Statistics Annual Report, 1969, 1970, 1971, 1972, 1973, 1974, 1975, 1976, 1977, 1978, 1979, 1980, 1981, 1982, 1983, 1984, 1985, 1986.

Ministry of Health and Social Affairs, Public Health and Social Affairs Statistics Annual Report, 1969, 1970, 1971, 1972, 1973, 1974, 1975, 1976, 1977, 1978, 1979, 1980, 1981, 1982, 1983, 1984, 1985, 1986.

Population Health Research Institute of Korea, Plan for long-term national development in preparation for 2000—population and public health medical sector, 1985.

Population Health Research Institute of Korea, Population, Public Health Index and Statistics, 1984.

Population Health Research Institute of Korea, Study of basic plan establishment for the primary public health medical treatment in preparation for 2000, 1986.

Population Health Research Institute of Korea, Workshop Report on Plan for Long-Term Public Health Medical Manpower, 1985.

Sociomedical Science Research Center, Hallim University, Medical Manpower Management—Study Report, 1986.

White, R. (ed.), Political Issues in Nursing—Past—Present and Future, vol. 1, New York, Wiley, 1985.

Yoo, Sung-Hung, Method Principle of Public Health Planning, Prevention Medical Science Room at Medical School, Yonsei University, 1985.

Yoo, Sung-Hung, Supply and Demand for Doctors in Korea, Report for the 25th Korea Medical Association Composite Academic Convention, 1987.

Section Two

Educational Goals and Implementation

This section was organized around students, faculty, and curriculum needs and levels. Presenters were asked to respond to the following:

1 Who are your students and where are they coming from? That is, what are their general characteristics based on demographics, socioeconomic status, scholastic achievement, parental careers, long-range career plans, etc.? Is there a problem in recruitment of students in your country? In your region what systems do you have to recruit and retain nursing students (support systems, financial and otherwise)?

2 What is the entry level requirement for admission to schools of nursing? Does this need change?

3 What educational level will best fit the needs for delivery of health and illness services in your country? Do you need more than one level of educated nurse? What has been learned from educational models in the United States that could or should influence the development of new models in nursing education in your country (your region)? Is there any way in which your thinking has been reshaped by experience in other countries?

4 What is the level of faculty preparation in your country now? What do you need? What changes must take place to achieve this (educational preparation, research skills, clinical specialization, etc.)?

5 What is the context of the learning environment for nursing education? What do you think ought to be the relationship among universities, schools of nursing in and out of universities, and clinical agencies where students obtain their experiences?

6 Is nursing education part of the mainstream of higher education in your country? If not, what ideas do you have for making nursing education integral in higher education?

7 How is the school of nursing contributing to the advancement of nursing knowledge?

8 What is it for which you see yourselves preparing (e.g., community health, primary care roles, hospital practice)? What are your major priorities and why? What are your "ideal" goals for number, types of programs, and deployment of nurses (by levels, generalization, specialization, etc.) to meet the health needs of your country?

9 Has the nursing/midwifery curriculum been revised recently to reflect the most recent health plan or goals in the country?

10 Do you have programs for nursing and midwifery, or are they integrated into one basic program for all nurses?

Nursing Educational Goals for the 21st Century: Canada

Jean Innes
Judith Oulton
Marianne Lamb
Shirley Stinson

INTRODUCTION

Chapter 6 is a unique and largely speculative document. Unique because it constitutes the first literature focused specifically on nursing educational goals in Canada for the twenty-first century; speculative because futuristic content, even that which is comprehensive in breadth and depth, must nevertheless be regarded as essentially tentative.

Three types of forecasting are outlined by Nutall (1976) in her article on nursing in 2000 AD in the United Kingdom: primary, secondary and tertiary. "Primary forecasting is in reality an extrapolation—with an expected continuation of events as they have happened in the past," whereas the secondary type pertains "to what ought to be—or what is thought to be—desirable," and tertiary forecasting "involves making a prediction on what will actually happen" (pp. 102–103). The forecasts about Canada presented in this chapter are largely of the secondary type. However, these forecasts are presented on the assumptions that the process of change is often very long and that some of the variables which "ought" to change over time may change very little or not at all.

An overview of the current nursing education picture in Canada is presented followed by important factors to be considered in developing and implementing educational goals. Examples of four Canadian educational goals and of beginning implementation endeavors are then highlighted.

Information about the country involved can provide a useful background in literature written for international readership, so here are a few highlights about Canada:

Canada became a dominion in 1867, under the British North American Act, which recognized Canada as having two official languages, English and French, and which enumerated powers on the provinces for health and education. (There are 10 provinces, plus the Yukon and Northwest Territories.) As such, goals such as nursing educational goals agreed upon at the national level, e.g., by national professional associations are ultimately subject to controls at the provincial level. Canada has a democratic government, entailing an elected parliament and an appointed senate at the national level and elected legislatures at the provincial level. It is a large country of 3.85 million square miles, thus it is somewhat bigger than Australia, and the United States, and smaller than the continents of Africa (11.5), Antarctica (5.5), Asia including forests, prairies and mountains. The population is over 26 million, of whom approximately two-thirds have English as their mother tongue and one-third have French. Public health services, hospitalization and medical coverage for the population were introduced through federal legislation and are provided and funded through provincial-federal arrangements. Currently, approximately nine per cent of Canada's gross national product is spent on health care. The principles underlying the *Canada Health Act* guarantee equal access to health services and health care. However, there are still "inequities" in several of the conditions which lead to "good health," such as sound nutrition, income, education and housing (Stinson, October 1988, p. 33).

Basic nursing education in Canada is achieved through the successful completion of either a diploma-level or baccalaureate-level program leading to eligibility for the designation of "registered nurse." Diploma nursing programs last from 2 to 3 years and prepare the graduate to practice at the bedside in hospital and long-term care settings. Generic baccalaureate nursing programs are usually 4 years in length and are designed to prepare the graduate to function as a generalist in a variety of health care settings, including community, occupational, and primary health care.

Diploma nursing programs are offered in all ten provinces and are housed in junior colleges, hospitals, and technical institutes. The length of program and entrance requirements vary from province to province and school to school, although programs are usually 2 or 3 years in length and require senior high school matriculation. In 1988, the number of admissions to the 110 diploma programs in Canada was 9,718 demonstrating a reduction of approximately 1 percent from 1987 (CNA, 1989). Recruitment is beginning to become a major problem in some provinces.

Generic baccalaureate nursing programs are offered in twenty-one universities across Canada and are an integral, recognized part of university systems. Most generic programs are 4 years in length; entrance requirements vary according to the general university requirements. Considerable flexibility exists within the policy framework of the university to admit nonmatriculated applicants and international students. Generic baccalaureate programs in 1988 admitted 1,862 students (CNA, 1989). Statistical data reveal an increase in the admission of students to generic degree baccalaureate programs in the past 10 years, and a stabilization of admissions to the diploma programs in the last 5 years (CNA, 1986). There are 5,485 students currently registered in generic baccalaureate programs in Canada. Attrition is estimated at approximately 20 to 25 percent.

In both these types of basic programs, students are usually enrolled on a full-time basis, and they come from urban, rural, and multi-cultural backgrounds. Most are female; it is estimated that 5 to 10 percent of all students are male. Although national statistics are not available, several provinces have observed an increase in the number of mature or adult learners in basic programs; many of these students have been prepared in another occupation and are married with children.

Generic baccalaureate programming accounts for the highest number of students prepared at the baccalaureate level. A second type of baccalaureate program, the post-RN program, is designed to meet the educational needs of the postdiploma student. This program is offered in all but one Canadian province. The number of admissions to post-RN programs has increased steadily since 1982. Currently, 5,169 post-RN students are enrolled in twenty-seven programs, the vast majority of which are offered in university settings (CNA, 1989). Increased demand for access to post-RN programs by practicing nurses is a major issue in continuing education in Canada. A serious need exists to expand the number of seats allocated to these programs and to accommodate the number of nurses wishing to pursue baccalaureate degrees. In many provinces access to distance education programming allows students to remain in their own off-campus locales and to be employed while completing the baccalaureate degree. Some university faculties offer only the post-RN programs and have specialized in offering off-campus distance education courses which can be accessed by students living in remote geographical areas or in other provinces.

Faculty appointments to clinical agencies and appointments of nurse clinicians and administrators to faculty positions is a common practice in Canadian university faculties of nursing. These joint appointments enhance communication between service and education, strengthen the knowledge base for nursing practice, increase the clinical research effort, and provide faculty members opportunities to maintain clinical competency.

All nursing programs consist of a blend of theoretical and clinical learning opportunities. Most entail a mix of classroom lectures, small-group seminars; independent learning programs (including computerized programs); and guided clinical experience to facilitate learning. Clinical practice of diploma students occurs primarily in hospital and long-term care settings. In addition to these settings, baccalaureate students also obtain clinical practice in primary health care, community health, and community-based agencies. Preceptors in nursing service areas serve as role models and provide supervised clinical practice.

In 1988, 12.7 percent of Canada's registered nurses held baccalaureate degrees; 47.3 percent of these nurses were employed in general duty or staff nurse positions in hospitals and community health (Statistics Canada, 1988). Fewer than 2 percent of Canada's nurses hold master's degrees, and only approximately 200 nurses in Canada are qualified at the doctoral level (Stinson, MacPhail, and Larsen, 1988). All programs need to upgrade the educational and clinical qualifications of faculty. Provision is made in most program settings for educational leave for faculty. In Canada eleven universities offer graduate preparation in nursing at the master's level. Access to master's programs is limited by lack of adequate resources.

FACTORS AFFECTING EDUCATIONAL GOALS AND THEIR IMPLEMENTATION

A number of major internal and external factors need to be considered in developing and implementing nursing education goals. External factors which have direct and/or indirect impacts on nurses and nursing practice, education, administration, and/or research which are essentially interdependent in nature include governmental health and social policy, structure of the health care system, economics, demographics, education, environment, information systems, public legislation, housing, value and reward systems, technology, perceptions of health and lifestyle factors (Oulton, September 1989; Rodger, May 1989). These types of interrelated variables have impacts on factors "internal" to nurses and nursing such as required nursing skills; development of philosophic, historic, and scientific nursing knowledge; consideration of numbers and kinds of nurse practitioners required; settings in which nursing takes place; autonomy of nurses; the service ideal of nurses; basic and ongoing socialization of nurses; nursing values and reward systems; nursing ethics and the economics of nursing (Stinson, 1969; Stinson, Field, & Thibaudeau, 1988; CNA, February 1988; Rodger, May 1989; Oulton, September 1989).

Educational goals must be congruent with the health policies of the country involved. Canadian health policy is defined in the Canada Health Act in accordance with the following principles: comprehensiveness, universality, portability, accessibility, and public administration. A provision in the act allows provinces to enact legislation that would permit nurses to serve as first point of entry to the health care system. Implications for nursing education therefore would include preparing nurses to work in a variety of settings with emphasis on community-based practice. This entails the need for nurses to have multiple assessment skills. The federal government has brought forward a framework for promoting health, entitled Achieving Health for All (Epp, 1986). In keeping with Alma-Ata Declaration (WHO, 1978), this document sets out important health challenges for professional health workers and implies clearly the need for nursing education to integrate both the concept of health promotion and the strategies to achieve health promotion into nursing curricula. Nurses must be prepared to be front-line advocates for health and be conscious of their role in creating social change and healthy public policy.

The economic climate of a country has a profound effect on the funding allocated for health care and education. In Canada, health and postsecondary education are cost-shared by provincial and federal governments, so large national deficits also markedly influence the amount of financial support made available to improve and extend nursing education programs (Oulton, September 1989). Further, the continuation of disproportionately high amounts of monies allocated to acute care institutions means only limited funds are available to develop and maintain community-based disease prevention, health promotion, rehabilitation, and support services programs.

Professional nursing associations are directing attention to health care reform aimed at shifting the emphasis from an illness- to a health-oriented system, in which nurses would play an important role in primary health care. Nevertheless, any such shift in emphasis must include recognition that care in both hospital and community settings will continue to be highly technical and increasingly complex.

CANADIAN NURSING EDUCATIONAL GOALS

Examples of Canadian nursing educational goals that follow from the internal and external factors include:

The minimal educational requirement for entry into the practice of nursing (in Canada) by the Year 2000 should be successful completion of a baccalaureate degree in nursing (CNA, 1982 April).

Practicing nurses in Canada in the 21st century should be educationally prepared in primary health care to function as first level contacts within the health care system and have access to continuing education to ensure a continued level of competent practice.

The educational and clinical qualifications of nurse educators should be upgraded.

Nurse administrators at all levels should be educationally prepared both in professional and corporate dimensions (CNA, February 1988).

GOAL IMPLEMENTATION

The establishment of generic baccalaureate education as the requirement for entry into practice requires flexible, innovative, creative, and collaborative approaches to educational delivery. Since education is a provincial responsibility, approaches developed by provinces are of necessity sensitive to the provincial economic and political climates.

Considerable progress has been made in all provinces despite the lack of full commitment by governments to support the entry-to-practice position. Nursing education leaders and representatives of professional nurses' associations in the provinces have concentrated their combined energies on the development of educational programs to meet the national entry-to-practice mandate rather than lobbying directly with government to secure support.

Two general approaches to implementation are being taken in relation to provision of baccalaureate education. The Collaborative Education Model (CEM) stresses an approach through which diploma and university faculties along with nursing service administrators create and implement a new 4-year baccalaureate nursing program. In this model, diploma programs cease to exist as diploma programs per se, and diploma faculty members become full partners in baccalaureate education. New administrative structures are being developed to accommodate changes brought about by collaboration, and faculties work together to develop and teach theoretical and clinical components. Collaborative models have been developed in three provinces. One CEM was implemented in 1989, and two are scheduled for operation in 1990.

In the Phasing Out Model (POM), all diploma programs are gradually phased out and the responsiblity for nursing education is transferred to universities. One province has adopted this model and has scheduled implementation for 1992.

Throughout these efforts, faculties and schools of nursing and provincial nurses' associations have benefited directly and indirectly from assistance provided by the Canadian Nurses Association (CNA), including the CNA's interpretation of the entry-to-practice position for other national-health-related organizations and the federal government; the establishment of a mechanism for provincial nursing counterparts to meet annually and to share goal implementation strategies; the publication of significant statistics about nursing and nurses and of newsletters containing pertinent updated information; and expert consultation to provinces on request.

In relation to the goal of primary health care, baccalaureate in nursing programs would be taught within a framework of primary health care. Clinical experience in primary health care settings (local, provincial, national, and international) would prepare graduates to function at a beginning level in multiple settings. Health promotion would be emphasized throughout the program, and principles of primary health care would guide the development of major curriculum components. Graduate preparation of clinical specialists in a number of primary health care areas would include nurse midwifery, women's health, and gerontology. Issues in continuing education for nurses have been identified as a priority of the CNA (1988); the development of a national certification program (CNA, 1986) and adequate provision of certificate courses in specialty areas (CNA, 1988) will continue to be important in preparing nurses for practice.

The goal of upgrading educational qualifications of nurse educators has been a key priority in Canadian nursing since 1982. Anticipation of fulfilling the mandate for entry to practice has made this a major goal in many faculties across the country. The shortage of clinically and academically adequate faculty, not only to practice nursing and teach but also to transmit, conduct, and utilize nursing research, is a major problem.

Of the approximately 600 nursing faculty members in university nursing programs (Stinson, Field, & Thibaudeau, 1988), fewer than 20 percent are qualified at the doctoral level (Stinson, MacPhail, & Larsen, 1988). Because of the need not only for doctoral preparation but for doctoral preparation *in nursing* "the nursing profession in Canada has made valiant efforts since the mid-70's to establish one or more PhD in Nursing programs in Canada." Although five university nursing faculties are actively seeking to establish such programs (the universities of Alberta, British Columbia, McGill, Montreal, and Toronto), none has yet been established (Stinson, Lamb, & Thibaudeau, in press). Implementation strategies include fund raising and seeking interdisciplinary and interorganizational support for Ph.D.-in-nursing programs and providing educational leave for faculty to become adequately prepared.

The role of the nurse administrator and standards for nursing administration were developed by the CNA in 1988. A major position taken by CNA—which is supported by a total of five national associations—is that all nursing adminstration positions require preparation in nursing at least at the baccalaureate level, which should entail preparation not only in professional nursing but in the corporate dimensions of nursing administration. Senior and/or complex nursing administration positions require at minimum a master's degree with preparation in both the professional and corporate dimensions (CNA, February 1988). "Currently, less than 20 percent of Canada's 30,000 nurse administrators hold baccalaureate or higher degrees." Further, very few of Canada's university nursing faculty members are adequately qualified to teach nursing administration (Stinson, 1989).

A national endeavor to increase the number of graduate nursing administration programs available in nursing administration was undertaken in 1989 by special provincial nursing committees made up of representatives of the five national associations, the CNA, Canadian Association of University Schools of Nursing, Canadian College of Health Service Executives, Canadian Hospital Association, and the Canadian Public Health Association. These associations also strongly support improved continuing education opportunities for working nurse administrators (CNA, Feburary 1988).

Nursing education for the twenty-first century challenges teachers, students, practitioners, researchers, and administrators to discover innovative methods to accomplish goals such as those set out here. The twenty-first century will see many changes, the first of which will be the end of such extensive emphasis on classroom teaching. Home computers will become standard, required student equipment. Satellite television will often bring teachers, patients, and students together in the comfort of patients' own living rooms. Some courses will be offered without students ever setting foot in a classroom. Independent clinical programs (via video and computer) will prepare students for entry into a variety of clinical areas, facilitating the application of theory to practice, and providing students with opportunities for individual skill development. Teachers, students, and preceptors will come together in dialogues to question, to demonstrate, and to participate actively in the learning process. Curricula will be process-driven, research-based, and oriented to critical thinking.

These authors hope that in the twenty-first century the world will become the clinical nursing practice arena, and nursing will develop a "world view." International exchange programs for nurse students and faculty will become common, and nursing research teams made up of international counterparts will operate throughout the world. Distance education will expand and extend to international sites, and multiculturalism will cease to be something nurses study and become something nurses live.

The future of nursing education in Canada will depend not only on educational goals and internal factors but also on external factors, including the public's respect and the respect of other health professionals and of politicians for nursing expertise in practice, education, administration, and research—and the extent to which nurses themselves respect this expertise.

REFERENCES

Canadian Nurses Association. (April 1982). *Entry to the practice of nursing: A background paper.* Ottawa.

Canadian Nurses Association. (1986). *Entry to practice newsletter. 5*(11), Ottawa.

Canadian Nurses Association. (February 1988). *The role of the nurse administrator and standards for nursing administration.* Ottawa.

Canadian Nurses Association. (1988). *CNA's certification program: An information booklet* (2d. ed.). Ottawa.

Canadian Nurses Association. (1989). *Statistics in admissions to Canadian schools of nursing.* Ottawa.

Epp, J. (1986). *Achieving health for all: A framework for health promotion.* Ottawa: Department of National Health and Welfare.

Nutall, P. (1976). Nursing in the year A.D. 2000. *Journal of Advanced Nursing, 1*(2), 101–110.

Oulton, J. (September 1989). *A vision for the future of nursing in Canada.* Paper presented at the Executive Nurses of Alberta Conference, Edmonton, Alberta.

Rodger, G. (May 1989). *Forging nursing's future. Nursing in the 21st century. A nursing perspective.* Paper presented at the meeting of the International Council of Nurses 19th Quadrennial Congress, Seoul, Korea.

Statistics Canada. (1988). *Registered nurses management data.* Ottawa.

Stinson, S. M. (1988). *Deprofessionalization in nursing?* Unpublished doctoral dissertation, Columbia University, New York.

Stinson, S. M. (October 1988). *Education of nurse administrators in Canada: Implications for practice, theory and research in nursing administration.* Paper presented at the Rockefeller Foundation International Health Care Management, Education and Research: Nursing Action Conference, Bellagio, Italy.

Stinson, S. M. (1989). Education of nurse administrators in Canada. In B. Henry, R. Heyden, & B. Richardson (eds.), *International nursing administration.* Philadelphia: Charles Press, pp. 112–125.

Stinson, S. M., Field, P. A., & Thibaudeau, M. F. (1988). Graduate education in nursing. In A. Baumgart & J. Larsen (eds.), *Canadian nursing faces the future.* St. Louis: C. V. Mosby, pp. 336–361.

Stinson, S. M., MacPhail, J., & Larsen, J. (1988). *Canadian nursing doctoral statistics: 1986 update.* Ottawa: Canadian Nurses Association.

Stinson, S. M., Lamb, M., & Thibaudeau, M. F. (in press). Nursing research: The Canadian scene. *International Journal of Nursing Studies.*

World Health Organization. (1978). *Report of the International Conference on Primary Health Care: Alma-Ata, USSR.* Geneva, September 6–12.

Chapter 7

Nursing in the 21st Century in Latin America

Esperanza de Monterrossa
Ilta Lange
Roseni Rosangela Chompré

In an analysis of the development of nursing in Latin America, three phases have been identified in the evolution of the profession in the region that can be related to important and significant historical periods (see Table 7-1). The major transformations, especially in this century, have been institutionalization and university-level education, resulting in a rise in the number of nursing schools and of graduate programmes at master's level and more recently a few doctoral programmes. And most countries have at least established directives for the preparation and use of nursing personnel.

Despite this progress, the quantity and quality of nursing personnel are still inadequate to solve health problems and to answer the needs of an extended health care service to meet the greater health demands of a rising population.

In most countries there is an important deficit of nurses as well as of nurses' aids. According to the Colombian Association of Nursing Faculties and Schools, in 1984 Colombia showed a ratio of only 0.3 nurses and 4.2 nurses' aids per 10,000 inhabitants. In Chile, in 1989 the ratio was 2.8 nurses and 23.8 nurses' aids per 10,000 inhabitants, and in Brazil in 1985, 1.9 nurses and 4.6 nurses'

Table 7-1   Important Periods in the Evolution of Nursing Practice and Education in Latin America

Characteristics	Repercussions	Nursing function	Performed by
Phase 1: Colonial period until independence			
—Nursing is organized and controlled by the Religious Orders.	—Greatest increase in health care delivery to sectors of the population, since the colonial times.	—Performance of activities related to patients' hygiene and domestic chores.	—Nuns or lay people (the majority women of lower social classes.)
Phase 2: End of 19th century until beginning of World War II			
—Development of Institutions for Education and Public Health Practices.	—Organization of systems for education and services. —Struggle to improve professional status. —Surge of professional associations. —Adoption of specific legislation.	—Control over recruitment and preparation of nursing personnel. —Direction of nursing schools.	—Nurses. —Surge of practical nurses. —Nurses' aids. —Helpers.
Phase 3: Beginning of World War II until present			
—Professionalization of nursing personnel. —Definition of national policies on nursing education. —Organization and structuring of Nursing Services within the health care institutions.	—Nursing programmes incorporated into the university level. —Nurses begin to specialize. —Creation of graduate programmes.	—Nurses carry out nursing activities and are responsible for nursing care. —Nurses are in charge of nursing services in institutions belonging to various levels of care. —Nurses control and direct programmes for the preparation of nursing personnel.	—University trained nurses. —Practical nurses. —Nurses' aids. —Helpers (personnel without specific training).

Sources: Souza, A.M.A. Development of Advisory Services of PAIIO: Impact on Nursing Education in Latin America 1940–1980 (doctoral thesis). Translation M.H. Alves. Ohio State University, Columbus, Ohio, 1982.

aids.[1,20,5] Added to the nurse shortage is the high concentration of professionals in urban centres, especially in hospitals.

In the preparation of nursing personnel, difficulties arise in a curriculum that strongly emphasizes curative care. Although some countries—e.g. Chile, Ecuador, Colombia and Brazil—have permanent organizations to establish regulatory mechanisms for the profession, the fulfillment of the norms and regulations for nursing practice as well as

education of the different categories of nursing personnel have not been completely resolved. At a 1985 meeting of "Leaders in Nursing" held in Caracas, the main problems of nursing in Latin America were analyzed, based on the following basic premises[10]:

1 The magnitude of the health problems requires prompt action to guarantee every man's natural right to good health.

2 Concomitant with the Latin American countries' rapid social change is a restructuring of health systems whereby health professionals are becoming social actors with scientific, technical, ethical and moral responsibilities.

3 Nursing issues can be better understood only through the study of the concept and analysis of human resources in health as a whole, of which nursing personnel is one component.

4 To improve the health care delivery for the population, it is important among other aspects, to assure the advancement of the various health professions and to develop leadership skills in the health professionals. Each country needs leaders with the potential to promote the desired changes, with expertise in their professional field, with ability to communicate and fundamentally willing to assume the risk that change implies. Leaders with these characteristics will have a comprehensive view of the health-disease continuum and of its social determinants.

5 Cooperation through networking is imperative in today's world. Nursing must thus interact energetically not only within its own profession but externally with other health care professionals, international agencies that work in this field and other development sectors at a national, subregional and regional level. In this way, the transformation processes will be accelerated.

On the basis of the above premises, the issues related to nursing in Latin America can be grouped into five categories: (1) human resources in nursing; (2) institutional development; (3) curriculum development; (4) Latin American nursing literature; and (5) recruitment of nursing students.

Based on these issues, the W. K. Kellogg Foundation developed a nursing strategy in Latin America, placing emphasis on institutional development of nursing schools and the training of nurse leaders for primary health care.

GOALS AND IMPLEMENTATION

Formal education in Latin America is structured into three levels: primary school (8 years), secondary school (4 to 6 years) and higher education (3 to 5 years). In the majority of the countries, the constitution establishes primary schooling as mandatory, and delegates this responsibilty to the state. Even so, the general situation in regard to education is critical in Latin America and results in a high number of illiterates, difficult access to secondary schooling and university education and a high rate of desertion at all levels (mainly in primary school).

This situation is aggravated by the existence of programmes that overlook the students' potential, deficient teaching conditions, inadequate preparation of teachers at all levels of formal education and poor incorporation of educational technology—all of which have direct repercussions on the preparation of the different categories of human resources in nursing.

Preparation of health personnel includes all the educational processes that are geared to train people to work as a team in the health field. In this definition we include all levels of preparation from the state-regulated formal educative process (in schools, colleges and universities) that prepare health professionals to the informal educative processes carried out mainly by service institutions that train personnel for work in the community,[21] and emphasize the teaching of procedures.

Nursing education is regulated in almost all Latin American countries. The variations are categorized in four levels:

- Nurses' aids, who, having completed two years of secondary school, are trained in educational or service health institutions;
- Technical training at the secondary and post-secondary levels;
- University education, with its basic mode and complementary mode; and

• Specialization programmes. A master's in nursing science exists only in Mexico, Colombia, Brazil and Chile, while a doctorate programme is offered only in two universities in Brazil.

According to Manfredi, graduate programmes in Latin America have not produced the expected formation of nursing leaders and researchers who can contribute to promote the changes required in nursing, perhaps because these programmes have not enjoyed the regularity required and because they have been designed according to characteristics of developed countries and not according to Latin American conditions.

THE CURRENT SITUATION

According to Souza, education for professional nursing at the regional level is characterized by a high degree of heterogeneity and complexity, which varies not only from country to country but also within countries themselves.[23] The first school of nursing in Latin America was founded in 1886 in Buenos Aires, Argentina.

During the '60s, some 70% of the existing nursing programmes were developed in Latin America. At that time nursing schools numbered 411, of which 52% were affiliated with universities, 21% with the ministries of education and 19% with the ministries of health. By 1985 the number of nursing programmes linked to the universities rose to 69%

Three-fourths of the nursing programmes are financed by the public sector, and since 1963 are mostly (91%) under the direction of nurses. In most countries the mandatory requirements for admission to the undergraduate nursing programmes is completion of secondary education.

Almost all Latin American nursing programmes have written objectives, many explicitly directed toward "forming professional nurses and contributing toward the improvement of health services". Most schools offer two-three-year basic nursing training, the title granted depending on each country's legislation. A university degree in nursing (equivalent to a bachelor's) requires four to five years of study. Some of these programmes are offered in a complementary mode of one-two additional years after the completion of basic nurses' training.

During the '60s nursing curricula were changed more frequently in line with general educational reforms in certain countries and proposals made by teachers, students and international advisors. Today, Latin America's current trend toward comprehensive medicine, preventive medicine, teaching-service integration and more recently intersectorial work are determining what nursing curricula should consist of. The W. K. Kellogg-sponsored projects, in particular, have contributed decisively to achieving the necessary curriculum reforms in dentistry, medicine and nursing.

The time allotted for developing the plan of studies in nursing schools has remained at some 33% dedicated to theory and 57% to practice, though it is believed that this proportion may have recently shifted to 40% and 60% respectively.

Of the nurse educators, 62% work full-time, and 76% of teachers from other professions are hired part-time. Some 44% of the teaching nurses are specialists or have a master's degree; only 2% have a doctorate.

The number of nursing graduates has grown slowly during the '60s and '70s. While the student/teacher ratio averages about ten to one, in some schools it is as low as three to one.

The conquests of institutionalization, the entrance of the nursing programmes into the universities and the creation of graduate programmes have represented a great struggle with the power groups in the health sector. The advancements have made it possible for nursing to have its own educational process, which has had strong repercussions in professional practice.

THE PROBLEMS

The progress in nursing education has not been made without accumulated problems, many associated with technology advances, particularly in education, and most greatly influenced by the economic and social crises plaguing their countries.

Some of the problems besetting nursing education in Latin America, identified at the 1985 "Leaders in Nursing" meeting in Caracas, are:

• The definition of the educational and occupational profiles is primarily limited to physicians, which means the community has a variety of health needs to which no one responds.
• The lack of planning in human resources for health care delivery.
• A low leadership potential among nursing faculty, which delays the processes of change in teaching institutions.
• As nursing teachers lack practice as health care providers, the teaching/learning process is mainly converted into the transmission of existing information.

For specific countries, some general problems in nursing education include:

• The training of "helpers" is limited in time and employs inadequate methodologies. As helpers represent a large percentage of the nursing personnel in many countries—reaching 63.3% in Brazil and 29% in Colombia—the situation requires an immediate solution.
• The curricula of nurses' aids programmes are a reduced version of the curricula of the professional nurse, transferring problems related to the teaching/learning process.
• The high desertion rate of nursing students in all countries reflects the low attraction this career exercises on young people, because of inadequate salaries, deplorable working conditions, low status and/or unattractive role models.
• The leaders of the numerous nursing programmes created in the '50s and '60s are now retiring and no efforts have been made to prepare new leaders who can assume the direction of these nursing schools and programmes.

Moreover, professionals must be prepared to respond to the population's growing health needs and demands, the reorganized health services and the progress in science and technology. But for nursing education to guarantee the preparation of such professionals, it must overcome the internal barriers and obstacles in the profession.

The W.K. Kellogg Foundation has supported many projects and programmes in Latin America that have contributed to the definition of policies and development of innovative educational and practice models in the health field. Nursing has benefited a great deal from these experiences, especially through its participation in interdisciplinary community-based, health projects that provide care to underserved urban and rural populations.

The W.K. Kellogg Foundation has developed an innovative model for training nursing leaders that has had a great impact on nursing in Latin America. The process is described below.

At the first 1985 meeting on leadership in Caracas, several strategies were proposed to contribute to the improvement of primary health care. Some of these:

• To encourage graduate education, especially at master's level.
• To develop specialization courses in mental health, adult health and occupational health.
• To develop continuing education programmes with emphasis on primary health care.
• To promote faculty exchange among the American countries.

• To organize traveling seminars that could contribute to professional exchange and broaden knowledge about community work.
• To create a Latin American Nurses' Association that would unite nursing schools and facilitate networking activities.
• To stimulate the publication and distribution of Latin American nursing literature.

NURSING POLES

In 1986 the School of Nursing of the Federal University of Minas Gerais surveyed Latin American schools to obtain information on their potential to develop graduate nursing programmes for inclusion in a catalogue of university-based nursing programmes. Later on, the same university organized a workshop to discuss leadership strategies in nursing for primary health care, based on the information obtained in Caracas in 1985. At this meeting emerged the concept of "Nursing Poles of Development", which were defined as strategically located places in subregions of Latin America with a potential for growth and institutional support. The objective of a developmental pole would be to contribute to the development of nursing in Latin America through projects designed to:

• Develop innovative models for primary health care, using the strategy of teaching-service integration.
• Incorporate the concept of primary health care into the basic curricula.
• Develop graduate nursing programmes with emphasis on primary health care.
• Develop systematic continuing education programmes for all levels of nursing personnel.
• Develop innovative technology to be applied in teaching and service institutions.
• Promote research and publication of conventional and non-conventional nursing literature.
• Encourage networking activities.

A parallel workshop was held for the purpose of discussing strategies to promote publication and dissemination of Latin-American nursing literature.

At the end of 1987 13 selected nursing schools were visited to obtain a more direct and overall view of the leadership capacity of these nursing institutions. And in 1988 a group of six nurses participated in a conference on "International Collaboration in Education, Practice and Research in Nursing" in Galveston, Texas, and then visited various doctorate programmes in the US.

In April 1989, the Nursing School of the Federal University of Minas Gerais organized two subsequent meetings: The first was a workshop to discuss the progress of nursing leadership proposals in Latin America; at this meeting, five institutions presented their proposals for the constitution of nursing developmental poles. At the second meeting ("Mobilization and Training of Leaders in Nursing") strategies to mobilize and train nurses as leaders for primary health care were discussed.

This seminar constitutes an example of networking activity in which information was shared and new groups of nurses were motivated to participate in the leadership process.

THE CALLED-FOR CHANGES

The health sector in Latin America requires a new technological composition to solve the current and future problems in covering the health needs of the population. This new composition should include:

1 Reorganization of the health service production systems based on the following principles:

• Universality: the guaranteed access to health care for the urban and rural populations;

• Equity: timely access to the health services and technologies;
• Hierarchization: a health service structured and organized according to levels of care;
• Regionalization: a managerial model that guarantees autonomy for decisionmaking at each level.

2 Use of appropriate technologies geared toward health promotion, disease prevention, recovery and rehabilitation.
3 Adequate preparation, use and administration of human resources, in both quality and quantity.
4 Community participation in development of health care delivery models through mechanisms that assure its continuity and representativeness.

But to be able to implement policies that seek to transform the health services, it is necessary that the health professionals develop innovative attitudes and behaviours through training. To achieve this condition it will be necessary:

• To prepare human resources for incorporation in the health care models.
• To develop pedagogical models that consider the educational characteristics and needs of the students.
• To define strategies for preparation of teachers.
• To reorganize the professional practices giving emphasis to multiprofessional and interdisciplinary work based on the essential criteria of timely and risk-free care for the population.

THE PERSPECTIVES

The mechanisms implemented by W. K. Kellogg have produced an impact on the preparation of leaders in nursing, and the results can be seen in the recent approval of the first pole of development in the University of

Nueva Len, in Monterrey, Mexico, and with the perspective for approval of five more developmental poles in the near future.

It is suggested that the efforts of national nurses' associations, national teaching and service institutions, and international organizations such as the PAHO and the W. K. Kellogg Foundation, among others, join to elaborate policies and strategies to attain a new model for nursing practice in Latin America, considering the following priorities:

• To establish innovative educational models for all levels of nursing that will, on one hand, guarantee the quality of health care for the population and, on the other, attract a greater number of aspirants to the nursing career.
• To develop teaching/service programmes that provide feedback to nurse educators and stimulate the creativity of students by means of their conscious and permanent participation in multiprofessional and interdisciplinary teams.
• To form teachers with a renovated view of the teaching/learning process, of the role of the nurse, and of primary health care.
• To promote the search for and the training of leaders who work in comprehensive teaching-service programmes in order to encourage positive role models for the students.
• To establish in the schools or faculties of nursing, plans for continuing education for nurse educators, according to the academic needs of the faculty and the health needs of the population, and seek strategies to assure their strict fulfillment.
• To orient the basic and post-basic study plans in the nursing schools toward primary health care so that they are relevant to the priority needs in health.
• To design a new model for preparation of nurses that transcends current institutional, economic and language obstacles, facilitates the sharing of experiences among different countries in Latin America and contributes to national and regional development.

• To provide nursing students with opportunties and experiences that will improve their capacity to exercise pressure on the educational system, assure relevant and accessible educational programmes and help them attain a greater mobility within the nursing profession.

• To define strategies for training nurses' helpers through the joint efforts of service and educational institutions, supported by nurses' associations.

The support of the W. K. Kellogg Foundation in the formation of nursing poles of development represents a concrete contribution to prepare nursing in the region for the next century. The work proposed by the developmental poles should have important repercussions on the training of nurse educators and therefore will have an impact on the models of education and practice of nursing.

The definition of an innovative model for master's and doctorate education through the organization of a consortium of nursing institutions in Latin America and the US should produce, in the medium- and long-term, the following results:

• The preparation of a greater number of nurses with a master's or a doctorate in foreign institutions.

• Exchange between universities in the US and in Latin America, with positive effects on collaborative and comparative research, in an atmosphere of mutual respect and based on the concept of bilateral exchange.

• The production of research about different realities and health problems in the region, and about the role of practice and education in the definition of nursing policies and regulations.

The efforts implemented at the present time to achieve the results of ''health for all'' in the next century should have as a final objective, the preservation of man on the basis of his right to live well, be happy and reside in a world at peace.

REFERENCES

1 Asociación Colombiana de Facultades y Escuelas de Enfermeria. (1988). *Actualidad y Perspectiva. Estudio Nacional 1984-1987.* Bogota.

2 Carillo G. (1989). *Formación de Recursos Humanos para la Atención Primaria.* Paper presented at the: II Seminario de la Red Chilena de Proyectos Kellogg. Santiago, Chile.

3 Carillo G. (1985). *La situación de la Enfermeria en América Latina.* En: La Enfermeria en Latinoamérica. Estrategia para su desarrollo. Memorias de la Reunión de Lideres de Enfermería. FEPAFEM, Caracas, Venezuela. 121-127.

4 Carillo G. (1989). *El Papel de los Centros de Technologia en Enfermeria. Pasado, Presente y Alternativas de Trabajo Futuro.* Reunión Latinoamericana de Enfermeria Universidad Federal de Minas Gerais. Escuela de Enfermeria Brasil.

5 Conselho Federal de Enfermagem. Associacao Brasileira en Enfermagem. *Exercicio de Enfermagem Nas Institucoes de Saúde do Brasil 1982-1983.* Vol 1 (1985), Vol 2 (1986).

6 Garzon N. (1987). Ejercicio Profesional de la Enfermera. *Enfermeria.* XXII (90/91):11-15.

7 Lange I. (1989). *Nursing leadership development for primary health care in Latin America.* Paper presented at the 16th Annual International Health Conference. National Council for International Health, Washington, D. C.

8 Lange I. (1989). *Strategies to prepare Latin American Nurses with Doctoral Degrees.* Paper presented at the Task Force Meeting: ''Movilización y Formación de Lideres de Enfermería para la Atención Primaria.'' Universidad Federal de Minas Gerais, Brazil.

9 Lange I. (1986). *Impacto de Programas Educativos en el Autocuidado de Pacientes Ambulatorios.* Informe Final. EPAS 3(2) 6-18.

10 Maglacas A., Ulin P., Ships C. (1987). *Health Manpower for Primary Health Care: the Experience of the Nurse Practitioner.* WHO/University of North Carolina, Chapel Hill.

11 Martine G. (1989). *O mito da explosão demografícia*. Cien Hoje. Rio de Janeiro, 9(51):28–35.
12 Meleis A. *Nursing Research: A Need or a Luxury*. Paper presented at Global Nursing Conference, Galveston, Texas.
13 Mendes, Dulce de Castro. *Assistencia de Enfermagem e Administracao de Enfermagem: a Ambiguidade Funcional do Enfermeiro*. Rev. Bras. Enf., 38(3/4):257–265.
14 Manfredi M. (1985). *Formación de Recursos Humanos en Latino América*. En La Enfermería en Latinoamérica: Estrategia para su Desarrollo. Memorias de Reunión de Lideres de Enfermeria. FEPAFEM, Caracas, Venezuela, 129–149.
15 Ministerio de Salud de Chile, Depto. de Recursos Humanos. (1989). *Tendencias del Personal de Salud para el siglo XXI*, Santiago, Chile. (Internal Document).
16 OMS. (1986). *Mecanismos de Reglamentación de la Enseñanza y la Práctica de Enfermería; Satisfacción de las necesidades de Atención Primaria de Salud*. Serie de Informes Técnicos 738. WHO, Geneva, Switzerland.
17 PAHO. (1986). *Las condiciones de salud de las Américas 81–84*. Publicación Cientifica 500. Washington D.C.
18 Pulido P. (1985). *Palabras de Bienvenida en:* La Enfermería en Lationoamérica: Estrategia para su desarrollo. Memorias de Reunión de Lideres de Enfermería. FEPAFEM, Caracas, 25–27.
19 Ramirez M. et al. (1987). *Problemática Profesional y Personal de las Profesionales de Enfermerí*. Enfermeria XXI (88–89): 8–13.
20 República de Chile. (1989). Diario Oficial Nro. 33429, Santiago, Chile. 25–58.
21 Santos I., Souza A. M., Vieira T. C. V. (1987). *Preparãsao de Pessoal Pelas Instituicões de Saude*. Brasilia.
22 Silva, G. (1986). *Enfermagem Profissional: Análise Critica*. São Paulo, Brazil, Cortez, 143.
23 Souza, A. M., Manfredi M. (1982). *Perspectivas para la Educación de Enfermeria en América Latina frente a la meta de Salud para Todos en al Año 2000. PAHO*.
24 Souza A. et al. (1988). *Estudio de Tendencia de la Investigación sobre la Práctica de Enfermería en Brasil*.
25 Souza A. M., Champré R.R. (1988). *International Cooperation: Experience of a local University in Brazil*. Paper presented at the Conference International Collaboration in Education. Practice and Research in Nursing. Galveston, Texas.
26 Styles M. (1985). *La Reglamentación de Enfermería*. International Council of Nurses, Geneva, Switzerland.
27 WHO. Leadership for Health for All. *The Challenge to Nursing: A Strategy for Action*. Tokyo International Encounter Conference. Tokyo, Japan.

Chapter 8

Nursing Education in China

Dai Yu-hua

The Peoples' Republic of China, having recently celebrated its fortieth birthday, follows the socialist course in development of health care and medicine. The figures in Table 8-1 provide a comparison of how far we have come in that time.

CURRENT STATUS OF NURSING EDUCATION IN CHINA

Nursing education started in 1888 in China when formal modern training of nurses replaced practice tutorships in nursing care by Chinese traditional doctors. In the century after the first nursing school was established

in Fuzhow, growth of programs was extensive, with 180 nursing schools created before 1949 and 373 schools established within the last 40 years.

Before 1949 only one college-level nursing program offering a bachelor's degree after 4 to 5 years of education was run by Peking Union Medical College (PUMC). That program began in 1920, graduating 264 nurses from 1924 to 1952 (see Table 8-2).

In 1952 medical education as well as nursing education at PUMC faced a big issue: whether to focus on the quantity of health care workers needed or the quality of their education. The final decision at that time was to have a

Table 8–1   Selected Health Statistics, 1949 and 1988

	1949	1988
Population	475 million	1.08 billion
Life expectancy, years	35	67.9 (F 71.6, M 67.0)
Prevalence of infectious disease per 100,000	20,000	80
Net increase rate in population, percent	16	14.3
Health institutions	3,670	205,988
Hospital beds	84,625	2,794,926
Medical personnel	540,000	4,670,000
Beds per 1000	0.15	2.30
Medical personnel per 1000	0.93	3.43
Physicians	360,000	1,480,000
Nurses	32,800	829,000
Medical colleges	22	119
Medical students	15,000	190,000
Vocational medical schools	180	553
Vocational medical school students	15,000	270,000
Traditional medical colleges	0	27
Traditional medical college students	0	30,000
Medical research institutions	4	332
Research workers	300	37,000

shorter curriculum, placing emphasis on the quantity of workers needed. The PUMC nursing school was reduced to and has remained a vocational technological school.

DEVELOPMENT OF MEDICAL EDUCATION IN PUMC IN THE LAST DECADE

After a suspension of 32 years, under the new policy of reform and openness, more and more medical and nursing specialists demanded the reestablishment of college-level nursing schools. From 1984 to 1988, eleven faculties for nursing schools were set up in different medical universities (three in Beijing, two in Shanghai, one in Tianjin, one in Shenyang, one in Xian, one in Guangzhou, one in Shandong, and one in Nanjing). There are about 300 students studying in these schools, with only two classes graduated by 1989. The curriculum for these programs is 5 years in length. Students are enrolled after they pass

Table 8–2   Graduates from Peking Union Medical College

	1924–1942	1952–1958	1964–1970	1987	Total
Medicine	310	297	506	30	1143
	1924–1949	**1950–1952**			
Nursing	219	45			264
			1960–1968	**1981–1986**	
Research fellows			117	578 (MM)* 16 (MD)**	711
Total	529	342	623	624	2118

* MM: Master of medical sciences
** MD: Doctor of medical sciences

Table 8-3 Reconstruction and Development of Medical Education at Peking Union Medical College

Initial year of program	Type of program
1978	Research fellow & postgraduate training
	Master of medical sciences (3 years)
1979	Medical students (8 years)
1981	Doctor of medical sciences
1985	Nursing college students (4 years)
1985	Evening school for adults (3 years)
	Laboratory techniques (3 years)
	Nursing (3 years)
1986	Medical laboratory technology (3 years)
1986	Establishment of graduate school
1986	Postdoctorate training program in medical biology
1987	Establishment of Department of Social Medicine and Public Health

national examinations for entrance to universities and colleges (see Table 8-3).

In accordance with PUMC's curriculum, the nursing education is divided into four periods. The first 3 semesters are spent in Beijing Teachers' College learning basic natural science and humanities. The second 2 ½ semesters are spent in basic medical sciences. The third 2 ½ semesters are clinical medical sciences and nursing practice. The students spend the last two semesters in PUMC hospital in a nursing internship.

The goal of the college-level nursing education is to produce qualified nurses who can teach, research, and administer nursing care, who are able to develop nursing in science rather than provide technical care. In other words, we hope to produce qualified nursing professionals and nursing leaders from this cradle.

To improve our vocational nursing education, we have to take the next step of continuing nursing education for the current nurses. In 1979 the thirty-fourth World Health Assembly proposed the ambitious goal of "Health for All by the Year 2000." This presents a great challenge for the medical schools as well as the nursing schools: to provide qualified

medical personnel in enough quantity and with appropriate quality to meet such a large goal.

Among China's 829,000 nurses are 650,000 produced after liberation. Basically, they are at a high school vocational level: 250,000 of these "nurses" did not have formal training. They are associate nurses doing nursing care work. A very small number of the nursing teachers are at college level, and most of them will be retiring soon.

Continuing nursing education has been implemented in the last decade in different ways:

1 *A 3-year evening school curriculum with over 800 teaching hours for experienced nurses.* Prerequisite requirements are working experience for more than 2 years and successful passing of a local examination sponsored by the municipal board of examination. No degree is conferred, but a college-level certificate for graduation is given at the end of the training with passing of the final examination. This system is welcomed by the working nurses for refreshing their knowledge and for learning to meet the needs of modern advancing medicine. This kind of nursing education enrolls students under 35 years of age.

2 *Credit accumulation by examination in different required disciplines.* There is no limitation as to time or the student's age in this plan. If the high-school-level nurse finishes twelve required courses, gets 75 credits, and successfully completes examinations that include clinical practice competency, she will be acknowledged as a college-level nurse and certified. Since this system is more flexible, it is welcomed by many nurses.

3 *Specified certificate for senior nurses over 35 years of age with more than 5 years experience in clinical nursing.* In this program the nurse can get 14 daytime courses within one year of off-position training. The program is comprised of more than 800 teaching hours of intensive study. If the nurse can finish and pass all the courses, she can get a specified certificate which qualifies her for employment as a college-level nurse. This new program just started in 1988.

4 *Teaching by correspondence with sixteen courses in a 3-year period.* Finishing these courses and passing the examination acknowledges the nurse to be at the college level.

5 *Special short courses.* Courses in intensive and coronary care nursing, geriatric nursing, psychiatric nursing, and other specialties are available.

6 *Special arrangements.* Recently we have been working with the Cumberland College of Health Sciences in Australia producing some special courses for educating physiotherapists among the general nurses.

FACING THE TWENTY-FIRST CENTURY

Although family planning is one of our most important national policies, China's big challenge is to control her population to under 1.2 billion by the year 2000. We have 1.1 billion in 1989, with 80 percent living in the rural areas. The one-child-per-family policy is still not well accepted by the rural population.

By the year 2000, our elderly population will reach 130,000,000. Our current physician-to-nurse ratio is 1:0.57, and the ratio of hospital beds to nurses is 1:0.29. The need for nurses is even more critical than the need for physicians.

Traditionally, nurses are not as highly respected as doctors, and Chinese girls prefer to learn medicine rather than nursing. We are trying to rectify our policies so as to make nursing more attractive.

More scholarships are being set up in nursing schools than in medical schools. Recently, Nightingale awards honored eleven outstanding pioneer nurses in China. There is an International Nurse's Day every year but no similar physician's day celebration.

Dr. Sawyer, the president of the China Medical Board of New York, helps China set up scholarships for nursing master's degree education for some brilliant young nurses. Another goal is to strengthen Chinese nursing education in patriotism and in the spirit of service and sacrifice. The improvement in both the quantity and quality of nursing education in China are still urgent.

"Health for All by 2000" is a great dream. China can improve its medical and health care work through hard effort, but the improvement will be gradual. China will walk steadily ahead and have a brighter future.

Chapter 9

Nursing Education in Korea

So Woo Lee

SOCIOECONOMIC DEVELOPMENT IN KOREA

Korea occupies a peninsula extending south from the northeastern corner of the Asian continent. The total land area of approximately 220,000 square kilometers is politically divided between north and south in a ratio of about 6 to 5. The total population in South Korea is estimated to be 40 million.

Along with a decrease in the average birth rate, average life expectancy has been on the rise, resulting in an annual population increase of 1.5 percent. Population density is about 406 persons per square kilometer, one of the highest in the world. The development of the small urban nuclear family has added to housing shortages, which have stimulated tremendous apartment house construction. Rapid economic development has brought about far-reaching social changes such as the breakdown of class barriers and an increase in demographic mobility. Urbanization is pronounced, and the general standard of living has risen considerably as indicated by a per capita GNP equivalent to $2032 in 1986.

These substantial improvements have resulted in expanded opportunities at all levels of education. Also, plans will be made to develop social welfare programs commensurate with the ability of the Korean economy to pay for them. Unions are organizing in most places of employment as well as in most hospitals.

Not only employees in industry but also health personnel want to be assured of such fringe benefits as severance pay, disability insurance, and paid leave.

As a divided nation as well as a newly emerging industrial country, Korea has faced many difficulties in an uncertain political and economic situation.

GENERAL EDUCATION

The benefits of modern education were extended to Korea toward the close of the nineteenth century when the royal court of the Choson dynasty decided to discard its closed-door policy and open the country to modernization through contacts with Japan, China, and the European powers. Interest among members of the Korean government in what was happening in the field of education in other countries, and in making use of some of the facilities for the benefit of Korean students, was first evinced in 1880 when a group

of fifty eight educators and other professionals toured Japan for about 70 days, visiting educational institutions of all types.

The first institutions of modern education were set up in Korea during this period (1882). However, the forcible annexation of Korea by Japan in 1910 impeded the independent development of modern educational institutions in Korea for the next 35 years. To perpetuate the Japanese colonial rule in Korea, educational opportunities for Koreans were severely restricted, and the level of education was generally suppressed.

Liberation from Japanese colonial rule in August 1945 provided a new starting point for education in Korea; the democratic way of life was introduced as the new basis of public education. The Republic of Korea has also had many educational reforms in educational policies, curricula, educational systems, and entrance examination systems since the first republic was established. The most revolutionary reforms are enumerated in Table 9-1.

Table 9-1   Important Education Reform and Changes

Year	Contents
1949	Promulgation of education law
1952	Free and compulsory education in elementary schools
1962	Abolishment of normal schools, to be replaced by junior (2-year) teachers' colleges
1968	Proclamation of the Charter of National Education
1969	Abolishment of entrance examinations for middle schools
1969	Introduction of preexamination system for college admission
1972	Opening of correspondence (2-year) college
1973	"Equalization" of high schools—reform of high school admission system
1974	Creation of the National Institute of Educational Research and Training
1979	Opening of junior (2-year) vocational colleges
1980	Educational reform of July 30: • Abolition of individual college examinations—replaced by uniform college entrance preexaminations • Establishment of graduation quotas • Weighing of high school academic records in college admission
1981	Establishment of scholastic achievement examination for college entrance (rephrasing of pre-examinations for college entrance) Teachers' colleges upgraded to four-year courses National Correspondence College (5-years) established Open college established Fifth revision of educational curricula

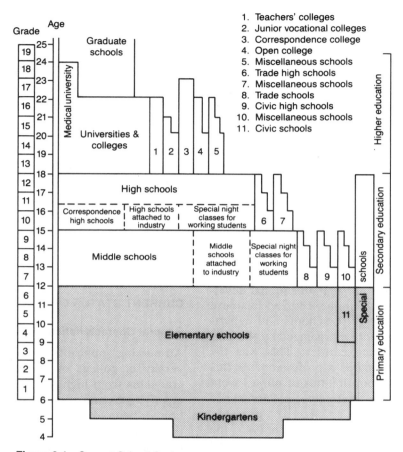

Figure 9-1 Current School System.

Since the Education Law was promulgated in 1949, a ladder-type school system of 6-3-3-4 has been in use (the current school system is 6 years of elementary school, 3 years of middle school, 3 years of high school, and 4 years of university or college). (See Figure 9-1.)

NURSING EDUCATION

Korea first became interested in Western medicine in the early 1900s. Medical care in Korea was available only to the wealthy and royalty and was administered in their homes by traditional medical practitioners. The vast rural population and ordinary people had care only from their families or traditional healers. The first modern Western hospital in Seoul was established in 1899 by the order of King Kojong. Since then health care in Korea has developed mainly in urban areas. Health care for rural areas continued to be under-developed until the Mother and Child Health Law was proclaimed by order of the Ministry of Health and Social Affairs in 1973.

Between the early 1900s and the late 1940s, there were no major changes in the development of nursing education and practice. From the beginning of nursing education in Korea, nurses and midwives were trained by Western missionary nurses at Christian hospitals or by hospital schools operated by the government. Nursing educational development owed its impetus to efforts of two distinct groups: government and the Christian missionary enterprise. In 1913 regulations concerning the education of nurses and midwives were proposed, and these regulations became law in October 1914. Qualifying examinations for nurses have been in place since 1914, testing for both theory and practice. The testing was done in each province until 1962. In 1962, the law was revised to require licensing which could be obtained by passing a national examination after graduating from a nursing school in either a 4-year or a 3-year program.

From 1910 to 1945 under the Japanese colonial rule in Korea, nursing educational development was mainly influenced by Japanese medical policy. In 1910, schools and departments of nursing were reorganized by the government as separate entities. This was the beginning of nursing as a profession. At this time the main responsibilities of nurses were giving medications, treatments, and assistance to doctors.

After liberation of the nation in 1945, the Nursing Bureau of the Ministry of Health and Welfare was set up to work toward the standardization of nursing education. However, until 1973, there was no standardization of entrance requirements nor of course length for nursing educational institutions. Until 1973 there had been two different educational systems for nursing: secondary school education and higher education. The former system was a high school nursing level (6-3-3), the latter system was divided into two levels: one a junior college level (6-3-3-3) and the other a university level (6-3-3-4). The nursing curriculum in the high school and junior college was the same length and content, differing only in entrance requirements.

In 1970, the government established a law for a professional school system. Thereafter, entrance requirements for nursing schools became equal to that of other professional schools, i.e., high school graduation and qualifying exams. The first students in a bachelor's degree program graduated in 1955 at Ewha. The first graduate program in nursing in Korea began at the master's level in 1960 at Ewha and at the doctoral level in 1978 at Yonsei. Since 1967, the Ministry of Health and Social Affairs initiated a program for nurse's aid preparation.

Concepts of modern nursing were introduced after the Korean war (1953) mainly from the United States. Nursing education related to modern concepts has stimulated the development of new nursing knowledge and clinical research.

CURRENT STATUS OF NURSING EDUCATION

General Characteristics of Nursing Students

All nursing applicants for admission to a university or college or junior college must be graduates from high school, have passed the qualifying examination for high school graduation, or be graduates of schools recognized by the Ministry of Education as equivalent to high schools. All applicants must take the college entrance examination administered by the government after they have selected a college and submitted application forms. Universities or colleges select their first-year students on the basis of the composite score of the scholastic achievement examination for college entrance, high school grades performance achievement, and an essay test administered by each university or college.

Most students first apply for a 4-year college or university and then, if they fail, may decide to take the junior college entrance examinations. The junior college entrance examinations are held after the 4-year college entrance examinations are finished. Some students will wait to take the university entrance examinations again the next year.

Who are the applicants for nursing? Women make up 99.9 percent of all applicants. Most applicants for nursing come from the middle or lower socioeconomic classes. Their parents are farmers or merchants or in trade and commerce, anxious to provide higher education for their children. Reasons young people choose nursing as a major are several: further studying abroad is easy, to become a professor, to get a job, to serve others, for variety of personal relationships, and ease in going abroad for a job. (See Table 9-2).

Nursing Faculty in Korea

It is frequently said that the quality of the faculty is the key factor for success in nursing education. Demands for nursing faculty are increasing, and the need to improve the quality of the faculty is most urgent.

Doctoral programs in nursing came into being to provide qualified nursing faculty. According to 1987 Ministry of Education data, professors of nursing with earned doctoral degrees account for 10 percent of the total faculty.

Government requirements for tenure at university are 200 points for published research. A single-author study counts 100 points, two authors count 70 points, three authors count 50 points, more than three authors, 30 points. A committee of the university selects the appropriate applicants and recommends them as faculty to the government for approval.

The Learning Environment for Nursing Education

All types of nursing education programs are operating within the mainstream of higher education. However, although nursing education as a profession should consider the supply and demand of staff in health delivery system, there has been no committee or consultation on a policy for demand and supply of the nursing workforce among the responsible organizations, the Ministry of Education and the Ministry of Health and Social Affairs.

The Ministry of Education has evaluated nursing schools only for academic affairs such as the number and qualifications of the students and faculty and for facilities for teaching

Table 9–2 Reasons for Choosing Nursing

Author	Year	No. of respondents	Reasons
Lee & Woo	1971	238	Employment abroad; devotion to society; variety of relationships
Kim	1973	—	Study abroad; having a service job; to get a job
Han	1973	160	Study abroad; interest and aptitude; to get a job
Ahn	1975	225	Advice from parents or teacher; employment abroad; interest and aptitude
Yoo	1975	476	To get a job; utilize for housekeeping; helping others
Yoo	1976	270	To get a job; interest and aptitude; utilize for housekeeping
Park	1977	149	Aptitude and interest; to serve others; utilize for housekeeping
Kim & Lee	1978	711	Employment abroad; continuous social life; guaranteed employment; good chance of good partner
Park	1978	—	Interest and aptitude; having a service job; advice from parents or teacher
Lee	1988	371	Idealistic humanitarian; social interaction; financial; professional: others

nursing. However, the Ministry of Health has focused on the licensing of registered nurses (RNs) and the legislation of RN activities. All the 4-year baccalaureate programs in universities use university hospitals for clinical practice in medical-surgical, maternal-child care, and psychiatric care. Community health nursing practice takes place in the public health centers operated by the government. There are many problems related to clinical experience for students of the 3-year junior colleges. Many junior colleges were established without connection to a practice hospital. With the exception of several schools with good clinical experience, most of the 3-year program schools have major weaknesses in the provision of practice. The faculty is continuously looking for government or private hospitals to provide clinical experience. If the college cannot find appropriate hospitals for practice, the students may not have the minimum experience necessary. Even if most clinical experience for physiological care can be found, psychiatric care experience is more difficult to obtain. Students use summer or winter vacations for 1 or 2 months of experience in psychiatric care at national mental hospitals or private psychiatric hospitals.

The 4-year bachelor program colleges, except the two colleges of nursing, are under control of the Dean of the College of Medicine, and thus do not have control over a budget for operating academic affairs. Requests for teaching equipment for the nursing arts laboratory and classrooms are handled by the university.

Curriculum and Teaching

Although the educational system has been stabilized at two levels, we are confronted with the problem that bachelor's degree nurses' and diploma nurses' functions have not been differentiated in practice settings, and no standards have been defined. Junior college education is aimed at nursing knowledge and skills for middle-level practitioners to serve national and social development goals. Bachelor's degree education provides skills to teach and to research nursing theories and to develop leadership ability. Credits required for graduation from junior college range from 120 to 138; from 140 to 160 credits are needed for the 4-year programs; 20 percent of the total credits must be in the liberal arts and 80 percent in professional subjects in the junior colleges; 30 percent in liberal arts and 70 percent in professional subjects for the 4-year programs. There is a wide range of curriculum subjects and credits.

The curriculum of both programs of nursing is structured to prepare students to practice immediately following graduation, except for midwifery. For midwifery, nursing graduates practice 1 more year in obstetrics. There are at present in Korea no post-RN baccalaureate courses. There are two degree programs in nursing: master's degree courses are offered at thirteen graduate schools of nursing, three schools of public health, and two schools of education. Doctoral degree courses are conducted at five graduate schools of nursing and two graduate schools of public health. For their degree, students major in nursing or public health. Table 9-3 illustrates the numbers of diploma and bachelor's degree nurses graduated from 1986 through 1990 (estimated).

Table 9-3 Number of Registered Nurses Graduating, 1986 to 1990

Year	Diploma	BSN	Total
1986	4,172	824	4,996
1987	4,616	863	5,476
1988	5,168	883	6,051
1989	5,440	887	6,327
1990 (est.)	5,440	913	6,353

Nursing Education and the Advancement of Nursing Knowledge

One of the primary goals of nursing education is to provide an environment in which the student can develop cognitive, affective, and psychomotor skills to practice professional nursing independently and collaboratively. Under the suppressive rule of Japan, Korean nursing education was far from achieving this goal. As Korea was liberated, education for nursing began to build nursing knowledge. Concepts from modern Western nursing were introduced after the Korean war (1953) from the United States.

Development in nursing service and education are complementary. One nursing education accomplishment in the 40 years since the nation's liberation is the contribution to the independence of nursing from the medical faculty. The educational contribution to nursing's clinical development is within the context of human resource development and the search for new knowledge and interventions in nursing.

The quantitative expansion of education was the pacesetter for nursing's clinical development as nursing's growth called for a variety of skilled practitioners in increasing numbers. In qualitative terms, education in nursing upgraded nurse's interventions toward quality care.

But the quality of education has not shown a commensurate improvement. The quality of education depends on the conditions for education, which include educational content, teaching methods, the quality of the faculty, physical facilities, financing, evaluation methods, and research. Schools are evaluated in terms of how they create a balance of these resources. Educational development of baccalaureate and graduate programs is contributing to the public image of nursing. The public is becoming aware of nursing as a profession as well as a science. Finally, nursing education is contributing to the adancement of nursing knowledge through research, health teaching, organizational strategies.

Health Care Delivery and The Role of Nursing Personnel

There are two health care delivery systems in Korea. One is offered by the private sector, the other one is conducted by the public sector. The private health care delivery system is mainly a hospital-based medical care service. The public sector provides community health services at health centers as well as medical care services at hospitals.

According to statistics of the Ministry of Health and Social Affairs (1988), private clinics and hospitals account for more than 95 percent of all medical facilities, employ 72 percent of the physicians, and include 72 percent of the total hospital beds. However, most private sectors are concentrated in urban areas. In Korea, although about 68 percent of the population resides in urban areas, 92 percent of the physicians and 86 percent of hospital beds are located in the cities. Thus access to medical care for the rural population is scarce. Moreover the health care problems faced by the rural population are complicated by geographical and socioeconomic conditions. Significant health problems in rural areas are inadequate maternal and child care, low immunization levels, unsanitary living conditions, inadequate acute disease care, and inadequate family planning services.

In response to these problems, the government established a special law for rural health care in 1981. This legislation included support for the training and development of professional nurses as Community Health Practitioners (CHP) to deliver public health services in remote rural communities. According to this special law, the CHP was specified as a registered nurse with 6-months additional training as a community health practitioner.

The 2000 CHPs have been recruited countrywide through local governments.

There are three other major health care problems. One is the health care of the urban poor. Another is the health care of the aged. According to a report of the Korea Institute of Public Health, the proportion of those aged 65 and above to the total population was 42 percent in 1985 and is estimated to approach 62 percent by 2000. The need for health and medical care of the aged is of major concern among social policy issues. The last problem is chronic health care as well as adult health. Recently, the incidence rate of noncommunicable diseases such as malignant neoplasm, hypertension, diabetes, cerebral hemorrhage, chronic liver disease, heart disease, and chronic kidney disease has been rapidly increasing. The causes for these increases are related to economic development, the improvement of household income level, and changes in life-style since the 1960s. The prevalence rate of such adult diseases is estimated at 1811 persons per 100,000 (1988, Ministry of Health).

In Korea, the medical security program is divided into three categories: medical insurance, medical assistance, and medical aid. The latter two are provided for low-income families as a part of public assistance programs. Legally, nurses are still hampered by laws and pressures which permit them to work only under the supervision of physicians. As a result, the potential role of the nurse in health promotion and disease prevention has not been developed. During the last decade modern nursing education has prepared the nurse to assume more responsibility, but the organizational structure of Korean hospitals and the attitudes of some physicians and administrators tend to limit the role of nurse to that of doctor's assistant. Nurse's aides are frequently employed at clinics or hospitals when, by law, RNs should be giving the nursing care.

Discussion

To enhance the effectiveness of nursing education, we must think again about what kinds of nursing education best fit the need of delivery of health care and the needs of the students. Although two types of basic nursing programs are available, the 4-year baccalaureate and the 3-year junior college program leading to a diploma, there is only one nursing license for graduates from both programs. This license is acquired after passing licensing examinations administered by the Ministry of Health and Social Affairs with questions selected from a national pool. This system contributes to conflict between nurses from diploma and bachelor-degree schools, since nurses from both programs apply to hospitals with the same license for staff nurse positions. There are also no differences in job descriptions for clinical nurses in the hospitals and clinics, and there is no credit given for the BSN degree. Despite the fact that they have as much clinical experience and more theory hours, nursing administrator's expectations or even the public's expectations of BSN nurses have been the same as for diploma graduate nurses. Should we not expect different job descriptions for graduates from the two different programs? Is it not the reality that Korea needs both technical and professional-level nursing at the present time? According to the national health plan, we need CHPs as the primary professional health workers. Since 1982, about 2000 nurses have been working in remote rural areas as CHPs. Most of them are diploma graduates. Most nurses in the public health centers are also diploma graduates. Remote rural area settings and poor working conditions (including a low salary and benefits) make the Public Health Centers unattractive to nurses with degrees, who tend to prefer university hospitals. When we think of how nursing education programs should reflect needs in national development in the economic, health and welfare systems, and the culture, at the moment we probably need both technical and professional levels of nurse preparation, but neither prepares nurses for quality clinical nor primary health nursing responsibilities.

All bachelor-degree programs in nursing, except for two nursing colleges, are under the control of the deans of the colleges of medicine. This system adds to the confusion of the public and students. The public as well as applicants who want to choose nursing as a major think of nursing not as an independent science but as a dependent technical occupation. Nursing education must be in independent colleges. This is necessary for the profession's autonomy and the development of nursing science within the discipline.

Four-year nursing programs have expanded and developed a great deal since the first generic university programs in the early 1960s to master's and doctoral level studies. One of the most important contributions to the establishment of baccalaureate programs has been made by the universities. Their financial support enabled schools of nursing not only to improve the quality of nursing education but also to contribute leadership for the health professions.

However, much development is still needed in order to provide progressive leadership in furthering nursing excellence nationally and internationally. University nursing education should concentrate its efforts on three areas: quality education at all three levels of study, faculty development in the areas of clinical specialties and nursing research, and continuing education.

First, the curriculum should be revised. The direction of change should be toward an integrated curriculum with an early introduction of professional nursing subjects, more elective courses, and provision of opportunities for independent study. For the successful implementation of a new curriculum, the opinion of students should be surveyed for what they want to change. This is to support the faculty belief that the primary aim of nursing education is to provide an environment in which the student can develop cognitive, affective, and psychomotor skills to practice professional nursing independently and collaboratively with special emphasis on self-discipline, critical thinking, and intellectual curiosity. Second, for faculty development, there are two focuses: development of clinical specialties, and upgrading the quality of nursing research. It is critical for nursing faculty to develop clinical competencies in the face of ever-advancing science in the clinical fields. It is also important for nursing faculty to have continuous clinical experience for professional growth and to set a model for nursing excellence through clinical practice. Nursing research centered on clinical phenomena should have a high priority for study by faculty. To further develop the nursing faculty's research capabilities, consultant services and overseas training in the field of clinical research in nursing, opportunities for cooperative research and participation in national and international academic conferences, and the development of a support system for faculty research will be necessary.

Finally, continuing education is necessary to maintain and improve the quality of patient care, to keep the nurse's knowledge and skills up to date with the latest nursing developments, and to stimulate and motivate nurses for the further development of nursing science.

NURSING EDUCATION IN THE FUTURE

Increasing demands will be placed on baccalaureate nursing programs to provide opportunities for diploma-prepared nurses to earn the baccalaureate degree. The demands could be met by change in government policy.

An increasing number of doctoral-degree courses will become available. University administrators and the public will understand nursing as a science and a discipline, but the clinical practice component may not be well understood unless nursing demonstrates quality of care. Nursing education will develop as a community-oriented preparation based on primary health care concepts as well as hospital practice. Nursing curriculum will focus on preparing professional nurses who are concerned with the health of individuals, families and the community.

To provide adequate clinical education for nursing students, strong affiliations between academic institutions and practice settings must be developed. Faculty should maintain clinical expertise and come to some agreement on a common knowledge base for the development of nursing education, practice, and research. Private and public funds supporting nursing research should be expanded. The Korean Nursing Association (KNA) should seek to resolve the most pressing issue related to nursing education by obtaining a consensus among the public, those in national socioeco-nomic policy development, and the relevant medical laws to support KNA's plan for the integration of the two levels of nursing education programs.

CONCLUSION

Korean nursing education is strongly influenced by educational models from the United States, and in the enthusiasm for developing nursing education, we would be unwise to adopt uncritically the system of another country. We must be selective to develop nursing education based on our country's culture, system of general education, economic and social development, system of medical and health services, and the needs of our communities. Moreover, the effectiveness of the implementation of nursing education goals depends on the development of nursing as an independent discipline and on taking the initiative to solve health problems in a variety of practice settings. Professional and academic autonomy is essential to develop nursing education within the mainstream of higher education.

Chapter 10

Educational Goals and Implementation in Pakistan

Patricia Scott

BACKGROUND

Pakistan has the highest per capita income among the South Asian countries, according to the World Bank (1985) report, at $390, compared to the lowest, Bangladesh, at $140, yet in 1985 Bangladesh spent 8 percent of its gross national product on health care and Pakistan that year spent 0.6 percent. In 1987–1988, the total health expenditure rose to 1 percent. There are far more doctors than nurses: 51,238 compared to 17,731, almost three times as many doctors. There are 54 beds per 100,000 population, compared to India with 75, Sri Lanka with 16, and the United Kingdom with 894. The world average is 1 bed for 290 persons; Pakistan's works out to 1 per 1,852. The nation's health has been improving however on the following indices: in 1982–1983 infant mortality was 98.5 per 1,000; it is now down to 80. The life expectancy was 58.6 years, now up to 61. Expected gains by 1992–1993 are: infant mortality down to 60 and life expectancy up to 63 (Economic Survey, 1988–1989).

Pakistan is divided into four provinces; the largest is the Punjab, then Sind, followed by the Northwest Frontier Province, and the smallest is Baluchistan. Karachi, the commercial capital, is in Sind. Islamabad, the diplomatic and government capital, is located in the Punjab, very nearly in the center of the country.

As in many nonindustrialized countries, statistics about nurses and nursing are not totally reliable for a variety of reasons, as is true for other statistics. Clearly, however, there is a desperate shortage in all areas. Sind alone in 1988 has 1,451 government posts sanctioned, with only 808 filled. A large (600 bed) hospital in Karachi has only 9 RNs. Nearly all nurses work in urban hospitals and clinics.

The Pakistan Nursing Council (PNC) is responsible for the education and regulation of nurses, midwives, and "lady health visitors." Midwives have a 1-year midwifery course; lady health visitors are midwives with 1 year at a public health school (the principals are doctors), and nurses have 3 years of general nursing, plus 1 year of midwifery which may be taken before or after the general nursing.

PNC requirements for entry into general nursing include that applicants be single and between 16 and 25 years of age. All students are required to live in. In exceptional circumstances older (or even more rarely, divorced) women are permitted entrance. Students study 3 full calendar years, with 1 month's leave per year and 1 week sick leave permitted. Excess absences must be made up before registration. The PNC has consistently voted against coeducation in nursing schools; there are three separate schools for males. Although required to take a year's specialty training in lieu of midwifery, male nurses complain they are seriously discriminated against because both "RN" and "RM" registration is required for class A qualifications, necessary for promotion to senior positions.

The PNC provides a uniform curriculum throughout the country for all three types of registered personnel. A content outline and the minimum number of hours are specified. Implementation varies somewhat as some schools give a greater number of hours than required. All are required to pass the regional examination given by the regional nurse examination boards. The RN examination is given in two parts: Part I after the first year and part II on completion of the third year. This system ensures that the same subjects with a minimum number of hours are taught in the first year, although there is some leeway in sequencing in the second and third years.

The language of instruction is officially English, as are the approved textbooks. In many cases, however, the students' and the teachers' command of English is weak, so many "explanations" occur in Urdu or another of the regional languages.

In 1989 there was a motion in PNC to raise the entry requirements to "interscience" for nurses. This would mean 12 years of education with the secondary years in the science stream. At present, students are accepted with "matriculation" (10 years of schooling) in either the arts or science stream, although most schools prefer intermediate certificates, either arts or science. The motion was defeated. We conducted a study in the summer of 1989 comparing achievement in our diploma program at the Aga Khan University School of Nursing with matriculation and intermediate certificates, both arts and science, and found no significant difference in the academic ratings among all four groups in the six classes which have graduated to date. Scores on English were more predictive of success in our program.

Recently the curriculum designed by PNC has been under revision. In 1987, the World Health Organization (WHO) sponsored a workshop to begin curriculum revision. In November 1987, a second workshop, funded by the Canadian International Development Agency (CIDA), was held in Islamabad, followed by a third in August of 1988. Two consultants from Canada were the facilitators. Since then a number of local workshops in several provinces have been held, funded by WHO, with representatives from all four provinces attending. The CIDA consultants are expected to return in early 1990.

The curriculum was last revised in 1973 but was never formally implemented countrywide.

NURSING STUDENTS IN PAKISTAN

As in many parts of the world, nursing is not recognized as a profession or occupation for young women from "good" families. A possible exception to this generalization is the Ismaili community, where his Highness, Prince Karin Aga Khan has repeatedly stated he wishes his spiritual daughters to become nurses. In any case, nursing students tend to come from poor families, from lower socioeconomic groups who have not been educated in the better schools. Most come from the urban areas where the school they attend is located, even though residence in the hostels is required. Young women in this culture do not go far from home; they return to their families on their days off. Another reason for the residence requirement is that young women do not go out alone at night, so shift work would otherwise be impossible.

Nursing students also tend to be at the lower end of the academic achievement scale: Although a minimum "second degree" pass is required for entry, those with better marks choose medicine, engineering, or other "higher status" careers.

The economic issue is important too, though not for the reasons usual in the West. Nursing education throughout Pakistan is not only free but in most cases rather generous stipends are paid, as much as some men earn in paying blue-collar jobs. It is not at all rare for the young student to be the only "wage earner" in the family in addition to the father. Families of rejected applicants plead for us to take their daughters so they are "provided" for. Free room, board, and "wages" are powerful incentives! Although this conclusion is no where supported by research data, when we opened a 4-year generic bachelor of science in nursing (BScN) program in one of the countries of the Middle East, we had 87 percent male students. The reasons given were that the females at the diploma schools were given stipends but the university charged tuition. The diploma programs were not open to males (an unintended effect was we had the university champion football team).

There has been virtually no research done in Pakistan on either nurses or nursing. WHO plans a major nursing workforce study within the next few months; Aga Khan University recently commissioned a two-part study on nursing and attitudes about nursing. The first part, completed in October was internal: the University Medical Center nurses (past and present), doctors, medical students, and administrative staff were surveyed. Part two will be conducted nationally. In this study nurses were found to be the most positive about nursing as a career, doctors least, with other personnel falling between the two (Holzemer, 1989).

The nurses in this study planned to continue work after marriage, although anecdotal evidence (newspaper reports, conversations) indicate the public perception is that nurses "cost a lot to train and only work for a few years." The Aga Khan University Hospital has only been open for 4 years, so it is too soon to say. Certainly visits to other hospitals throughout the country have a predominantly young, unmarried staff. Christians and Ismaili (Shia Muslims) are disproportionately higher in numbers according to their distribution in the population.

NURSE TEACHERS

Three colleges of nursing in the country train nurse teachers. The course is a 2-year post-RN certificate course in "Teaching and Ward Administration." The teachers in those colleges have a certificate as their highest academic attainment. One college has expert advisors from Japan with master's degrees. In September 1989 one nurse returned from the United Kingdom with a master's degree to teach at the second. There are very few nurse teachers with bachelor's degrees in the entire country. To the best of my knowledge, there are two Pakistani nurses in the country with master's degrees: the second is actively employed in health work but not in nursing service or education. Approaches have been made to several universities to offer bachelor of science (BSc degrees; Karachi University refused, but at least two others do take RNs and after four courses (English, Urdu, religious studies, and national studies) confer a BSc, but not in nursing. There is talk now of conferring BSc degrees for all nursing schools, since "it is a 4-year course with midwifery." One university is reportedly considering awarding master's degrees to nurses "as long as their teaching staff has at least one masters-prepared person employed." A master's degree in English is suggested as the most likely "masters" to be available for staffing nursing master's programs. Many are opposed to proceeding in this manner, but those who believe higher degrees are a pass-key to progress are gaining acceptance.

In November of 1988, the Aga Khan University opened a 2-year post-RN BSc in nursing program. This is the first one of its kind in the country. The philosophy and goals were carefully formulated to address the needs of Pakistan and an Islamic society. Our university has six Pakistani nurses with BSc degrees, four in the diploma program and two assisting in the degree program. Thanks to the generous assistance of CIDA and the British Overseas Development Agency (ODA) we have four doctorally prepared nurse faculty from abroad, two masters-prepared, and one very experienced British nurse tutor with a BSc equivalent, for our thirty-nine students. The

assistant director of our school, a Pakistani nurse with a BScN from McMaster University in Canada, has been very active in the PNC, working on the revision of the diploma curriculum.

Unfortunately, for most of the rest of the country the teachers are too few in number and ill-prepared to teach or design curricula which are appropriate to the health needs and the culture. Considering where nursing has come from since the inception of Pakistan as a state (there were fewer than ten nurses in the country), phenomenal progress has been made. However, from the beginning those who have worked to establish nursing professionally as consultants from abroad, have been "foreigners, unfamiliar with national traditional patters, cultural values, and religious beliefs" (Kamal, 1984, p.13). The Pakistani nurses who have since come into leadership roles have been greatly influenced by the early role models as well as the fact that those who have earned higher degrees have all done so in the West. "The ideologies," Kamal states, "of these countries." Nursing professions were inadvertently imported, defects and all, into situations with totally different health needs, cultures, perceptions, values, and resources. "Unfortunately, long after the initial unavoidable conditions and necessities, the pattern still continues." (Kamal, ibid.)

That "westernization" continues is illustrated by the students in a fundamentals of nursing class who take basins, soap, towels, gowns, and wash clothes with them when they go to their affiliation in another hospital which lacks adequate supplies and equipment. Several efforts by the expatriate director to persuade the faculty to teach students to teach patients hygiene with whatever is available have so far been ineffective. In our own degree program where I teach a first-year course in "advanced concepts," I find I am continually reminding students to assess with their five senses *first* and confirm or validate with technology; to intervene with their own hands and intellects and skills *first* before proceeding with medicine and machines.

NURSING NOW

From about the early 1960s, nursing in this part of the world has struggled with varying degrees of success to compete on an equal basis with nursing in the West, particularly in the United States, with an emphasis on higher education for nurses. All the countries in the eastern Mediterranean region, with one exception, now have basic diploma nursing programs in general nursing. One country has opted for an associate degree program instead. In addition, seven countries have basic degree programs, three countries have post-RN degree programs, four have master's programs, and two have doctoral programs in nursing.

As I see it, the major problem is that too little consideration has been given to the appropriateness of the transfer of technology *and* knowledge. Technology—such as that required for heart and liver transplants—has been superimposed on what is basically, in Pakistan at any rate, a farming society. We need to develop skills for dealing with diversity, we need to increase our effectiveness as nurses in training for managing cultural differences and understanding human behavior (Harris & Moran, 1979). Anatomy and physiology, chemistry, physics, and other "hard" sciences are doubtless the same over the world, but genetic diseases and predispositions to certain conditions change from country to country, as do the common disease conditions caused by lifestyle and environment, to say nothing of infectious diseases. Our teaching is just beginning to recognize these factors because our textbooks are printed in St. Louis and Philadelphia and London and San Francisco.

In the social sciences we are even further afield. Turkey has published a great deal in social research in the last 15 years; some studies on family structure are percolating through to us from the Middle East, but we have few books on social science for Pakistan, and, except in our program, they are not used as texts.

Nursing models have been developed almost exclusively in the West and therefore have limited utility in this part of the world. Theories are not normally developed by nursing students at the BSc level; not too many models appropriate for practice are developed on the master's level. In practice, the few teachers who are interested and able academically are so overburdened, carrying such heavy workloads and such large numbers of students, that they have no time for scholarly activity. Or perhaps, as in one school I have personal knowledge of, one teacher teaches all subjects for all 3 years of the general nursing program. Doctors "guest-lecture" a good deal, and courses are divided into such topics as "medicine" and "medical nursing."

The wonder is not that nursing in this part of the world is so far apart from the West, but that, all things considered, it is so close! This is not to imply for a moment that I believe the Western model is one we should follow in Pakistan: Simply, it is the model available.

A major issue in criticism of nursing by the medical staff in our institution is that the nurses are inappropriately assertive. When the pediatric census was full, one of the surgeons needed to admit a child with a ruptured appendix who had already been to two other hospitals. The young nurse in charge, barely 2 years out of the diploma program, refused because "we have reached the limit." It does little good to explain to the chief of surgery that the nurse is exhibiting "advanced beginner" behavior and will progress, probably, to "expert" in another 10 years or so! The nurses we have are spread too thin and have no appropriate role models themselves to mentor them through their early years after graduation when their clinical judgment skills need such tender loving nurturance.

Patients complain mostly about not receiving personal service; emesis basins aren't emptied, sheets not smoothed, dirty dressings not removed, water not given. A student explained the reason for some of this: "everyone except the very poorest families have someone else to 'pick up' after them and do 'the sweeping.'" They literally don't *see* these things. As poor as nurses are, and as low in status, one frequently hears them speak of their household help. Perhaps our ideas of what a nurse *should* do need reevaluating. As long as the job gets done, must a nurse do tasks in Pakistan which are reserved for strictly menial laborers? In the West homemakers do all those "dirty little jobs" around the house. In Pakistan, they don't. Forcing nurses to do these jobs reinforces in the public's mind the idea that nursing is part of the servant class. I gave my sweeper a raise, many years ago, only to discover that promoted him out of the "sweeper" category, and he wouldn't wash my floors anymore. Hospitals in Pakistan frequently have "ward boys" who wash bedpans and scrub floors.

The concept of *caring* is another major issue in Islamic cultures. Perhaps *caring* as we know it in the West is inappropriate among strangers in other cultures. Western insistence on wearing name tags and introducing oneself to patients and their families causes major difficulties when "brazen" behavior of young women is considered an invitation to inappropriate advances.

And although one supports the objectives of primary health care (PHC) and "health for all by the year 2000," and although nurses are definitely desperately needed in the community, when you have nine nurses for all three shifts 7 days a week for 600 patients, who will *you* release for the funded PHC program for which you've been asked to provide a candidate?

The first year our degree program opened we had fifty applicants for the twenty seats; we accepted twenty, and lost two for financial reasons. This year we accepted thirty; two were also accepted in U.S. schools and declined admission to our program; we are told six others could not obtain release from their employers. The class has twenty-two members. Short courses offered in North America and Great Britain have repeatedly not been accepted by Pakistani nurses, as the government institutions have felt the already short-staffed wards and schools could not be depleted further.

These are not all the problems facing the emerging profession in Pakistan, but perhaps they are the most significant in terms of barriers to the full development of the profession. In summary:

• Recruitment and retention are hampered by the poor image and low status and by the traditional role of women, complicated by the nature of the tasks required and cultural values regarding relationships among strangers.
• Education is hampered because the teachers themselves lack the theoretical background and the necessary expertise in curriculum development and clinical supervision skills (many teachers have never been clinical practitioners themselves). In addition, students are generally used to staff the hospitals. There are too few nurses. There are also too few teachers.
• Research to advance nursing knowledge is nonexistent; those few prepared to carry out research have major and overwhelming other responsibilities.
• There is only one very new BScN program in the country. Unlike other nurse education, there is a relatively high cost to attendance, which includes loss of financial support to their families as well as paying tuition and fees. If nurses leave employment without having their resignations "accepted,"

they lose pensions, gratuities, and other benefits.

PREPARATION FOR CHANGE

Harnar (1989, p. 14) has suggested, in the context of Pakistan, that it is useful to look at an adaptation of Lewin's model for change: unfreezing, moving, and refreezing, in understanding what happens when innovations are attempted. (Table 10-1).

Harnar queries whether the problem with attempting to develop health care services, particularly primary health care, in many countries might not be due to implementers and planners rushing to the integration stage without first securing the earlier stages. I suggest nursing has erred in the *moving* stage: Textbooks, movies, television, international consultants, visits, and some study by nurses abroad, have all contributed to an awareness and arousal of interest. If heart transplants can be done to save lives in the West, why not here? Physicians (who have more resources available, for a number of reasons) are trained abroad, and the machines and technology are only a plane trip away; they can be flown in almost immediately. A limited *trial* would soon show that nurses require more knowledge and special skills to do the follow-up care. What usually happens? Doctors teach them. Now physicians are very good indeed at what they do—but what they do isn't nursing. So they can't teach nursing. And nursing, usu-

ally, gets one more black mark. I hear constantly "our nurses need to be better," yet no evaluation has been scientifically carried out to actually determine what it is we aren't doing well; whether those things are, or should be, nursing tasks; and, in terms of priorities, what should be changed first, what second, and so on. At this stage of the development of nursing in Pakistan, it is crucial to discover what nurses do, what they should do, and what changes need to be planned for, tried out, evaluated, and integrated. Medicine still dominates in health care in Pakistan; nurses are given very little say (if any) in policy or planning decisions. To bring nursing into the decision-making arena, even for its own education and practice, the education of a critical mass of nurses needs to be brought to a par with that of physicians. It is unrealistic to expect a physician with postgraduate degrees and wide experience to deal as a colleague either with someone who, though experienced, lacks the cognitive and scientific background, or is 23 years old and has earned a bachelor's degree but has no clinicial experience at all. Senior nurses' treatment of interns in the West is too well known to need a clearer drawing!

PREPARATION FOR LEADERSHIP

With a population of over 100 million (some sources say up to 120 million) no time can be lost in increasing the numbers of nurses. In the United States, the introduction of the 2-year

Table 10-1 The Harnar Model for Gaining Acceptance of Innovations

Change	Steps in acceptance of innovations
Unfreezing	Awareness—involves information sharing
	Interest is aroused with new knowledge
Moving	Trial—limited efforts to try out new ideas
	Evaluation of the trials and outcomes along with more widespread trials
Refreezing	Acceptance of the innovations as a real need
	Integration of the innovation into the system.

associate degree program enabled bedside nurses to be prepared in two-thirds the time. In the United Kingdom, the handwriting seems to be on the wall with Project 2000; nursing is moving even more rapidly into institutions of higher education. One would venture to predict that not too far down the road associate degree (2-year) programs will be introduced there as well. In the Middle East, Bahrain is already educating bedside nurses at the associate-degree level.

I would propose a two-pronged approach to both the problem of leadership and increasing numbers of caregivers: the introduction of a pilot program enabling Pakistani students to earn an associate degree in nursing in two years, and the rapid development of a minimum number of bachelor's, master's, and doctoral national nurses. There must be sufficient numbers not only to carry out educational programs and conduct research but to support each other in interchanging ideas and concepts so that a truly culturally appropriate national system of nursing and nursing education can be formulated which is economically feasible. Again, in the beginning, foreign expertise will most likely be required. There are, however, a number of enclaves in academia where culturally sensitive and aware leaders are helping to mentor younger scholars. There is also a likely pool of Pakistani nurses in North America (both Canada and the United States) who might be enticed to return if the working conditions including salaries, benefits, and academic rank were competitive. One of the chief reasons for the "nurse drain" is better employment opportunities elsewhere. Pakistani nurses are paid better in even the oil-poor countries of the Middle East than in Pakistan.

Nurses selected for advanced education will need to be sponsored not only for tuition fees and living expenses but in many cases will require additional funds as well, since they nearly always are major contributors to the support of their extended families. The programs which have been successful in attracting nurses to advanced study have been those which pay a major proportion (if not all) of the salary as well as other expenses. Very few understand the significance of the nurses' salary in the entire extended family's economy. Advanced degrees will not only provide the academic background to develop a national nursing identity but will more than any other measure elevate the status and image of nursing. A doctorate is honored in whatever field, and education is highly honored in this culture. A degree is a big plus for upgrading image. In Jordan, university students are placed in majors according to their secondary school ranking: For example, top students are assigned to medicine or engineering. Nursing, once at the bottom, has moved up to third or fourth place because students are choosing it; as many stated, "It's a degree, and you always have a job."

With nurses prepared to speak on an equal basis with other health care planners, they will gradually begin to do so; we see this happening in other parts of the world, and for the same reasons.

During the time that national nurses are being prepared abroad, expert advisors need to be working side by side with national nurses who remain in positions of leadership. The often-quoted reason for hiring expatriate nurses *instead* of nationals "because the national nurse is not prepared" will never change until something radical is done to prepare national nurses. Short-term non-degree study or observation tours are useful in their way (and essential for awareness and awakening interest), but in most cases both awareness and interest are well established. The problems of nurses and nursing are identified by even very young Pakistani students as I have described them. In class, a few months ago, students were given an exercise to assess the nutritional status and physical fitness of each other. We expatriates gave ourselves a pat on the back when the group's spokeswoman started her report by saying, "you have to realize these standards were set for Western women, and we need to establish our own norms."

Nurses who go to study abroad should go to carefully selected, academically sound university programs with special interests and expertise in mentoring students from this part of the world. Financing should be sufficient to enable them to conduct their research in their countries. I would go so far as to suggest the thesis and dissertation advisors should examine candidates in their own countries. This procedure would enable the national nurse to serve as a role model for scholarship and academic rigor in her own setting as well as increasing the community of ideas on the home front. Nursing and other leaders from the home institution should sit on dissertation committees. It is these people to whom the new PhD is going to have to sell her leadership. It is these colleagues who will (and can) raise the "reality questions" most dissertation committees never hear about.

Once a small cadre of educationally prepared and experienced nurses are in place, continuing education programs need to be fostered which enable national nurses with leadership abilities to be involved in planning, decision making, and policy statements. The failure of workshops in the past is due, I believe, to the lack of follow through. Occasionally a project gets as far as a small trial, but very rarely, in this country at least, does a careful scientific evaluation take place. Evaluation, so far, has been the most difficult part of the scientific process to teach. Much of the reason is probably culturally determined: socially it is difficult. Critiques are extremely difficult processes for students, and any mark less than an A is likely to bring on floods of tears. We have found it necessary to have a 2-week orientation in which we continually

deemphasized marks and encourage learning for its own sake. Culturally it is not appropriate to recognize error; probably no expatriate can teach how to do this.

In addition to the evaluation phase, the expert needs to be in place for advice, support, and feedback as the trials, with appropriate modifications, are carried out on a wider scale. Except for small single-task or single-skill projects, without follow-up the activity departs with the consultant. I have seen numerous workshops on "The Nursing Process" conducted. With no one in the setting with a thorough understanding of how to implement and evaluate the use of the process itself, the staff end up knowing what the words mean, but it's like teaching people to drive a car by showing them one and having them read the owner's manual. It takes considerable practice. And if you learn to drive only on Main Street in a small town in the desert, you're in big trouble on the streets of San Francisco or Karachi or in the Alps. You are not really a good driver until you've mastered driving in a variety of conditions on a variety of surfaces.

Most of these comments have addressed nursing education, because I believe at this time, at this stage of development, nurse educators have the greatest opportunity to have the greatest impact on changing. However, nursing service personnel must be included to as large an extent as possible to avoid widening the gap between service and education which is as alive and flourishing in Pakistan as anywhere else. One advantage is that in most institutions, the director of the hospital nursing services is also in charge of the school. This is a unique opportunity for clinical practice and academia to develop together. It is unlikely that other sectors are going to seek out nursing during this developmental stage; nursing leaders in training must seek intersectoral collaboration. We have to prove ourselves before others will recognize we have something to offer.

Government planners, physicians, and other concerned departments and individuals are well aware of the problems identified. If the Harnar model of introduction, trial, and integration is followed, there is good reason to expect a successful outcome. It has been successful in several places in Asia in primary health care. It needs to be tested in a broader arena.

REMOVING THE BARRIERS

Many barriers identified are social, economic, and political. Nurses need to be educated to be able, in every sense of the world, to hold their own with the decision makers. Funding (which is a must for increasing not only available educational opportunities but *access* to those already available) is rarely allocated with any input from nursing. Although it is simplistic to suggest that education will alleviate all the problems, as an educator I do firmly believe that everything helps, and education cannot be downgraded. Even family planning efforts in Asia and the Middle East are more effective where literacy rates are higher.

A major barrier to higher education for nurses is access: With the worldwide shortage of nurses and current efforts of all continents except Africa to recruit Pakistani nurses abroad, we should establish, as soon as an applicants' pool is large enough, a master's program in nursing in Pakistan. Since financing and recruiting the qualified faculty will present a major problem, I believe, in its early years, a floating faculty of short-term experts should be set up. Few students take more than one or two courses from any one professor, so the argument for lack of continuity doesn't hold up. There would need to be a consistent philosophy to which the faculty subscribes and administrative continuity. Would it not be exciting to have experts from around the world gathered, semester by semester? Why should they not bring their masters and doc-

toral students with them? Should not countries in the third world be hosting international students?

By the same token, I believe one solution to the unequal allocation of nurses lies in the *where* they are educated. Rural areas cannot support nursing schools. Those families either brave enough or desperate enough to send their daughters away rarely get them back—and if they do the young woman is unprepared to practice where she lives. I would suggest traveling schools—teachers could travel from region to region on a rotating basis; families might permit them to go for a few months (or two or however—these are just ideas); another teacher would come, and so on. We certainly have no evidence to suggest taking four or so subjects at once is any more effective than one (or two, or three) at a time. Perhaps two teachers, or even three, could go at once. The major advantage would be the nurses would remain in their communities, and, if you have the right teachers, the education would be tailored to the needs of the communities. It would be essential to include learning and practice activities related to health care from the very beginning. Perhaps one could start with activities normally carried out by community health workers—pre-natal and infant monitoring, and so forth.

Whatever strategies are finally adopted, nurses must be careful to "mind their own business." A colleague in primary health care studied what community health nurses were doing and her report stated, "They were wearing everyone's hats but their own" (Herberg, 1989). If nursing doesn't soon begin to be involved in making decisions about its own future, the decisions may well be taken out of nursing's hands. Allocation of resources and various political decisions have never really been in nursing's hands, but there are rumblings from governmental sources now that since nursing is not solving nursing's problems, some new mechanism should be established.

It is also high time that we in nursing stopped trying to place blame for our failures: "They won't let us," "They expect this," "They won't accept that." We must spend our energies more productively. We need to clearly separate power issues from gender issues. Nurses often say they can't do anything because they are predominantly women. Let's go further and say we are impeded because we lack *power*. Sri Lanka, India, and now Pakistan have had women as heads of state. People can be educated to exercise power. Leadership skills are not confined to men. Barriers within nursing must be withdrawn at the same time we try to eliminate barriers in other arenas.

CONCLUSION

There is no clear evidence that Western models of education or practice have proved effective in solving the problems of human response to illness, which is the chief concern of nursing. There is considerable evidence that education and research improve the quality of service, education, and health. Education improves the capacity of all people to be involved in decision making and the development and implementation of health policy. Policy-making bodies of all nations are composed of educated leaders. It is time for nurses to take their places in these bodies. We have already lost too much time.

REFERENCES

Benner, P. (1984). *From novice to expert*. Menlo Park, CA: Addison Wesley.

Diers, D. (1990). To profess—To be a professional. *Journal of Nursing Administration, 16*(3), 25–30.

Harris, P. R. & Moran, R. T. (1979). *Managing cultural differences*. Houston, TX: Gulf.

Herberg, P. (1989). *Analysis of the role of the CHN in primary health care in the Katchi Abadia*. Unpublished manuscript. The Aga Khan University School of Nursing, Karachi, Pakistan.

Holzemer, W. M. & Amarsi, Y. A. (1989). *Nursing at the Aga Khan University Medical Center*.

Kamal, I. T. (1984, November). *Perspectives in nursing toward the year 2000*. Paper presented at the WHO conference on Nursing Manpower Development, Bahrain.

Khan, N. (1989, February). *Nursing care in hospitals of Pakistan*. Paper presented at the Pakistan Academy of Medical Sciences Conference, Karachi, Pakistan.

Lee, M. B. (1989). *Pilot study on meanings and expressions of care in Pakistani Muslims experiencing and giving care in a critical care unit - A proposal*. Unpublished manuscript.

Lee, R. (1989). *Factors predicting academic success: a comparative study*. Unpublished manuscript. The Aga Khan University School of Nursing, Karachi, Pakistan.

Majid, A. O. (1988). Health and health care facilities in Pakistan. *Economic Review, 20*(8), 23–24.

Rajwani, R. (1989, February). *The problems of nurses in Pakistan*. Paper presented at the Pakistan Academy of Medical Sciences Conference, Karachi, Pakistan.

Sarwar, S.M. (1989). World health versus Pakistan [sic] health. *Economic Review, 20*(8), 27–30.

Scott, P.A. (1984). *Social networks of Turkish women: Dimensions of relationships*. Unpublished doctoral dissertation. University of California San Francisco, San Francisco, CA.

Chapter 11

Some Thoughts on Education in Hungary

Klára Sövényi

When I received the honorable invitation to think freely about the training objectives and methods of implementation of nurses of the twenty-first century, the first thing that occurred to me were Abraham Lincoln's words. "If I knew where we are, it would be easier for me to tell what to do and how to do it."

The following are ways of approaching the future:

- Prediction
- Free outlining of "desirable" future
- Foreseeing the effects of the present situation projected into the future

I mainly used the third method, but naturally took the positive or negative effects of the numerous influencing factors into consideration; what is more, I must confess, that the outlining of the desirable future also mixed into my thinking. My prime factor was, that if one is given the possibility to dream of the future, one should first look back on the past and study the present, as they had their roots in the ideas of dreamers of the then future.

Let us now have a look at the realities of present rooted in the past and consider the principal problems that characterize nursing and training of nursing personnel. I should like to stress, that my experience and information have been gained first of all in European countries and mainly in Hungary.

The representatives of some European countries summarized the European problem, its causes, and means to overcome it as follows: There is increasing need for nursing in all countries, therefore nursing has become a crucial issue. However, the number of nursing personnel who would be able to satisfy nursing needs is on the decrease. Two methods can make nursing needs equal nursing personnel. One method characterizes affluent countries, namely that they can afford to pay for qualified nursing personnel from foreign countries and thus are able to maintain the level of care. Characterizing less affluent countries, the other method consists of dressing employees "in white coats" to ensure the personnel, thus giving up the quality of nursing completely.

As to the underlying causes, let me mention only a few:

• Insupportable workload, especially in hospital nursing
  • Low wages
  • Lack of other benefits
  • Inappropriate training
  • Unfavorable image of nursing
• Lack of esteem in society and within the health sector

From these issues, I shall mainly tackle training but will often link it to the practice of nursing, as theory is rooted there.

"One learns from one's mistakes," goes a Hungarian saying. What mistakes did we make in the training of nursing personnel? I found the following "mistakes" in the course of the past of nearly half a century:

• First we trained the nursing personnel at short "cram" courses, thus we only made quantitative developments. This was our first mistake.
• Later we succeeded in extending the duration of training, which resulted in improved quality, but we failed to fit the training of nursing personnel into the Hungarian school system. This was our second mistake.
• When finally it became possible, we took the training of nursing personnel down to the secondary school level, which was too low in fact. I think this was our third mistake.

• This came about, when the foundations of professions had to be laid down rather early, due to demographic causes. "Semifinished" nursing personnel were trained on the secondary school level; these personnel had to acquire further skills in addition to doing their work to perform their duties on a higher professional level. In addition, it was decided that the other part of the nursing personnel would be trained exclusively in the frames of on-the-job training, thus they were employees and students at the very same time. The skills and knowledge they were able to acquire in this way were determined by the personal and technical conditions of the given workplace, which of course, might be either positive or negative. In the frames of this type of training, the nurse is only prepared for what "there is" and does not even think of what there should be. These nurses are definitely not the vehicles of nursing in the future.

Another important factor in the training of nurses is the content of teaching, which even today consists mostly of medical knowledge. It can well be said, that we train "minidoctors" rather than highly qualified nurses. However, it is stongly related to the fact that neither nursing, nor nursing personnel has found its genuine social mission. Any investigation of the training of nursing personnel will raise the issue of nursing as an independent discipline, as it is strongly linked to the problem of autonomy, which is essentially a basic criterion of being a discipline. It is well known to all of us that in numerous European countries, nursing is still a "maid-servant" of medicine. There not being possibilities for academic training, ambitious and dedicated young persons either do not choose to be nurses, or if they by chance come here, they practice the profession for a very short time only. They are attracted by professions offering possibilities for further education and thus they quit nursing. As in nursing, the avenues for progress are rather limited in several countries, young people from higher social strata hardly opt for this profession. In Hungary, those choosing nursing as a career come from social strata of lower, or at the best, medium educational level. All these causes result in the failure of the nursing personnel to stabilize and in their inappropriate educational level.

Studies we have conducted reveal that the nursing personnel is renewed every 6 to 8 years with very low average age. Currently, nursing is like filling a leaky sack at the mouth while it is leaking out at the bottom.

The issue of shortage of nursing personnel will only be solved in the long run in countries where it will be possible to obtain the highest level of qualification in the given country in nursing, including the doctor's degree in nursing. Not only the level of training but also financial remuneration has to be similar to other professionals with higher-level education, e.g., doctor-nurse-teacher.

Realizing the negative aspects of training, Hungary recently has decided to raise the level of training of a part of nursing personnel to the academic level, equivalent to other university degrees. It would include first and foremost those who can work with great independence in public health care (PHC), on the level of family medicine and in special areas of clinical nursing (e.g., oncology). This group will then yield, after postgraduate education, nursing managers, nursing instructors, and, thinking in the long run, nursing researchers.

After having outlined some of the problems nursing faces, a few questions turn up as a matter of cause:

• Will nursing be needed in the next century; if yes, in what form?
• Will training be needed, if yes, what will be its objectives and content?
• Shall we be able to identify the place and relative autonomy of nursing among the disciplines?

• Will nursing be one-level or not?
• Will nursing be institutionalized or not?

If the answer to the above question is yes, still another question turns up: What shoud be the bases for developments in the next century of nursing and of the training of nursing personnel? Some trends are beginning to be clear:

• Hospital-centered, rather passive health care is being replaced by PHC-oriented, active health promotive, disease preventive and rehabilitative care.
• In nursing, that has so far been exclusively patient care, health care is also gaining ground.
• Technology-centered care will shift toward care centered on the patient.
• Mainly disease-centered nursing provided as a routine by nursing personnel who have been trained by a self-made, self-taught, watch-learn method and who are mere executors of the doctor's instruction will be replaced by highly qualified nursing personnel who have been trained for their new role as well as by direct nursing based on scientific bases, from which all families and communities will benefit.

Principal questions related to the training of nursing personnel in the twenty-first century include:

• What tasks do we prepare them for?
• What shall we teach to them?
• Who shall teach?
• On which level or levels shall the nursing personnel be trained?
• Shall the disciplines be based together, or shall we continue to provide the current more or less specialized training?
• What should the nursing attitudes be in the next century?
• In what structural frameworks will knowledge and novel nursing attitudes become manifest?

These questions are very important because a training system introduced today will display its positive or negative effects after a period of about a decade only. Thus, it takes about a quarter of a century for the effects of a "change in the training system" to be felt. This is a very long period if we have to face the negative effects of training.

The key to training of nursing personnel required for health care delivery of the next century lies in demography, factors determining health status, and socioeconomic and environmental factors. Principal characteristics that are already known in Europe include:

• Changing social structures, increasing or stagnating number of the elderly and lonely persons; negative lifestyles of young persons.
• Growing number of the chronically and mentally ill.
• Increased quantity of tasks of a surgical nature.
• Growing number of problems caused by social changes (alcoholism, drug abuse).
• "Four major killers" continue but newer diseases also appear (e.g., AIDS).
• Society revolts against uniform and institutionalized care and demands individualized care.

These are the principal factors that determine the individuals' health needs and within them nursing needs. We must plan the training of nursing personnel so as to make it relevant in both content and form to these factors.

Training and education of nursing personnel of the next century should meet the following demands:

• It should be community-oriented, while serving treatment.
• It should further develop the skills to establish personal contacts and communication within the professional staff and with the community to be served.
• It should motivate for positive nursing attitudes.

• It should make the importance of the role of nursing personnel recognized in shaping future health.
• It should train in a way that nursing and the word *nursing* should not be associated solely with hospitals, patients, diseases, but with continuous follow-up care and health.
• It should prepare for research and the practice of nursing science.
• Training and education should take on a dual role and influence both instructor and student.

The attainment of this system of objectives requires a change in attitudes. We have to reevaluate and expand our knowledge of people, community, health, health promotion, environment and its positive and negative effects, factors endangering health, healthy lifestyles.

Training programs have to be formulated to be appropriate for getting the mastery of all this. We have to teach the methods to shape positive health, which is socially determined, but at the same time is a good mirror of the structure of the individual's personality.

We have to become familiar with the complicated methodology of preventing substance abuse. We have to shoulder the roles of active health educators and health promoters together with "trend-setting," because only in this way can communities be made to change their lifestyles.

The key issue of the entire desired process of change is that those who are responsible for training nursing personnel should accept and be able to transmit that health is a genuine value, and they should include this value in their value system. This value system should also include that the individual is responsible for his/her own health and that of his/her fellow citizens and that no one else can protect health against the individual.

One of the most difficult but also the most important tasks is the elaboration of a method that will enable the nursing personnel to transmit health-centered programs and to raise the interest in and responsiblity for health. Namely, it is not an easy task to teach the hygiene of work, eating, sleep, rest, and amusement as well as the lifestyle rules of the different ages, to adhere to the hygienic rules of mental and intellectual life as well as to control diseases we caused ourselves (obesity, alcoholism, smoking, drugs, etc.).

The first step, however, is that we ourselves accept the essence of the change, include the notion of "health is a value" in our value system and raise the theory and practice of prevention and health promotion to a rank. In the training programs of the future, priority will have to be assigned to the principle that if we implement the knowledge related to healthy lifestyles, it will in itself lengthen the life of some population groups by years. We have to train in a way that would-be nursing personnel may recognize this existential interest and may be able to transmit it, as it plays a significant role in improving the quality of life. Especially we, nurses, should not forget that health of tomorrow is in the hands of man of today.

So far, I have mainly dealt with the implications for training of health nursing. This, of course, does not mean that I would completely reject the need for hospital nursing in the next century. This is not the case. In hospital care, nursing related to "surgical activities" will most probably get into the foreground. The number of homes providing "nursing only" is likely to increase. However, one will have to reckon with very special nursing responsibilities, e.g., care of AIDS patients (at home or in institutions).

When thinking of training in the future, we should not disregard the differing interests of economy and education. The economy, including the health sector, requires first of all specialized knowledge. In contrast, education keeps the acquiring of convertible knowledge to the fore. In my opinion it would be of great benefit for humanity, too, if we could reach a stage in the next century, when professional knowledge of different types would be built on a unified health-motivated body of general knowledge.

Today, a student, a would-be nurse is likely to have the feeling that society consists of sick people only, because this is what the teaching material reflects. Undergraduate education in medicine and nursing could bifurcate after common bases, allowing for passage until a defined term of training. An intermediate solution would be to run training facilities for nursing personnel as faculties of medical universities with teaching programs built on each other. We are trying our hand at this model.

Irrespective of what the basic training for future nursing personnel will look like, a system of postgraduate education providing a special and new body of knowledge must be built (e.g., training of managers, instructors). However, these will have to be framed by a lifelong continuing education system, the main objective of which is to prepare for new challenges.

In this accelerated world, there is not much time to be spent on educational experiences, therefore we have to hatch plans, the implementation of which is consistent with challenges of the next century.

Challenges to Practice

This section covers a broad range of issues in primary care, gerontology, midwifery, and other areas and is organized around the following questions:

1 What are the current constraints affecting the practice of nursing in your country (too few RNs, too little education, too dominated by other professions, not allowed to practice in manner educated, legislation)?

2 What geographic and resource allocation or availability factors affect the ability of nurses to provide good nursing care in your country?

3 What are the rewards or benefits allotted nurses who provide services in rural or remote areas?

4 Who are the predominant providers of primary health care in your country or region? Are nurses prepared for primary health care delivery?

5 What legislation in your country fosters or constrains the practice of nurses, and what recommendations would you make for change?

6 Do you have a need for and a plan for utilization of clinical nurse specialists in health delivery in your country?

7 Do you have problems obtaining a sufficient number of nurses for any particular practice setting (long-term care, hospitals, primary care, community health, etc.)? Do you have a plan for addressing these problems? What gets in the way of the proposed solution?

Chapter 12

Midwifery and Safe Motherhood

Barbara Kwast

The human right to enjoy successful pregnancy and childbirth and to regulate fertility safely is still denied millions of women today. The magnitude of maternal mortality and morbidity is witness to this social unjustice.

The World Health Organization estimates that at least half a million pregnancy-related deaths occur each year. Most of the women who die in pregnancy and childbirth are poor and live in remote areas or city slums. Their deaths are accorded little importance and fail to enter registers. Unless we are educated and sensitized to this major human tragedy of unnecessary loss of life and relate this to our current strength and activities, maternal mortality alone will destroy 7.5 million women between now and the onset of the twenty-first century.

Developing countries see between 50 to over 800 maternal deaths per 100,000 live births. This is about 200 times higher than the figures of between 5 and 300 in developed countries. It was against this background of gross disparity that the Safe Motherhood Initiative (SMI), was launched at the Safe Motherhood Conference in Nairobi in 1987. It was cosponsored by the World Bank, WHO, and the United Nations Population fund (UNFPA). A call to action was unanimously adopted to reduce maternal mortality by 50 percent in one decade.[1] The World Health Assembly adopted the resolution on maternal health and safe motherhood in the same year.[2]

To meet the goal of reduction of maternal mortality by 50 percent, an integrated approach to maternity care is needed at all levels of the health care system. Midwives are indispensable members of the maternal health care team and a vital link in the hierarchy of the maternity services.

An estimated 50 percent of deliveries in the developing world are now supervised by a trained birth attendant. Such supervision varies widely among regions and countries. In some countries this figure may be as low as 5 percent.[3]

THE SAFE MOTHERHOOD INITIATIVE

The Safe Motherhood Initiative is a global process and implies advocacy and information, development and technical support, changes in health practice, education and research. SMI has to become an integral part of the health services.

The urgency of SMI's goals can be well understood when the population pyramids of developed and developing regions are compared (Figure 12-1). In the first diagram there is a demographic reality of negligible population growth. In an aging population, both curative, often in health institutions, and promotive care is an important need. Paradoxically, women in the reproductive age group (15 to 49 years) constitute 25 percent of the population in both developed and developing countries. Because the total fertility rate (TFR) in developing countries is twice that of developed countries (1.8 to 2.1 compared to 3.4 to 4.0) more frequent childbearing occurs with a concomitant increase in the population under 15 years of age, to about 33 percent. Countries with high fertility rates have high mortality rates. Examples are Zimbabwe and Kenya with a TFR of 6.6 and 8.0 for 1985 to 1990, respectively. Vast energy and effort needs to go to health promotive care through primary health care (PHC), emphasizing the 'M' in MCH. Cuba, Sri Lanka, and Singapore have TFRs of 2.1, 3.1, and 1.9, respectively and have achieved a remarkable fall in maternal mortality ratios.

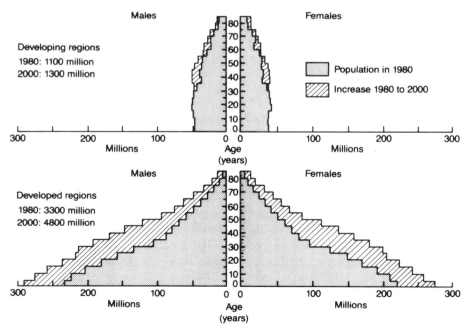

Figure 12-1   Population by Age and Sex (1980 and 2000).

Under the umbrella of the Health for All Strategy, the four major elements of SMI are:

• Adequate primary health care and an adequate share of the available food for girls from infancy to adolescence; family planning universally available to avoid unwanted or high-risk pregnancies.

• After pregnancy begins, good prenatal care, including nutrition, with efficient and early detection and referral of those at high risk.

• The assistance of a trained person for all women in childbirth, at home as in hospital.

• Women at high risk, and above all, women in the emergencies of pregnancy, childbirth, and postpartum, must all have access to the essential elements of obstetric care at the first referral level.

Primary prevention is a major key to SMI. The big problem facing nursing and midwifery is to get the services to the women at the grass roots. If we want to give full effect to the strategies of safe motherhood we have to ask at least four questions about midwifery.

1 Where are the midwives in maternal and child health (MCH)?

2 Is the midwives' education appropriate to fulfill the goals of safe motherhood?

3 What does it take to meet the requirements of the maternity care team?

4 To what extent can midwives themselves change the situation?

PROBLEM STATEMENT

The definition and situation of the category of health worker referred to as midwife or nurse-midwife varies between countries, and more importantly, appears to be changing, not necessarily for the better. Although there may be some variation between countries, the following appear to be the major midwifery patterns (see Table 12-1) in different countries:

Shortage and Inadequate Distribution of Midwives

Workforce planning in developing countries generally aims at the figure of one midwife per 5,000 population, that is, approximately 200

Table 12-1 Major Midwifery Patterns

Category of personnel	Prerequisite training/ education	Midwifery training	Other nursing training
Nurse (master of science nursing)	B.Sci., Nursing	2 years	Integrated
Nurse (B.Sci., nursing)	Secondary	4 years	Integrated
Midwife	Secondary	3 years	None
Nurse-midwife (registered)	Secondary	1 to 1.5 years	3 years
Nurse-midwife (registered)	Secondary	6 months	3 years
Enrolled midwife (nonregistered)	Primary/ some secondary	2 years	None
Nurse-midwife (nonregistered)	Primary/ some secondary	1 year	2 years
Auxiliary nurse-midwife	Primary/ some secondary	6 months	2 years

deliveries per year.[4] Even though nurses and midwives make up more than 80 percent of training health personnel, there exists a serious shortage of midwives globally. This situation is especially significant in parts of Africa and Asia. Two scenarios, one in each continent, illustrate the issues: Country A in South Asia with 80 million population and a birth rate of 45/1,000 would expect 3.6 million births per year. There are 213 midwives in the service. This yields a midwife:population ratio of 1:375,586 or 1 midwife per 16,901 births. Eight percent of deliveries take place in institutions. Maternal mortality is between 400 to 600 per 100,000 live births.

Although traditional birth attendant (TBA) training is extensive, there are not enough midwives to support the primary level. Nor are they available for even emergency obstetric care at health centers or for essential obstetric care at first referral level. Thus, the concept of a maternal health care team cannot be realized.

In Bangladesh and India, however, the physician:population ratio is higher than the nurse-midwife:population ratio. This indicates that most of the maternal and child health services are provided by auxiliary health personnel who have less training. This in itself presents a problem for the management of pregnancy-related life-threatening complications.

Country B in Africa with a population of 42 million and a birth rate of 45 per 1,000 would expect 1,890,000 births per annum. The number of nurses was 1,896 in 1984, giving a nurse:population ratio of 1:22,151 or one nurse per 997 births. Maternal mortality figures range between 600 to 1,000 per 100,000 births. Setting aside North Africa and southern Africa, the number of physicians per 10,000 inhabitants is also very low. It is also generally true that countries which are poor in human resources have high maternal mortality ratios.

Even where the situation is somewhat better—for instance one nurse-midwife per 2,000 population in Kenya, one per 3,000 in Uganda, one per 3,000 in Nigeria, and one per 5,000 in Malawi—the disparity between urban and rural staffing is great. The numbers are insufficient for adequate village services or constructive supervision. In many of these countries 80 percent of the poulation lives in rural areas where the majority of babies are born, TBAs, where they exist, cannot cope with the isolation. Even where rural maternity centers exist, many do not have a midwife or are closed because of lack of personnel and equipment. Thus, for the twenty three countries in Africa for which data are available, seven would be considered adequately staffed and sixteen would have a need for 21,000 additional trained midwives.[5] An example of the range of human resources available, as reported by countries, for maternal health and safe motherhood are presented in Table 12-2.

Health Services and the Community: The Interface

The women who die unnecessarily from pregnancy-related causes are rural or disadvantaged urban women. Services for their care are either not available or too costly to use; these women are too distant culturally from the highly educated health professionals, making it difficult to communicate, and care is therefore unacceptable. The midwife could respond to the needs of women during the reproductive years. Unfortunately she works mostly in hospitals, in towns, where other colleagues are available and often providing care of a nature that could be delegated to other health workers. Relatively well educated and sophisticated, she is often out of touch with rural women and rarely willing to work among them.[6]

Health services need to respond to the catastrophe of maternal mortality and morbidity in two ways: through primary maternal health

Table 12-2 Human Resources and Maternal Health and Safe Motherhood

Country	Midwives per 1,000	OB/GYN per 1,000	Coverage-trained attendant
Algeria	0.5	0.21	14.7
Benin	1.9		44
Botswana	8.9	0.02	79
Burkina Faso	0.8		12
Burundi	0.1		
Cameroons	0.5	0.01	10
Central African Republic	2.5		65.7
Chad	0.1		24
Gambia	16.1	0.06	80
Ghana	10.5	0.05	73
Guinea-Bissau	3		
Liberia	2.2	0.03	86
Madagascar	3		62
Malawi	6	0.00	59
Mauritania	21		22
Mauritius	25.3	0.59	84
Niger	0.6		46
Nigeria	7.7	0.05	
Rwanda	1.4		
Senegal	1.6		40
Sierra Leone	7.7	0.08	25
Togo	5.3		
Zimbabwe	6	0.08	69
Argentina		2.09	
Bahamas	21.7	0.54	99
Barbados	93.3	1.32	98
Bolivia		0.29	17
Brazil		1.19	73
Canada		1.90	99
Chile	24.1	0.79	95.3
Colombia		0.45	51

Country	Midwives per 1,000	OB/GYN per 1,000	Coverage-trained attendant
Costa Rica		0.58	93
Cuba	4.9	0.59	98.7
Dominica	26.8	1.14	96
Dominican Republic		0.66	98
Ecuador		0.35	26.9
El Salvador		0.27	34.7
Guatemala		0.31	51
Guyana	19.7	0.14	92.5
Haiti	0.3	0.11	20
Honduras		0.17	50
Jamaica	41.8	0.95	89
Mexico		0.49	87
Nicaragua		0.21	41
Panama		0.57	83.3
Paraguay	1.6	0.57	21.9
Peru	2.9	0.19	44.2
Trinidad & Tobago		0.78	90
USA		7.12	99.7
Uruguay	20	1.00	
Venezuela		0.51	82.1
Bangladash	0.4	0.01	5
India	10.1	0.29	30
Indonesia	15.4	0.07	30.7
Sri Lanka	6.1	0.22	86
China	3.5	0.00	93.4
Fiji	59.9	0.09	97.5
Malaysia		0.43	86.7
Papua New Guinea		0.04	31
Philippines	5.2	0.18	53.9
Rep. of Korea	5.3	1.06	77.2
Samoa	8.3	0.20	95

care at village, dispensary and health center level and through essential obstetric functions at first referral level.

A WHO Technical Working Group (TWG) in 1986 defined the functions of primary care in the family and the community as prenatal screening; screening for high risk; primary and secondary prevention of certain conditions; treating such conditions as anemia before they become so serious as to threaten safe childbirth; health education; counselling; and domiciliary delivery by trained persons for women who desire it and who are not at high risk.[7]

To reduce maternal mortality also means discussions with communities and their leaders. It means sharing expertise and adapting knowledge so that local problems can be exposed locally and solutions sought locally. Villagers have much more idea of resources locally to solve problems and are often in a position to make arrangements for emergency and routine transport should removal to hospital or regular midwife support of TBAs be appreciated as necessary by them. Examples include the building of maternity waiting homes which give shelter to women at high risk during the last few weeks of pregnancy.[8,9] The consequence of maternal death falls heavily upon a community. Any proposals to reduce these deaths will be enthusiastically welcomed if understood and within the means of the people. The midwife, properly trained could be the key to the solution of such problems.

Highlighting the grave problem of most rural women of access to life-saving procedures in emergency during childbirth, the same TWG defined seven groups of essential obstetric functions which are life-saving in relation to the major causes of maternal mortality: surgical; anaesthetic; medical treatment; blood replacement; manual/assessment functions; family planning; and management of women at high risk. Table 12-3 shows the

Table 12-3 Health Services and Health Personnel

Level	Category
Village/community	TBA
	CHW/PHW
	MCH AIDE
Dispensary	Health assistant
Health center	Enrolled N-M, medical assistant, health assistant
District hospital	Registered N-M, enrolled N-M, clinical officer, physician

placement of midwives and other health workers in relation to primary and referral level.

Primary prevention is a major key to SMI. The big problem facing nursing and midwifery is to get the services to the women at the grass roots. To allow delegation of midwifery services to the traditional birth attendant or other community health workers will not produce stronger midwifery services in the long term. By definition, TBAs do not have the theoretical knowledge to extend their skills very far. Many countries do not have TBAs or other community health workers. However, until an adequately acceptable fully qualified midwife is available for every delivery, TBAs cannot be ignored where they exist. The trained TBA bridges the social and communication gap between the urban midwife and the rural population. Success demands that the midwife herself is made capable of taking responsibility for this training and the essential follow-up. Since the midwife must deal with problems referred to her by the TBA, the former must have the additional skills and facilities to deal with those referred problems effectively and locally. It is essential that the midwife is fully backed up in these endeavors by good working conditions, support services and continuing education, decent housing, and provision for her own children to receive education.

In many countries the enrolled or auxiliary nurse-midwife functions both at primary and secondary level. However, increasingly she is used for hospital services or her training has been abolished altogether. This leaves a serious gap that cannot be filled either by TBAs or by registered or degree-level nurse-midwives.

Basic Midwifery Education

Maternal mortality has many facets—social, political, educational, managerial, as well as clinical. To make an impact on the present unacceptable levels of maternal mortality, midwives must be able to act independently on all these levels. Each individual midwife, appropriately trained, equipped, and supported could do much to reduce maternal mortality in her own area. Her education therefore needs to encompass the philosophy of the role we ascribe to her.

The sphere of practice of the midwife was defined by the Joint Study Group of the International Federation of Gynecology and Obstetrics/International Confederation of Midwives (FIGO/ICM) as long ago as 1972.[10] It is important to reiterate that each midwife as a practitioner of midwifery is accountable for her own practice in whatever environment she practices. The midwife has a unique professional and legal responsibility. The definition includes the educational and practical prerequisites for the safe motherhood strategies. The midwife is already trained in the provision of many of the essential obstetric functions in developing countries and can perform others under emergency circumstances. Midwifery training should thus be considered among the highest priorities in the development of human resources for safe motherhood.

The apparent resistance to the fulfillment of her designated role when rural areas in Africa suffer from increasing loss of physicians while medical education has expanded considerably is an obvious contradiction. Increased medical education has led to considerable restriction in the sphere of practice of midwives trained in teaching hospitals thereby not equipping them fully to practice confidently where there is no doctor.

Content of Training Midwifery education generally still relies on a concept of training in a microcosm of individual maternity care rather than on education and a perception of a wider public health context with emphasis on promotive and preventive health. Except for a few countries, lack of awareness of the magnitude of maternal mortality and morbidity as well as restrictive or nonexistent regulatory mechanisms for training and practice have insufficiently prepared midwives to expand their role with technical skills to deal with obstetric emergencies. Concepts of problem-solving and team management are not yet widely practiced. Much training in the developing world is patterned on (if not governed by) rules and teachers trained in the developed world with standards of education and practice designed for different circumstances.

To meet the needs of primary health care systems, nurses should innovate and participate in interprofessional and intersectoral teams for health development; they will increasingly become managers of primary health care teams, supervising nonprofessional workers and monitoring health service activities.

Mwale stated that primary health care manages to be both exciting and frustrating. She suggested that Malawi needs more nurse-midwives who are generalists who can work in curative, preventive, and promotive health. This concept has led in many developing countries to an integration of nursing, midwifery, and public health training, where midwifery is no longer recognizable as a specialist entity to the detriment of maternal health care. A community health nurse without proper midwifery training is incapable of answering to the needs of 25 percent of the population when she or he is responsible for a community. It is of the utmost importance to consider population dynamics and priorities when structuring curricula and considering adoption of foreign training programs, rather than adaptation or innovation.

Midwifery Tutors   There is a dearth of midwifery tutors. Many countries cannot afford to train their own midwife teachers. The teacher-training institutes of the developed world often refuse to take as students those without educational and professional experience equivalent to their own. Where acceded to, this equivalency distorts the development of appropriate national training for midwives. The teachers trained overseas find themselves incapable of developing programs based on national realities and perpetuate the inappropriateness of midwifery training for national situations. Unfortunately, education for the midwife tutor diploma was well established in several countries in Africa, but has been discontinued. One of the reasons given was the unacceptability of diplomas for career development.

With the modernization of nursing education and the desire for basic and postbasic degrees, expansion of midwifery knowledge and practical skills has lagged when compared to other subjects. There are too few midwifery tutor training programs. What there is often includes insufficient theoretical and clinical midwifery education as part of a two-year bachelor of science nursing degree. In those developing countries where such programs exist, the future tutors are derived. This brings us full circle: The situation is perpetuated; nurse-midwives themselves respond reluctantly to the more extended role of the nurse-midwife. Where students may be trained in modern obstetrics, tutors may lag behind.

This creates tension between the clinical and training setting resulting in withdrawal by tutors from clinical teaching. These dilemmas have been outlined to me by appointed midwifery tutors who have received no additional education to prepare them for the task.

Midwifery Training Schools   Although the number of nursing schools in many countries has increased considerably, midwifery training schools have not expanded proportionately. They therefore could not absorb the necessary number of midwifery students. Furthermore, the provision of basic equipment and supplies such as teaching models, overhead projectors, and relevant educational materials has been severely neglected in many parts.

Refresher Courses   Hardly any country in the developing world insists on or organizes refresher courses or continuing education seminars in midwifery. "Hands on" experience to gain additional clinical skills would not only benefit midwifery practice but would be much welcomed by practicing midwives who feel that they have been neglected for too long, that they are the forgotten resource.

APPROACHES TO TRAINING FOR SAFE MOTHERHOOD

The development of the human resources for safe motherhood can no longer be left to an *ad hoc* process. Training for safe motherhood must be based on the actual national needs and adapted to local circumstances. There is no single international prototype for such training, although certain principles should be followed in the development of such programs. The process of development of a training strategy and program involves a critical assessment of program need and staff and system performance within the entire structure of maternal-health-related services. Such a program must account for the communities' perspective, particularly that of the most disadvantaged groups of women. In addition to a technical content, training programs need to be socially oriented and include such critical areas as sensitivity to and knowledge of community-perceived needs, team participation, clinical and program problem-solving skills, and communication skills.

Depending on the available human resources, the level of knowledge and skill among existing and anticipated staff, and the nature of the problems confronting those concerned with maternal health and safe motherhood, several training strategy options are available to national program managers. Training could be directed at any one combination of the following:

• Expanding the number of specific functions and/or categories of health workers
• Strengthening knowledge, skills, and the performance levels of specific technologies
• Improving the management of the system of care in terms of such skills as planning, monitoring, supervision, and evaluation
• Sensitizing the various levels of staff to the communities—particularly women's—perspective and involvement in care

Although training of the health workforce necessary for providing essential obstetric care to the population must be planned in the context of specifics in each region or country, some aspects of training can be developed globally and adapted to these different settings. Knowledge and technical skill alone are not sufficient in applying the various technolgies, techniques, and procedures for maternal and newborn care. The needs and technical content of training are closely linked to attitudes of health workers. Both the selection and training of health workers at various levels of the system must account for the social responsibility of the health worker and hence his or her sensitivity to the needs and perceptions of the community.

As countries recognize the need for upgrading the knowledge and skills of their staff they have also experienced the problem of their staff being overextended by training courses and workshops, with the consequent and continual disruption in the provision of services. Consequently, training strategies need to be oriented to the principle of minimal displacement of staff and maximum on-site tutorial training, including the planning, management, and evaluation ("program or community-side" training) as well as the technical content and quality control of the care provided (practical clinical training). Distance learning, or correspondence courses, will need to be used more frequently for the updating of technical knowledge and the strengthening of managerial skills of health workers.

Given the level of education, training, and experience of qualified midwives, they clearly have a critical role in clinical care and in the management of district-based maternal health programs. Such midwives are already training in the provision of many of the essential obstetric functions and can perform others under emergency circumstances. Furthermore, midwives are more likely than many medical officers to remain in the rural areas. Midwifery training should thus be considered among the highest priorities in the development of human resources for safe motherhood.

THE MATERNITY CARE TEAM

For a maternity care team to be effective the organizational environment must foster team work. Effective teams operate with clearly defined goals and expectations. Their leaders lead by example and not by job titles alone. Leaders plan and make decisions in groups but are allowed a great deal of personal freedom. They communicate and share information. They set high standards and acknowledge one another's contribution and support.[12] Traditionally, work and educational environments have not been team-oriented and problem-solving, but rather hierarchical and authoritarian.

The Safe Motherhood Initiative, perhaps more than any other initiative so closely related to life and death, requires team building and working effectively with other team members enhancing each others's role through mutual respect. The role of the midwife in the team is crucial. She (sometimes he, where male midwives are acceptable) is the lynch-pin in the maternity service. Her interdependent and independent role as a highly skilled practitioner in midwifery, extending to certain areas of gynecology, family planning, and child health, must be clearly understood. In addition she has an administrative, managerial, and educational role which requires critical thinking and leadership qualities.

The definition of a maternity care team will depend on the notion of our work confines and may differ between urban and rural areas. In an urban teaching center, the team would consist of the obstetrician/gynecologist, nursing/midwifery officer, nurse-midwife (registered and enrolled), public health nurse, community health worker, nutrition workers, social workers, and the community. When a senior nursing officer in charge of a maternity unit in Africa was asked about her role in the maternity team, the answer was: "The midwife sets the climate for midwifery practice in the department. She is the specialist in normal midwifery, recognizes the abnormal and institutes emergency management until referral or medical aid can be obtained. While the obstetrician is the leader of the team, the midwife needs the leadership qualities to coordinate the team work. The midwife needs to set the tone because of the continuous rotation of 'outsiders' in the department, referring to expatriate staff in countries which do not have enough national obstetric manpower.[13] Even when that need is fulfilled, a teaching department will always have students, interns, and residents who rotate. Continuity of standard patterns of care therefore rest on the shoulders of senior midwives in the team." She added: "since Alma Ata midwifery has broadened—the midwife works *with* the community and is no longer viewed as taking care of patients in there for those who are out there." That particular department had an organized postnatal home-visiting service staffed by public health nurses.

In the rural area the team would probably be expanded to include: the district medical officer/clinical officer, district public health nurse, enrolled nurse-midwife, medical assistant, health inspector, TBA, CHW, VHW, the community.

Harman and Kesby recently reported on a study carried out by the Institute of Child Health, in The Gambia, Zambia, and Kenya on the changing role of nursing management in relation to primary health care (PHC).[14] That study on issues related to the Alma Ata Declaration. For a maternity care team to work effectively in a PHC system, the health centers form the pivot between the health care organization and the community. This does not work in reality in many countries both in Africa, as shown in Harman's study, and in southern Asia. Supervision of community health workers is often exercised from the district level, bypassing the health center. Interviews with staff of the different health units on their understanding of team function revealed a horizontal team concept and loyalties within their own unit, while each member of the team is accountable to vertical lines of management from a higher level.

The fact is that new policies and directions still come from central level. There, initiatives from nurse-midwives are limited as they are excluded in many countries from the health team in development planning that affects the health of people and delivery of health services. A midwife's task in the team must take in more than caring for individual women if maternal mortality is to be reduced. The midwife needs to be politically and socially aware and able and confident to interact in any sphere where decisions are taken about the welfare of women.

The recently established emphasis of WHO on strengthening district health systems (DHS) in relation to PHC provides an essential mechanism for dealing with problems so far resistent to solutions such as maternal mortality.[15]

CONCRETE ACTIONS AS A START TO SOLUTIONS

The Midwives' Action

How far have midwives come since Nairobi? Within six months of the Safe Motherhood Conference in Nairobi in 1987 a collaborative precongress workshop of ICM, WHO, and UNICEF was held on the theme "Women's Health and the Midwife—a global perspective."[16] About forty midwives, mostly from developing countries, took a long, hard look at the midwives' role in maternal health—the existing situation and the probable future. The participants produced an action statement on the changes needed if midwives around the world were to be effective partners in the drive for a reduction of maternal morbidity and mortality by 50 percent in the year 2000. Implications for change were considered relative to education, the roles and functions of midwives, administration and management, and midwifery research.

Educational Change Midwifery education needs to be diversified and each country should not be guided in this process by any factor other than the national status of women's reproductive health. Midwives endorsed the concept of primary maternal health (as set out above) to be essential in their education.

Changes in Role and Functions of Midwives Reduction of maternal mortality where it is most serious can only be effected if the midwife is helped to be accountable for her own actions and assume the role of specialist when life-saving care is to be performed in the absence of any specialized medical staff. District and subdistrict levels are the most appropriate places for her to work in the developing world.

The management of obstetric first aid should be the responsibility of all trained midwives. Where no other services of a specialist nature are available, the midwife must be able to safely remove a placenta, skillfully give intravenous injections and set up IV infusions, initiate prophylatic antibiotic therapy for women in danger of sepsis, treat eclamptics, perform vacuum extractions, etc. This is really not new. These procedures are used, even by lesser trained health workers. Postpartum hemorrhage is the major cause of maternal mortality and the highest cause for referral from the community in many countries. In Bhutan, the health assistant, 18 months trained, walks 8 hours up into the mountains to remove a placenta to save a life. In Bangladesh, the midwife in a rural area, called in the middle of the night for an eclamptic primigravida, gives emergency resuscitative care, administers intravenous valium, sets up an intravenous infusion; only at the end of the night can the woman be carried to the nearest transport, which is a boat ambulance 1 hour's walk away from the village. In Malawi, midwives have been taught to perform vacuum extractions from inception of registered midwives training, and regulations to this effect cover their practice. What seemed to be an appropriate suggestion 10 years ago has now become a commitment for action by the midwifery and obstetric community. Social justice for maternal health requires the development of an effective maternity service which combines a firm grasp of the essentials with confident flexibility about their practical application.

Sequelae of obstructed labor result in wreckage and social disruption which are indescribably miserable. The use of the partograph as an early warning system for cephalopelvic disproportion is used in several countries in the remotest health centers or maternities with good success. A recent initiative in Ghana showed tremendous energy and enthusiasm of midwives to learn management of labor with this tool. This is probably one example where success depends on a team approach in maternity care where all members can demonstrate leadership skills.

A positive team approach will promote integration of essential obstetric functions without apportioning blame to those who tried but were ill-equipped to do so.

The midwife's role in helping families to ensure that each child is a wanted child implies that she must be able to prescribe, initiate, and monitor contraceptive activities that have been selected by the family as most appropriate to its situation.

Administrative and Managerial Changes Midwife managers must be developed, and all should be equipped to identify priorities and appraise the human resource situation and the distribution thereof in order to make proposals for a more equitable service.

Midwifery Research Each midwife should be able to collect, analyze, and interpret information at the level at which she functions. Basic epidemiology and statistics must be incorporated into education programs to monitor and evaluate their practice and make necesary changes. The Safe Motherhood Initiative has initiated teams of which midwives are members in operations research and will be a partner in authorship of subsequent publications of results. The Carnegie Corporation and the Center of Population and Health are partners with university teams in Ghana and Nigeria.

The Decentralized Education Program of Advanced Midwives (DEPAM)

A decentralized education program in midwifery and neonatal nursing science is described by Garde, in South Africa, as a development of the highly successful advanced diploma in midwifery and neonatal nursing science (ADM) which is based at the College of Nursing King Edward VIII Hospital, Durban.[17]

The new program will contain many of the features of a distance learning program. This new venture is envisaged as a decentralized, rather than a distance learning program because much of the educational experience is of a practical nature; the program will thus require facilitation by practitioners skilled in the art of midwifery and neonatal nursing science. The shift in emphasis is to a truly learner-oriented program in which the teachers will take on new responsibilities as facilitators and providers of liberating structures within which the student will gain sufficient self-confidence to become increasingly self-directed. The length of the course is 18 months but can be extended to 30. The course design will be problem based with the teaching designed to take place around a series of paper and practical problems. A series of paper problems based on real patients and covering the whole curriculum as defined in the ADM will be cosigned. Throughout the course advanced knowledge from the natural, biological, and social sciences as well as from the educational field will be acquired by the students in relation to cognitive, effective, and psychomotor skills in advanced midwifery and neonatal science.

The advanced diploma midwives will at the end of the course be able to administer midwifery and neonatal nursing services and participate in clinical teaching of these subjects at an advanced level and act as a clinical consultant. Midwives, doctors, and other members of the health care team will be involved in this program as facilitators of learning. They will maintain and enhance their own skills. The effectiveness of the course will be judged not only on whether students reach an acceptable level in a series of assessments but also by the graduate's effect on maternal and neonatal health markers through her training effect on the primary health care team and the community. This innovative education program is also advocated for medical training to prepare to face the risks and hardships of the isolated rural challenge.

Team Problem-Solving Approach

Remarkable results have been shown in reduction of maternal mortality through district team problem-solving efforts assisted by WHO in India, Malawi, and Malaysia.

What follows is a scenario of one style of management development with the potential to provide a variety of benefits to health service administrations. This approach is rooted in the premise that staff have considerable potential for self-development and service improvement if placed in the right circumstances. Frequently, senior program managers have to improve health service performance without being able to add substantially to the existing resources of staff and facilities. They must therefore call upon their staff at all levels to devise local solutions to many of the problems which inhibit the delivery of their services, both in coverage and quality. Maternal health and safe motherhood is a general area of concern which many governments are now turning to in their efforts to further develop the health services. Much improvement in health service management might be generated through team solutions, including improved supervision, strengthened and simplified recording and reporting, and improved patient referral procedures.

In one district in Malaysia deaths from postpartum hemorrhage accounted for 70 percent of all maternal deaths in 1985, and the overall maternal mortality was 320 per 100,000 live births. In its efforts to reduce maternal deaths particularly those from postpartum hemorrhage, an obstetric flying squad was instituted. At the time of evaluation 9 months later, there had been no deaths from this cause in nineteen cases, compared to seven of the ten maternal deaths in 1985.[18]

In Malawi, five multidisciplinary teams comprised of a total of five to eight doctors, midwives, nurses, medical assistants, and sanitarians each analyzed and developed a solution for an important problem currently being experienced in the delivery of maternal, child health, and family planning care.[19] One district team addressed maternal mortality from ruptured uterus. The lessons learned released a new conviction among health workers of the benefit of a maternity care team. The problem-solving approach was experienced as helpful for project formulaton and action health system research. The approach helped release the tremendous energy of community participation with information to reduce the dimension of the problem. Advocacy was so vibrant that safe motherhood became a theme for the university's theater for development.

The ICM/WHO Subregional Workshop in Ghana

The ICM/WHO subregional workshop on 'Enhancing National Midwifery Services' was hosted by the Ghana government and Ghana Midwives' Association. Five West African countries (Ghana, Liberia, Nigeria, Sierra Leone, and The Gambia) participated in teams of obstetricians/gynecologists, midwives, and health planners to draw up implementation plans for enhancing national midwifery services. The priority for the country-specific plan was extracted from the action statement formulated during the collaborative ICM/

WHO/UNICEF precongress workshop in the Netherlands in August 1987.[20] The process of the project formulation brought together various techniques and approaches for health service planning. Participants even used tools such as force field analysis and commitment planning. The follow-up so far shows very encouraging progress at country level after presentation to the national Ministry of Health. The Rockefeller Foundation sponsored this workshop and provided a fine example of cooperation between bilateral and nongovernmental agencies and national governments. A similar workshop for francophone West Africa is to take place in Burkino Faso in January 1990.

Other Efforts

In closing I would like to mention some examples of established maternity care teams which are truly inspiring.

In Lusaka, the urban maternity units have been organized into a properly functioning system. As a result deliveries in the Lusaka Teaching Hospital have been remarkably reduced. A nurse-midwife supervisor visits all clinics regularly, and the obstetrician overseeing all clinics provides constructive supervision and education. The partograph is in use, and the clinics have a radio system connecting them to an ambulance for emergency referrals to the teaching hospital.[21]

In the West Kiang district of The Gambia maternal mortality remained constant at about 2,000 per 100,000 births between 1951 and 1975. From 1974 onward, a physician and a midwife provided 24-hour emergency cover. No pregnancy-related deaths occurred between 1975 and 1983, even though sixteen would have been expected, estimated from the current maternal mortality in rural Gambia.[22]

In the Matlab Family Planning and Health Services Project (FPHSP) in Bangladesh, four registered nurse-midwives have been employed in two subcenters covering a popula-

tion of 25,000.[23] The midwives provide a 24-hour cover in shifts. They visit homes to provide prenatal care, delivery service, and family planning. If called upon they give support to the TBA. Such circumstances of work need more than commitment—they need courage. The midwives have to understand and cope with traditions that do not easily support maternity services or even a professional who is female.[24,25] These midwives are highly respected by their team. Field supervisors make regular visits, supplies are available, and the medical profession is concerned both for midwives' welfare and practice. Acceptance of the midwives is growing in the community. Management protocols for obstetric complications in the village are in use by the midwives. One year after the start of MCH strengthening with maternity care, results are impressive. While TBAs never called CHWs or family welfare visitors (FWV) during deliveries or when complications arose, 23 percent of the pregnant women in the area called the midwives during labor, and 58 percent had a postpartum visit—preliminary counts indicate a 40 percent reduction in maternal mortality in the area covered by the midwives.

Our conference offers us an opportunity to look back and to survey what lies ahead. While midwifery is in a crisis, the goal of safe motherhood is before us. The reduction of maternal mortality requires a vision interpreting our times and finding new solutions. We are at a threshold where on the one hand the output of midwives is worrying and on the other hand their services are needed more than ever. Saving midwifery would change the experience of childbirth for millions of women from misery to joy.

REFERENCES

1 Mahler, H. (1987). The Safe Motherhood Initiative: a call to action. *Lancet*: 668–70.
2 World Health Organization (1987). Maternal Health and Safe Motherhood. Resolution of the World Health Assembly, WHA 40.27.

3 World Health Organization (1985). Coverage of Maternity Care. Document FHE/85.1. WHO, Geneva.

4 Kwast, B.E. (1979). The role and training of midwives for rural areas. In Maternity Services in the Developing World—What the Community Needs. Proceedings of the Seventh Study Group of the Royal College of Obstetricians and Gynaecologists, Ed. R. Hugh Philpott.

5 World Health Organization (1988). World health statistics annual. Geneva.

6 Bentley, J. (1987). Maternal mortality and morbidity—a midwifery challenge. Paper presented at the ICM/WHO/UNICEF Pre-Congress Workshop; Women's Health and the Midwife—A Global Perspective. Document MCH/PCW/87.5 Rev 1. WHO, Geneva.

7 World Health Organization (1986). Essential Obstetric Functions at First Referral level. Document FHE/86.4 WHO, Geneva.

8 Farnot Cardoso, U. (1986). Giving birth is safer now. *World Health Forum* (7), 348.

9 Kwast, B.E. (1989) Maternal mortality: Levels, causes and promising interventions. *J. Biosoc. Sci.,* Suppl. 10, 51–67.

10 Maternity care in the world. 1966 International Survey of Midwifery Practice and Training. International Federation of Gynaecology and Obstetrics and the International Confederation of Midwives. Oxford; New York, Pergamon.

11 Mwale, T. (1985). The role of the nurse/midwife in Primary Health Care. *Medical Quarterly. Journal of the Medical Association of Malawi,* 2 (2), 48–49.

12 Reedy Johnson, C. (1986). An outline for team building. Training. BNA Communications Inc. Rockville, MD 20850.

13 Morewane, D.V. (1989), personal communication.

14 Harman, P. (1989). The changing role of nursing management in relation to primary health care. Book of Abstracts, ICN, 19th Quadrennial Seoul Congress, Seoul, Korea.

15 World Health Organization (1988). From Alma-Ata to the year 2000. Reflections at the midpoint. Geneva.

16 World Health Organization, (1987). Women's Health and the Midwife—A Global Perspective. Document WHO/MCH/87.5. WHO, Geneva.

17 Garde, P.M. (1989). Aspects of the Decentralized Education Programme of Advanced Midwives (DEPAM). Westville, South Africa.

18 World Health Organization (1987). Economic Support for National Health for All Strategies. Fortieth World Health Assembly, Background Document A40/Technical Discussions/2, Geneva.

19 World Health Organization (1988). District Team Problem-Solving. Report of a workshop. Liwongwe, Malawi October 21–30, 1987. Document FHE/87.8. Geneva.

20 Hornby, P. (1989). Enhancing National Midwifery Services. Report of an ICM/WHO West-African Sub-Regional Workshop. International Confederation of Midwives, London.

21 Tyndal, M. (1988), personal communication.

22 Lamb, W.H., Lamb, C.M.B., Foord, F.A., & Whitehead, P.G. (1984). Changes in maternal and child mortality rates in three isolated Gambian villages over ten years. *Lancet,* iii, 912.

23 Faveau, V., Koenig, M.A., Chakraborty J., & Chowdhury, A.I. (1988). Causes of maternal mortality in rural Bangladesh (1976–1985). *Bulletin of the World Health Organization,* 66 (5) 643–652.

24 Ajma Begum (1988), personal communication.

25 Faveau, V. (1988), personal communication.

Chapter 13

The Challenges of the Practice of Nursing in Latin America

Esperanza de Monterrossa
Ilta Lange
Roseni Rosangela Chompré

The practice of nursing may be defined as a set of actions carried out by different levels of nursing personnel directed toward promotion of health, prevention of illness, recovery from disease, and rehabilitation. In the majority of Latin American countries, the labor force in nursing, predominantly female, constitutes the largest contingent of health workers. In Brazil, for example, 51 percent of the health labor force are nursing personnel (Conselho Federal de Enfermagem, 1985).

Although nurses comprise a high percentage of health workers, the quality of their education has not been given equitable attention. This may be the reason for the heterogeneity in composition and preparation of the nursing labor force.

The rapid spread of health services that began in the sixties, especially the extension of services into rural areas, forced many countries, by political directive, to hire a great number of people without specific training to perform nursing tasks. In some countries, therefore, illiterate nursing personnel are carrying out the less complex nursing activities such as transport of patients and physical comfort measures. Because of the lack of available positions for better qualified personnel, these workers have assumed ever-increasing responsibility for nursing care.

Political directives have had strong repercussions on nursing practice, especially on the internal organization of nursing's work and relationships with others in the health sector. Perhaps the most important repercussion has been the composition of the nursing labor force, whose workers have education ranging from incomplete elementary schooling to university graduation.

The different groups of health workers carry out nursing care through complementary actions on different levels of complexity. In Latin American countries, no clear relationship exists between the complexity of the nursing action and the degree of preparation of the nursing personnel who perform the action. In the majority of these countries, the practice of nursing is primarily exercised by nursing assistants (or helpers) and nurses' aides.

Nursing assistants or helpers are trained in a process of "learning by doing." They have very low basic education, and many are illiterate. Various nations have policies demonstrating concern for this situation, and some are attempting to train these helpers or at least not to hire new ones with such low educational preparation.

In 1983, in Brazil, according to the data of the Conselho Federal de Enfermagem (1985), nursing helpers constituted 63.8 percent of the labor force in nursing. In Colombia, nursing assistants represent 29 percent of the nursing personnel; in Chile nursing assistants are 20.8 percent of nursing personnel but perform only minor nursing activities such as transport of patients, cleaning of patient units, and transport of laboratory samples, because of strict regulations of the Ministry of Health (Ministerio de Salud de Chile, 1989).

Nurses' aides, in contrast with the helpers,

have a general education of at least 2 years of high school and 1 year of specific technical training. In the great majority of countries, schools for the preparation of nurses' aides are under the supervision of the Ministry of Health. Typically, nurses' aides constitute the largest percentage of the nursing labor force. In Chile they comprise 69.7 percent of the nursing force, in Colombia, 57.7 percent; however, the figure in Brazil is only 32.2 percent.

Nurses' aides perform, in the absence of a nurse, all nursing care activities including administration of parenteral medication, arterial punctures, immediate postoperative assistance, as well as coronary and intensive care nursing. They have a key role in community work, taking active part in decisions that affect the health of the population. They are in charge of administering rural health posts, giving direct patient care, and referring patients to other health services when necessary.

In contrast to helpers and aides, nurses are prepared at the university in programs varying from 3 to 5 years. In some countries, 3-year programs prepare nurse technicians who act as nurses. In Latin America, there is a scarcity of both nurses and nursing positions in all levels of care (primary, secondary, and tertiary). The deficit is most notorious at the primary level of care.

Because of this situation, nurses often give priority to bureaucratic and administrative responsibilities, including the training and supervision of auxiliary personnel; they delegate most direct patient care to the nurses' aides (Chile and Colombia) or nursing helpers (Brazil).

At present there is a tendency to increase the presence of nurses in community health services. Nurses also work in hospitals and outpatient clinics, in public as well as private sectors. The private practice of nursing is not widespread, but several groups own placement agencies. In these agencies, nurses prepare nursing helpers to take care of newborns

A version of this chapter appeared as "Nursing in the 21st Century in Latin America: Part II—Nursing Practice," in *International Nursing Review*, vol. 37, no. 3, 1990, pp. 274–279.

and elderly people in homes and institutions. They hire nurses' aides to give care in homes and to act as private aides for specific patients in hospitals. They also hire nurses as supervisors for home care aides and to provide direct patient care when necessary.

The highest percentage of nursing personnel are not involved in these placement agencies but work in hospitals. The expansion of health services has increased the number of available positions in these acute care institutions.

The primary level of health care is still not considered important, and this situation is reflected in the practice of nursing. Traditionally, control of the working process has been in the hands of physicians, a hegemonious professional group. It is urgent that functions of the nurse be broadened to offer health care to the entire population. The educational system and health services still reflect a practice model centered on the curative process, but nurses are demonstrating greater awareness of and motivation to assume health promotion and disease prevention.

In general, nurses do not work at their maximum potential (clinical, educative, administrative, research) due to legal, administrative, educational, and social restrictions (OMS, 1986). There is incongruency in many countries between the capacity the nurses have to contribute to the goal of "Health for All," especially through primary health care strategies, and the functions and activities they practice.

The range of activities that nurses are permitted to carry out vary from country to country and depend on the presence or absence of physicians in the places where they work. In the more remote regions with no doctors, nurses make diagnoses, indicate treatment, and perform minor surgery. In the absence of a physician and nurse, these actions are executed by the nurses' aide.

In Latin American countries there is no clear differentiation between roles of nurses and auxiliary personnel. In hospitals different situations exist:

• *No nurses in the hospital.* The physician or an allied health professional is responsible for patient care; occasionally a lay person has the responsibility.

• *Only one nurse is employed, and she does administrative tasks.* Direct patient care is carried out by nursing helpers or nurses' aides.

• *Nurses present only during the day.* When present the nurse carries out administrative activities and some of the more complex nursing procedures; at night these activities are delegated to auxiliary personnel.

• *Nurses present 24 hours a day, 7 days a week.* This situation exists mostly in university or public hospitals and in large private hospitals. The nurse exercises clinical, administrative, and educational roles, and functions of nurses and helpers and aides are clearly differentiated.

PROBLEMS ARISING IN PRACTICE

Nursing practice differs greatly among Latin American countries. The degree of development of nursing practice generally is related to and determined by the economic, political, and social conditions of each country. Major differences include the composition of the nursing labor force, the social status of the profession, the capacity of the various groups of nursing personnel to organize, and the educational level of all classes of workers.

In spite of these differences, nurses in Latin America share common problems which will be the focal points of practice for the next century. Among them are the following:

• *The inadequacy of professional practice.* "When the various documents of the international and national health organizations are reviewed, from the past decade to present times, a very important role is assigned to the nurse within the Health Services. There has also been great discussion about her new role.

However, when we observe the reality of the practice of nursing in Latin America, we find that there is a great distance between the theoretical declarations and the objective reality: the greatest market for work is still the hospital with the consequent urban concentration of human resources and with traditional role models'' (Carrillo, 1985). In essence nurses scarcely participate at primary levels of care.

• *Lack of professional identity.* Nurses have little autonomy in the exercise of their profession as a result of the concentration of power in the medical profession. However, nurses are beginning to understand that their work constitutes an important element for necessary teamwork in health and that their identity should be the result of the uniqueness of their role and their competence in health care.

• *Lack of recognition of nursing practice as essential in the health institutions.* The lack of recognition is expressed in limited opportunities for professional promotion, low salaries, long work schedules, and a lack of participation in decision making. No regulations support the development of leaders in nursing. This situation is reflected in a lack of new initiatives, interference with the professional role, and deterioration of nursing practice due to limited opportunities to keep updated through advanced study.

• *Lack of critical analysis of health care delivery systems on the part of nurses.* Nurses do not assume an active role in searching for models of nursing practice that better respond to the health needs of populations.

• *Nursing as a predominantly female profession.* Women's positions in nursing reflect the social problems of the Latin American woman, including discrimination on social and work levels, low salaries, lack of opportunities for professional preparation, excessive demands for home responsibilities not shared with the husband, and responsibility for biological reproduction without sufficient social support.

• *Imbalance between nurse-to-nurses'-aide ratio and the nurse-physician-to-population ratio.* In most Latin American countries the labor force in health is concentrated in the hands of physicians, nurses' aides, and nursing helpers. There is inadequate geographical distribution of human resources in health according to health personnel and levels of care. The ratio of auxiliary personnel, nurses, and physicians to population strongly compromises the quality of health care. Health policies bear little relationship to existing conditions.

• *Poor working conditions.* Working conditions are influenced by the inadequate physical structures of the health services, often older facilities which have been adapted to service health care. These physical structures don't fulfill the minimal comfort and maintenance requirements for health services delivery. Many buildings have inadequate control of air temperature; they lack rest rooms; and they have no coffee shops or sitting areas for personnel or clients. There is little protection of personnel health for those working in the institutions, a critical situation with the increase of patients infected with HIV.

• *Deficiencies in services, equipment, and materials.* These deficiencies are obvious at all levels of care both in quantitative and the qualitative aspects, influencing directly the quality of health care and the job satisfaction of the nursing personnel. These deficiencies also constitute a risk for both the patient and personnel and are recognized as the most important source of stress among nursing personnel according to a study carried out in Chile by Ramirez et al. (1987).

• *Low salaries.* In the majority of Latin American countries, nurses (except for faculty in the public sector) receive lower salaries than other professionals in the health sector with similar academic preparation and similar work hours. The power distribution has encouraged distinctions and privileges regarding income and professional prestige favoring certain hegemonic professions to the detriment of others with less power to negotiate and defend their rights (Conselho Federal de Enfermagen, 1985). Salaries of nursing personnel are so low that they are forced to work double shifts to satisfy basic needs of their families.

• *Inaccessibility to continuing education programs and difficulty achieving teaching/ service integration at the operative level.* In most health services, no professional development policy integrates continuing education. This creates a distance between nurse educators and clinical nurses. Although teachers have greater access to bibliographical information that may facilitate self-learning, they have not contributed significantly to development of in-service education models to update nursing personnel.

The problems identified here affect nursing competency as well as the quality of health care. In a report of the Federal Council of Nursing of Brazil (Conselho Federal de Enfermagen, 1985), Klegon observes that the social influence of a profession creates internal and external dynamics. The internal dynamics concern how the work is carried out by the professionals; the external dynamic has to do with prevalent conditions in the social structure which enhance or undermine the social significance of the profession. In spite of all the problems, nursing in Latin America is valued by the health institutions mainly because it represents more than 50 percent of the health sector labor force.

From the perspective of nursing personnel, their ability to contribute to the recovery of patients, the quality of communication between nurse and patient, especially with the socially deprived, and the opportunity for team work are reasons for job satisfaction. All these satisfiers are inherent in the nature of nursing practice. This helps us understand the strength that nursing has retained and the satisfaction one gets from the capacity for self-development and the opportunity to overcome external obstacles.

PERSPECTIVES ON NURSING PRACTICE FOR THE TWENTY-FIRST CENTURY

The present conditions in Latin American countries require that governments take a stand with respect to social policies. Within this context, the health sector should respond to the needs and demands of the population with innovative policies and models that will help increase the capacity to offer all services to the population with high efficiency and quality.

As a social profession, nursing should work to overcome the difficulties that have accumulated over time. Nursing needs a new participative attitude; it needs to collaborate in the construction of new models for health care delivery.

Garzon (1987) points out that a profession requires a specific body of knowledge and abilities, a system of values, beliefs and attitudes. All these characteristics are acquired through academic preparation, professional socialization, and work and life experiences. According to the author, the practice of professional nursing includes the following elements:

• A definition of the scope of the professional practice and its relation to other professions and occupations
• Academic preparation and training
• Legislation and regulation of professional practice
• Research for progress in scientific and technological knowledge and the formulation of its conceptual and theoretical framework
• Professional code of ethics
• Permanent professional development
• Authority and power for self-regulation and self-direction
• Communication, relationships with the community, other professionals, technicians, and aides who work in the health field
• A correct image of the nature of its services
• Professional organization

Within this conception of professional practice, the International Council of Nursing has defined the following objectives: to develop nursing leadership for primary health care; to work on nursing regulations in each country; to establish standards to guide nursing practice, education, and research.

The challenge for nursing in the next century is to adopt the perspective that all people have the right to live in dignified economic, social, and healthful conditions.

The nursing role should be extended in the traditional health institutions (e.g., hospitals, convalescent homes, outpatient clinics) and in other settings (e.g., schools, industries, work places in general, and private homes). The practice of nursing for the next century should contribute to controlling the ecosystems, to correcting the work processes insofar as they cause health risks to the workers, to preventing problems that are inherent in the populations' aging process, and to developing care models to serve large populations.

The practice of nursing should be conceived of as an integral part of the work organization in health, contributing to scientific and technological advancements. Nursing practice should be based on the current concept of the health-disease continuum, giving strong emphasis to the primary health care strategy, to the self-care concept, and to health promotion and disease prevention at the individual, family, and community levels. The success of a new model for practice in health will be based on its capacity to promote inter- and intra-disciplinary relationships, taking into account the health needs and demands of the population.

Nursing should participate in the determination of policies for the Health Services, taking into account the most urgent problems of the population and formulating control measures for present and future health risks such as those related to AIDS, nuclear contamination, and environmental pollution. Nursing support for decisions in the Health Services that address the high costs of health delivery, the need for timely access for the population to Health Services, and the need to assure availability of comprehensive health care of good quality and free of risks.

The health team should have a new composition. The training of all persons in the health sector who do not already have specific work preparation is essential. The first priority is the training of nursing helpers in those countries where helpers act as nurses' aides or even as nurses. This level of nursing personnel needs to have higher basic schooling as well as to receive specific technical education which would permit a career promotion to higher nursing categories (nurses' aides and nurses). With strategies of this type and with the broadening of the nurses' role, the number of nurses could be increased for the next century. Thus, quantity and quality of the nursing team would be improved simultaneously.

The preparation and administration of human resources in nursing should be addressed. Deficiencies in the present preparation of nursing personnel have to be considered when defining strategies for the improvement of nursing practice to respond to the health needs of the next century. Simultaneously with the design of a model for practice, a new model for the preparation of nursing personnel must be developed which incorporates the health needs of the populations and considers:

• A new curriculum based on the social concept of health, using a problem-focused, teaching-service integration strategy
• The various characteristics of the students of the next century, who must be active, creative agents, with capacity for criticism, social commitment, a high degree of independence and self-sufficiency, and with greater experience in the use of technological resources
• The need for continuing education programs for nurse educators seeking clinical and epidemiological competence and social commitment
• The selection of teachers according to criteria which guarantee their commitment to the

changes required for a new model of practice and education

• The development of graduate programs at master's and doctoral levels to prepare leaders willing to assume the process of change

• The establishment of continuing education programs incorporating educational technologies that permit large-scale training of nursing personnel in the health services

• The evaluation of teachers, through application of objective criteria, permitting detection of persons whose performance is inadequate and whose atittudes do not favor change

The development of science and technology should be fostered. For the next century, nursing must participate in technological progress, incorporating and developing technology adequate to a new model for practice that contains a component of systematized evaluation.

Nursing will use research as a tool to better understand and explain the situations which are pressing the profession and also to find solutions to health care problems. According to Meleis (1988), significant and useful research should aim at improving nursing care in the entire world and at increasing nursing knowledge, giving credibility to the nurse and to her patients.

One nursing research track should investigate how to help people to take care of themselves, how to increase their sense of well-being, how to help them achieve greater independence and responsibility for themselves. Other areas of research suggested by Meleis are the adequate distribution of human resources to provide quality health care; the reduction of risks; beliefs, attitudes and behavior which foster health promotion and health self-care; concepts of health and disease in different ethnic groups and cultures; studies on community mobilization and participation; and interdisciplinary coordination.

To improve the quality and quantity of nursing research and to respond to the demands of the next century, the Latin American nurse should establish strategies for collaboration in research with her peers and with other disciplines.

Nurses should participate in the regulation of practice, formulating policies that permit them:

• To practice the extended roles foreseen for the coming decades

• To preserve their integrity and their specific professional role within the multiprofessional work in health

• To ensure an adequate preparation of the different categories of nursing personnel according to the complexity of the activities they are supposed to perform

• To establish relationships with other sectors of the society

According to Styles (1985), the scope of nursing practice as defined by law is usually more restrained than the capacity of nurses and the needs for services that the public has. Regulations should be established for nursing practice in each country to ensure that nursing personnel have the necessary qualifications for work. It will also be necessary to establish regulations regarding disciplinary measures within nursing practice.

Apart from specific nursing regulations, general regulations for health personnel will also affect nursing; for example, norms must be established to ensure safety and minimal comfort on the work site.

The progress that can be achieved in nursing practice will depend to a great extent on the organizational capacity of nurses. Improvement and strengthening of the national nursing associations will increase the participation of nurses in government organizations, principally in the health and education sector in the different countries in the region.

Nursing should also prepare for a conscious participation in social movements and in organizations that propose the transformation of health and education services. This participation will include a review of the role of women in society.

Meleis (1988) points out that the images for the future include:

• Universal, international collaboration, with an overall perspective but culturally adapted
• Regulated practice which prevents others from invading nursing's professional domain yet avoids confusing others concerning what nursing is and what it is not
• Nurses with the power to control their own practice and with the commitment to construct health care models which bring a maximum of well-being to large populations

Finally, the nurse for the next century should have a strong commitment to the construction of peace in Latin American countries and in the entire world.

THE W. K. KELLOGG FOUNDATION AND THE DEVELOPMENT OF NEW MODELS IN NURSING PRACTICE

Nursing in the twenty-first century has been considered in many of the programs, projects, and institutional activities in which Latin American nurses are currently participating. The W. K. Kellogg Foundation has given much support to institutions and to groups of Latin American nurses for the development of innovative models for education and practice of nursing. These projects have strengthened nursing leadership development in Latin America, invigorated institutional development of nursing schools, and broadened the professional role of the nurse.

In 1975, the Pan-American Health Organization (PAHO), in an agreement with the W. K. Kellogg Foundation, created the Latin American Center for Educational Technology for Health (CLATES), with headquarters in the Federal University of Rio de Janeiro, Bra-

zil. One goal of this center according to Carillo (1989) is "to contribute to the improvement of nursing personnel, the preparation of faculty, curriculum development and the design of instructional materials." These achievements are based on the teaching-service integration strategy and seeking nursing participation in primary health care.

Among the strategies for fulfilling these goals, CLATES proposed to support 15 to 20 centers for educational technology in nursing schools in different countries of the region. Only 8 were established, however, located in the following countries: Mexico (Monterrey), Costa Rica (San José), Colombia (Cali), Ecuador (Quito), Peru (Lima), Chile (Santiago), and Brazil (Belo Horizonte and Salvador).

These local technology centers in collaboration with CLATES prepared a great number of Latin American nurses through courses, seminars, and encounters, placing great emphasis on the participation of nursing in primary health care.

The work carried out by the local technology centers in their headquarters (schools of nursing) has stimulated nurse educators and clinical nurses to assume active roles in primary health care programs. The work also initiated discussions in the nursing schools about curricular changes needed to prepare students to act in primary health care.

Several nursing schools have initiated community-based, teaching-service integration programs, a first step in creating practice models based on the primary health care concept.

The following projects are supported by the W. K. Kellogg Foundation:

• The Project for Comprehensive Health Care at the Federal University of Ceara, Brazil, where a health care model was implemented to serve women during pregnancy, delivery, and immediately after childbirth. Appropriate technology was developed, and the knowledge and experience of lay midwives was incorporated into health care delivery for rural and marginal urban areas. This project was a great success in the recovery of cultural values for the served population, and it established a model for childbirth in the home and in "delivery houses" using appropriate technology.

• Project to Improve Life Conditions of the Peasant, University of Guanajuato, Mexico. This project established a nursing practice model for primary health care in close articulation with the area of agriculture. Work was done with underserved rural populations, offering comprehensive care to achieve adequate growth and development of the children and to assist pregnant women. This project included education, sanitation, housing, and help in the organization of women. The school for nursing of Irapuato, University of Guanajuato, had the leadership role in this project, and the model for practice has been incorporated into the nursing plan of studies. At the present time several nursing schools of the university participate in an interdisciplinary project which includes participation of schools of engineering, nutrition and agriculture among others.

• The Transectorial Program for Community Action at the Federal University of Minas Gerais, Brazil, is a multidisciplinary project with the participation of the schools of medicine, dentistry, psychology, and nursing. The project carries out activities in the marginal areas of the capital of the state of Minas Gerais and in rural areas. Nursing assumes a leadership role in developing the primary health care model targeted to children, pregnant women, and adults. The effective participation of nurse educators, students, and clinical nurses establishes a practice model which is being incorporated into the health services as well as into the curriculum.

• The Health Self-Care Education Project of the Catholic University, Santiago, Chile, is a project which developed a nursing practice model that incorporates education for self-care as a permanent component of health care delivery (Lange 1986). This model has been extended into a multidisciplinary health care model which has been recognized by the Ministry of Health of Chile as useful to improve the quality of care in the primary health care services of the country. To achieve adequate implementation of this model at the national level, the Ministry of Health has included health self-care education in the continuing education priorities of the health personnel who work at the primary care level. This model has also influenced nursing education and has been incorporated into the curriculum of the school of nursing of this university.

• The Comprehensive Mother-Child Care for Community Development in Bogota, Colombia, is an interdisciplinary project with emphasis on mother-child care. It has been carried out since June 1989 in a marginal community in the southeast section of Bogota. The purpose of this project is to develop three models: one for health care, another for management, and a third for education, all of which will hopefully promote changes in the quality of health care, in the expansion of the role of nursing, and in the preparation of health personnel. The project requires inter-institutional work, self-management by the communities, implementation and development of a system of reference and counter-reference, and the incorporation of the self-care concept as a fundamental tool in primary health care.

Currently a new social order is developing in Latin America. In the new order civil institutions are strengthened and the role of the state is being redefined. In this context, health stands out as one of the emerging social priorities, and in this context the time is right for nursing to improve its contribution to the health of Latin America and to upgrade its practice.

REFERENCES

Carillo, G. (1989). *Formación de Recursos Humanos para la Atención Primaria*. Paper presented at II Seminario de la Red Chilena de Proyectos Kellogg. Santiago, Chile.

Concelho Federal de Enfermagem. Associacao Brasileira en Enfermagem. *Exercicio de Enfermagem Nas Institucoes de Saúde do Brasil 1982–1983*. Vol. 1 (1985), Vol. 2 (1986).

Garzon, N. (1987). Ejercicio Profesional de la Enfermera. *Enfermeria*. XXII (90/91): 11–15.

Lange, I. (1986). *Impacto de Programas Educativos en el Autocuidado de Pacientes Ambulatorios*. Informe Final. EPAS 3(2) 6–18.

Meleis, A. (1988). *Nursing Research: A Need or a Luxury*. Paper presented at Global Nursing Conference, Galveston, Texas.

Ministerio de Salud de Chile. Depto. de Recursos Humanos. (1989). *Tendencias del Personal de Salud para el siglo XXI*, Santiago, Chile. (Internal Document).

OMS. (1986). *Mecauismos de Reglamentación de la Enseñanza y la Práctica de Enfermeria; Satisfacción de las necesidades de Atención Primaria de Salud*. Serie de Informes Técnicos 738. WHO, Geneva, Switzerland.

Ramirez, M. et al. (1987). *Problemática Profesional y Personal de las Profesionales de Enfermeriá* Enfermeria XXI (88–89): 8–13.

Styles, M. (1985). *La Reglamentación de Enfermeria*. International Council of Nurses, Geneva, Switzerland.

Chapter 14

Challenges to Practice: Midwifery

Margaret Brain

" . . . Midwifery is a profession different from but complementary to nursing. The role of the midwife can be said to be substantially different from that of the nurse in that a midwife potentially has a greater professional independence as the level of decision-making is of a different order. The midwife is expected to have diagnostic skills relating to both mother and baby that are at one level similar to the obstetrician, and indeed that there is an overlap of skills between the two." This statement is found in the report "Project 2000—A New Preparation for Practice" published in 1986 by the United Kingdom Central Council for Nursing, Midwifery and Health Visiting (UKCC).[1] This is the statutory body set up in the United Kingdom to establish and improve standards of training and professional conduct for nurses, midwives, and health visitors.[2]

Midwifery throughout the world is one of the oldest professions. Early references are to be found in the first two books of the Holy Bible describing events which are said to have taken place in the second millenium B.C. Childbirth has been universally regarded as a female mystery in which women have special knowledge and understanding. It has a history independent from medicine and from nursing. In English the word *midwife* means "with woman," and from earliest times women have helped women at the time of childbirth.

It was not until the early seventies that an international definition of a midwife was agreed. This was accepted by the World

Health Organization (WHO), the International Federation of Gynaecology and Obstetrics (FIGO) and by the International Confederation of Midwives (ICM). The definition continues to be widely used in legislation and by professional organizations throughout the world today:

> A midwife is a person who, having been regularly admitted to a midwifery educational programme, duly recognised in the country in which it is located, has successfully completed the prescribed course of studies in midwifery and has acquired the requisite qualifications to be registered and/or legally licensed to practise midwifery.
>
> She must be able to give the necessary supervision, care and advice to women during pregnancy, labour and the post-partum period, to conduct deliveries on her own responsibility and to care for the newborn and the infant. This care includes preventative measures, the detection of abnormal conditions in mother and child, the procurement of medical assistance and the execution of emergency measures in the absence of medical help. She has an important task in health counselling and education, not only for the patients, but also within the family and the community. The work should involve antenatal education and preparation for parenthood and extends to certain areas of gynaecology, family planning and child care. She may practise in hospitals, clinics, health units, domiciliary conditions or in any other service.

LEGISLATION IN THE UNITED KINGDOM

Legislation regarding the practice of midwifery was first found in Europe in the Middle Ages. In 1881 the Midwives Institute was founded in London by a group of far-seeing women. The Institute was to become the Royal College of Midwives that we know today. Those early pioneers believed the answer to the appalling conditions surrounding childbirth and the high maternal and infant mortality rates lay in proper training for midwives and their control by legislation.[3] Years of professional rivalry were to follow—between midwives and doctors, between midwives and nurses, and between supportive midwives and others. Many abortive bills came before Parliament, and it was not until 1902 that the Midwives Act was passed. DeVries, in his book *Regulating Birth,* differentiates between legislation which is "hostile" and that which is "friendly."[4] Hostile legislation is one where the profession is controlled by another profession and friendly legislation is where the governing body set up is formed within the profession or occupation. He describes legislation in three states in the United States.

The 1902 Midwives Act could in this sense be described as hostile legislation. It set up the Central Midwives Board (CMB) which was formed of sixteen doctors and as a great concession of one midwife representing the Midwives Institute. The CMB along with the General Nurses Council were abolished with the setting up of the UKCC by the 1979 Act referred to earlier. Current legislation requires the UKCC, on which sits a majority of nurses, to refer all matters relating to midwifery to its statutory Midwifery Committee on which there are mainly midwives. The Act states "the Secretary of State shall not approve rules relating to midwifery practice unless satisfied that they are framed in accordance with recommendations of the Council's Midwifery Committee." However, the government recently commissioned a review of the roles, function, and organization of the UKCC and the four national bodies for England, Wales, Scotland, and Northern Ireland. The report was published in August 1989 and is now out for consultation.[5] Implementation of the recommendations would have far-reaching effects on nursing and midwifery. The question of whether combined legislation is good or bad for midwives and midwifery will again be raised. In the world today legislation relating to midwifery may stand alone, may be incorporated with medical or nursing legislation, or may be part of comprehensive legislation covering all health care professionals. In some countries midwifery has ceased to be a separate profession and is seen as a branch of nursing. Some countries or states are in the process of drawing up legislation such as in Ontario, Canada, to introduce midwifery into their health care system. Their legislation will cover all health care professionals including midwives; midwifery will have its own governing body which in due course will be "friendly." The occupation of midwifery includes, in some places, more than one category. In addition to the qualified (registered) midwives there may be lay or empirical midwives who may or may not be required to hold a license. Even where licenses are issued, not all such midwives choose to obtain one. This is not the complete picture. Still large numbers of women go through pregnancy and labor with no care by trained personnel. Latest estimates show that only 58 percent of the births in the world are attended by trained personnel. This means that in 1985 56 million babies were delivered with the help of untrained traditional birth attendants, family members, or by the mother alone.[6]

In this context trained personnel includes physicians, nurses, midwives, trained primary health care and other workers, and trained traditional birth attendants. These worldwide figures hide the real problem. In the developed world nearly all births are attended by trained personnel, but the coverage in the developing world varies enormously. Some of the world's lowest rates are found in South Asia and parts of Africa, where the rates may be under 10 percent and even as low as 2 percent (Somalia). WHO estimates that half a million mothers die in childbirth each year—99 percent occurring in developing countries. Women in developing countries run a risk of dying in pregnancy or childbirth which is 50 to 100 times greater than that of women in the developed world.[7]

European Economic Committee

With the signing of the Treaty of Rome in 1970 creating the EEC a further dimension in midwifery legislation was introduced. The Treaty gave freedom of movement to workers within the member countries and so the task of reconciling the training and practice of individual professions began.

In 1980 the Midwives' Directives were signed to become binding on the nine member states by January 1983.[8] This gave time for the individual countries to carry out the necessary adjustments to their own training programs. The Directives also covered the setting up of an Advisory Committee on the training of midwives "to help ensure throughout the Community a comparably high standard of training of midwives." The EEC Advisory Committee is composed of three "experts" from each member state—one each from practice, education, and the competent authority. From the twelve countries the United Kingdom is the only one whose whole delegation is composed of midwives. In others teaching may be represented by obstetricians and the competent authority by a solicitor, administrator, or civil servant.

These Directives are also binding on all new countries joining the EEC. One of the most recent countries to join is Spain. They are having special problems at the moment because their government did not negotiate a time lapse for implementation. As a result all midwifery training has been suspended, and no new students can enter training. It is likely to be another 2 years before the problem is resolved.

Legislation a Help or a Hindrance?

Legislations brings with it rules and regulations about who can practice and about the scope of that practice. It is usually designed to protect the public and as such must be acknowledged as a help. But legislation may also be designed to protect the interests of other professional groups. Midwives can be, and indeed are, sometimes seen as a threat to the livelihood of doctors.

Legislation brings respectability and status and the potential to set standards. It prevents anyone setting up in practice without the appropriate training. However, DeVries suggests that those who continue to practice outside the law in the United States have a very strong commitment to their work and to their clients. Legislation can cause the occupation to become another legitimate career opportunity, and the numbers practicing then increase. Many take up the new profession to earn a living.

Some will find practicing within National Health Services restricting and will opt for independent practice. A small number of independent midwives practice in the United Kingdom today. In March 1989, 32,739 midwives had notified their intention to practice of whom only 31 were in independent practice. Legislation in the United Kingdom, as far as midwives are concerned, is enabling and not restricting. The Code of Practice which complements the legislation states "each midwife as a practitioner of midwifery is accountable for practice in whatever environment she practices."[9] The Code goes on to spell out the individual midwife's responsibility for acquiring competence in new skills when her practice so requires.

However, midwives themselves sometimes use legislation as a reason, or maybe an excuse, for not doing certain things. They use it as a constraint on their practice. "The law does not allow me to suture," "am I covered if I put on scalp electrodes?" etc. These queries show a lack of understanding of the legislation. Each midwife should have in her possession a copy of the Rules[10] and the Code.

In some places legislation is restrictive. For example, in the Phillipines midwives are finding it increasingly difficult to practice when the law forbids them to give any intramuscular injections. Today the use of oxytocic drugs by injection for the treatment of post-partum hemorrhage is widely accepted.

The Way Forward

Legislation that is archaic and no longer appropriate for the delivery of modern health care must be revised and updated. Leaders in midwifery need to be involved at policy and decision-making levels and need to be educated to enable them to function at national and state (provincial) level. They need to be involved in task forces, committees, and working parties looking at any aspect of maternity care. The understanding of the management of change is vital for all leaders.

The management of health care in the United Kingdom has undergone a profound change since the introduction of general management principles. The converse of this introduction has been the widespread obliteration of functional management. The professional leading and managing his or her profession is a gradually disappearing being. The change from chief nursing officer to chief nurse advisor has resulted in ill-defined roles and little ability for decision making. Midwifery services throughout the United Kingdom have additionally seen the post of head of service pushed further down the hierarchical structure to a point where she or he often has little authority to negotiate with the twin powers of doctors and managers. In most cases this down-grading has been accompanied by lower salary levels.

Although the short-term problem presented by this has been the alteration in local "power" relationships there is a long term effect that can extend well beyond the United Kingdom and other developed countries. For a profession to attract those with the potential to lead and to push innovation, it must offer positions of real authority matched with appropriate remuneration. If these posts are not available, gradually the dynamic entrant, with potential for development toward leadership, will opt for other professions. This will not only be of disadvantage in the country concerned.

The Royal College of Midwives is currently giving aid in the form of leadership and expertise to developing countries anxious to improve professional education and thus professional standards. This must be a role for professionals from the developed world, and at present we have the midwives with skills to meet this challenge. But will we have it in the future if all leadership potential is suppressed or only allowed to flourish at local level?

CHANGING DEMANDS OF WOMEN, NEW HOSPITAL RULES AND REGULATIONS, AND MEDICAL STAFF PROBLEMS

The last 20 years or so saw great changes in the way birth is regarded and conducted in most parts of the Western world. The place of delivery changed so that the vast majority of deliveries take place in hospitals. Pregnancy and childbirth have become medical conditions, and the use of ever-increasing technology and intervention has became the norm. Pregnancy was seen as pathological until proved otherwise, that is, after the event. Once the place for prenatal care and for delivery was changed from the home to the hospital, the practice of midwifery automatically changed, and the women's participation and that of the midwife diminished.

Recently society has seen some changes. There is greater interest in "natural" lifestyles. Women are demanding more natural childbirth. The experience for many now is a once-only experience, and pregnancy is no longer seen as an occupational hazard of marriage or of being a woman. For many it follows a positive decision to have a baby and is seen as an important life experience. There is a feeling that with modern hospital obstetric care something is missing. In searching for this extra dimension midwives are being sought out because of their known sensitivity and acceptance of pregnancy as a normal physiological event.

There has been a small increase in the number of home births, but the demand is for a birth which the woman herself controls no matter where it occurs. The word *birth* is preferred to "delivery," which has overtones of a mechanistic passive process. The woman wants continuity of care—she wants the same midwife to care for her throughout pregnancy and labor—she does not want unnecessary drugs or intervention—she does not want to be delivered—she wants to give birth. One must, however, remember that some women are content for their pregnancy to be managed, and they do not wish to participate in this way. Today's midwife must be able to care for this woman equally well.

Hospitals are organizations which have to be managed. Doctors are seen as the natural boss. In the main they and they alone have admitting rights or hospital privileges, and women become patients and are admitted under the care of an obstetrician. Hospitals develop protocols which can be restricting, e.g., all patients will be monitored with an electronic fetal monitor throughout labor. This blanket instruction takes no account of the individual woman's needs or the clinical judgment of the midwife. It has usually been drawn up by medical staff with little or no input from senior midwives. Many other hospital routine practices have psychological implications, including who may be present at the birth, contact between mother and baby at birth, rooming-in arrangements, feeding schedules. There may also be rules relating to shaving, enemas, birth positions, and episiotomy.

All these issues are of deep concern to today's mothers and today's midwives. Many of these protocols/procedures are not based on research and will vary from hospital to hospital.

The Way Forward

Midwives have become more aware of the need to base their practice on research recently both in the United Kingdom and internationally. Since 1978 annual Research and the Midwife Conferences have been held in the United Kingdom and the proceedings published.[11] Each year they attract more applications. Many of these research projects have been brought together in a recent book entitled *Midwives, Research and Childbirth*.[12] The second International Conference of Maternity Nurse Researchers in Jamaica in 1988 brought together 90 midwives, nurse midwives, nurses, and others involved in maternity care to share ideas and make research findings available for a larger audience.

Research into clinical midwifery practice is a fairly recent phenomenon. Practice has developed with little or no research. Textbooks have repeated traditional care with no references. For the future midwives must know not only what to do and how to do it but more important why they do it. By questioning what is done midwives can build the body of knowledge on which practice must be based.

To meet the changing needs of women and to speak with authority against hospital and medical routines, midwives need knowledge and skills to effect change. They, of course, also need an attitude which is sensitive to the need for change and a commitment to carry it out. Some hospitals have created birthing rooms within their labor suites. They have concentrated on decor—curtains, carpets, domestic furniture, and lighting. However, this is only part of the answer. Ellen Hodnett (Canada) has looked at the effects of continuous supportive care on childbirth outcomes.[13] The women involved said that the most important factor in their birth experience was the

quality of the support relationship. They were very clear that the physical environment had little impact on their satisfaction with their birth experience.

Continuity of care schemes are being developed in many parts of the United Kingdom. These schemes involve teams of midwives from five to seven who, together, give total care through pregnancy, childbirth, and in the postnatal period in the home or in the hospital to a group of women.[14] These teams are proving very popular with women and with the midwives. The midwife gets to know the women in her care and has the opportunity to use all her skills. The scheme provides flexible working hours which allow time for a normal family life. Midwifery leaders are needed to negotiate in the setting up of such schemes.

Who owns hospital beds? Should the practice whereby doctors alone have admitting rights in government-provided hospitals continue unchallenged? Midwives should take the lead. They have a statutory right to autonomous practice in the United Kingdom and yet frequently cannot achieve this where doctors claim full authority over beds. The provision of true midwifery beds could solve many of the problems of accountability and decision making found today. Some midwives have negotiated the use of beds, but this is by kind permission of the medical staff.

THE CHALLENGE POSED BY SHORTAGES

The availability of human resources fluctuates with periodic rises and falls in the birth rate. Other factors over which more control might be exercised include long-term decision making on education, skills preparation, and skills utilization.

For the past 5 years the United Kingdom has experienced a national shortage of midwives. Closer examination of this shortage reveals that the shortage is getting worse; that it is not regionally uniform, with no recruitment difficulty in some places but a considerable problem in others; that the "pockets of shortages" move, so that one region's success in recruitment is at the expense of another. These regional problems in the United Kingdom could demonstrate a future similar difficulty in the EEC with each constituent country comparable to the United Kingdom regions. Free movement of midwives could enable those countries with impending workforce problems, notably, the United Kingdom and West Germany, to recruit actively elsewhere. What midwifery in Europe must learn from the United Kingdom is that movement within an overall shortage only moves the shortages around. Such movement does not solve the problem and other solutions are needed. European incentives on recruitment and retention and on workforce planning may become increasingly necessary.

In the United Kingdom, in common with many other countries, recruitment and retention in midwifery is a more complex issue than for other professions in that midwives are usually doubly qualified. Entrants to the profession must be recruited from another already qualified group nursing, and midwives can choose to return to nursing practice.

Midwives must look at making midwifery attractive. Using a modern "yuppie" concept, we must market the profession. We must accept that the young of today do not like the strait-jacket that a hierarchical system imposes and they do challenge accepted practices. Professions that cling to outdated structures and rote-learned activities will not succeed against others in the scramble for recruits.

The United Kingdom is bracing itself for a demographic time bomb, as already the projected shortage of 18 year olds, to peak in the 1990s, becomes apparent. Alongside this and crucial to the provision of health care, the percentage of the elderly in the population is increasing. Discussion on the effects of this have been largely confined to the need for a reappraisal of nursing needs. Midwives must also not be complacent about this problem.

Open-ended spending on health care, whatever political stance a government might take, will never be achieved and is probably not desirable. Where, however, there is a total constraint upon the amount a country is prepared to spend on health care, and within that "global budget" one group clearly begins to need more and more resources, other groups will, of necessity, be losers. Maternity care might find itself a loser, and it may become very difficult to challenge this as caring for our old becomes more imperative. We should begin now to look with imagination at ways of meeting and maintaining standards of care in a future climate where our resources may be more and more constrained.

We must examine, as a matter of urgency, our own role, what support we need to fulfill that role, and the extent to which roles which overlap with fellow professionals waste human resources. We must also examine our practice. Is everything we do necessary? Is it wanted by the consumer? Becoming "leaner and fitter" does not necessarily go hand in hand with decreased standards. It might just lead to some improvements.

THE CHALLENGE FROM LITIGATION

It is not necessary to detail the problems that are being experienced in the United States as a result of the explosion of litigation—these have been widely debated and highlighted through professional and other media outlets.[15] Although not on the same scale, litigation is increasing in the United Kingdom. Opinions are mixed about whether it will become as pernicious as in the United States. Also well known is that obstetrics has been particularly hard hit. Midwives as well as obstetricians increasingly feel that their practice is being conducted in a "goldfish bowl"—

scrutinized from all sides as increasingly the practitioner is caught up in potential legal claims. The rise in such practice in the United States has as much to do with an altered activity amongst the legal profession as it has to do with poor obstetric and midwifery practice, and, of course, we have little power over the way lawyers wish to conduct themselves. Solutions to the problem can be identified. Some of these solutions help the health profession but do little to aid the health care consumer. If litigaton levels become unacceptably high, the health care professional can opt out. It is now difficult in some parts of the United States to obtain the care of an obstetrician—there just is not one available. Nothing would stop midwives who decide they could not face the anxiety of potential litigation from leaving practice.

Such midwives might even change their practice to the extent that they allow all their right to autonomic decision making to pass to the obstetrician or general practitioner. But these are not real solutions, because they do not serve the consumer's real needs for both an obstetric and a midwifery service. There are ways open to health professionals, however, that would begin to minimize litigation risk at the same time as safeguarding the right of individuals to obtain compensation if they have been damaged.

Where a trusting relationship has been built up between health care professional and client, it is much less likely that the client will wish to sue his or her carer. Particularly, the cases where damage has occurred, not as the result of another's action but by chance, are unlikely to be brought vexaciously. It is also becoming clear that when clients receive a full explanation of what has occurred, including, where necessary, an admission of fault, they are then much more likely not to proceed to legal action. Trust and openness must be engendered in the professional-client relationship. The midwife with professional

contact with clients over a period of months has the opportunity for this. This process must be encouraged by the adoption of systems that support much greater continuity of care than at present is offered in most parts of the United Kingdom.

As professionals we must not suppress the right of our clients to compensation anymore than we must condone poor practice. Concurrent with the need for developing a climate where litigation does not thrive must be the support for easier compensation for medical accident victims and an active and open "policing" of professional standards. No-fault liability or similar mechanism should be actively supported alongside an urgent reappraisal of professional conduct mechanisms.

THE IMPACT OF GOVERNMENT PHILOSOPHY AND ITS CHALLENGE TO PRACTICE

The past decade has been characterized, in much of the Western democratic block, by the adoption of radical, right-of-center economic policies. Of great interest, also, is the embryonic move of Eastern bloc countries toward a free-market economy approach. In the United States, health care has traditionally been provided as a market commodity, but very recently, with the publication of the United Kingdom government's White Paper for Change in the National Health Service, market systems are being proposed for United Kingdom health care. What we as health professionals must decide is how far these new philosophies will constrain our ability to provide the standard of health care we believe is appropriate. This is not easy as it requires certain skills that previously we have not had or have not developed—the skill to understand complex economic and financial argument, the ability and willingness to accept and manage welcome change, and the political power to negotiate over areas where we believe proposed change to be fundamentally flawed. We must learn to build alliances where previously we have not recognized our friends, and above all we must learn to reject professional self-interest where change is clearly for the good of the people we serve. Midwives are not unique in questioning the premise that health care can still be universally provided by the adoption of a more market-dominated approach.

Neither are we alone in welcoming United Kingdom proposals for greater self-audit by health care professionals or in recognizing the need for great efficiency where needed in health care provision. Our clients, women, however, although numerically the majority display many characteristics of minority groups. Women are politically relatively inactive even in Western democracies, and they tend not to organize themselves to achieve desired goals. The midwifery profession, therefore, must recognize the specific role it has to play in ensuring the high standards of care it has achieved and in safeguarding the provision of health care, including maternity care that is appropriate for women. If it does not we could find that our practice is "constrained" not by the needs of our clients but by current fashions in economic thinking.

THE CHALLENGE OF PROFESSIONALISM

Characteristic of midwifery in the second half of the twentieth century has been the aspiration toward professional status. To understand this aspiration and to evaluate whether we are moving in the right direction, consider what we are or to what we should be aspiring. Western professionalism developed in the nineteenth century. The parameters of professionalism—elitist, self-governing, self-taught, determining its own body of knowledge and entry requirements—were all laid down last century, as was a recognition of those occupations that were considered the professions, notably medicine, the church, the law. A few

others have been added to the list, whereas others aspiring to the label, midwifery amongst them, still have not achieved universal recognition. Two conflicting views exist over the professions, one which sees them as altruistic and offering service, the other which sees them as narrow, protectionist and elitist. Professionalism in this second sense is at present being challenged in the United Kingdom not only by social thinking and others but by government. Particularly, the government is scrutinizing professional restrictive practice both in its changes to the restrictive practice legislation and in the way it is attempting to deal with the legal profession. This leaves our "profession" somewhat at a crossroads.

It is probably true that the aspirations toward professionalism displayed by midwives are for acceptance under the nineteenth-century rules of the game. We do perhaps adopt arguments of exclusivity and elitism that are a century out of date. Perhaps we should use the approaching new century to reject old-style restrictions and to develop more open approaches. Perhaps we should forget aspirations toward professionalism in favor of really defining what is needed of us in today's society. So often the veil of professionalism obscures client's real needs. Professionalism and consumerism do not always accord, and consumer need should be paramount. It could be to our advantage that midwifery has not fully espoused professionalism: We could be the ones to lead toward consumer-centered care.

CONCLUSION

Health for all by the year 2000 will only be achieved by the full use of all health care professionals working together. Rivalry between different professionals must cease, and each must recognize the role of the other. The position of midwives needs to be recognized and utilized in all areas of maternal and child health. In this way the international initiatives for safe motherhood may become a reality.

REFERENCES

1 Project 2000—A New Preparation for Practice. United Kingdom Central Council for Nursing, Midwifery and Health Visiting, London, 1986.
2 Nurses, Midwives and Health Visitors Act 1979. London HMSO.
3 Behind the Blue Door. The history of the Royal College of Midwives 1881-1981. B Cowell and D Wainwright. Bailliere Tindall, London.
4 Regulation Birth. Midwives and Medicine and the Law. R G DeVries, Temple University Press, Philadelphia, 1985.
5 Review of the United Kingdom Central Council and the Four National Boards for Nursing, Midwifery and Health Visiting. Peat, Marwick, McLintock, 1989.
6 Coverage of Maternity Care, second edition, WHO, Geneva 1989.
7 Preventing the tragedy of maternal deaths. Report on International Safe Motherhood Conference, WHO, Nairobi, 1987.
8 Official journal of the European Communities. Legislation. Volume 23, February 11, 1980. Luxembourg.
9 A Midwife's Code of Practice for Midwives Practicing in the United Kingdom. United Kingdom Central Council, second edition, 1989.
10 Handbook of Midwives Rules, UKCC, May 1986.
11 Research and the Midwife Conference Proceedings. Annual publication. Nursing Research Unit, Kings College, London.
12 Midwives, Research and Childbirth. Volume 1, S Robinson and A Thomson, Chapman and Hall, London, 1989.
13 Conference Report: Maternity Nurse Researchers, Jamaica 1988. Midwifery 1988, volume 4, pp. 140–143.
14 Midwives Chronicle, March 1988, pp. 66–70, Team Midwifery in Everyone.
15 Malpractice Issues in Childbirth Proceedings, Milwaukee, Wi, 1985 Forum, International Childbirth Education Association.

Challenges to Practice in France

Genevieve Dechanoz

Chapter 15 presents the challenges to practice in France for the next decades, following the guidelines given. I will not address the issue of midwifery since, in our country, midwives do not belong to the nursing profession but to the medical profession.

The nursing profession in France had for a long time to face several challenges. As in many other European and Latin countries, nursing has developed under the influence of the religious orders; up to 1968, many nuns were still working in hospitals, nursing schools, and health centers holding most of the key positions in nursing.

Despite this situation, nursing began to expand and progress under several conditions:

• A new training program for nurses was set up in 1961 and up-dated in 1972 and in 1979 to meet the European agreements signed by France in 1967 and to fit the evolution of medicine.

• With the help and support of WHO, the International School for Nursing for French-speaking nurses opened in 1965, which educates nurses to get master's degrees and helps them prepare doctorates, thus introducing university education for nurses and training the leaders of the profession.

• Two other programs for master's degrees have been opened for nursing managers and nursing teachers by the Assistance Publique of Paris and the University.

Since 1965, nursing has really developed well in France, trying to become a much more autonomous discipline. But if a lot of nurses agree with this new conception of nursing,

155

some are still reluctant and stay, technically, curatively oriented.

This evolution of nursing is not well accepted by most doctors in the hospitals, presenting many difficulties.

CURRENT CONSTRAINTS ON NURSING IN FRANCE

About 290,000 nurses are working in different settings in France (Appendix 15-1) and at present we see a new important lack of nurses. We had such a situation in the 1970s, but the multiplication of nursing schools at that time and an increase of the salaries had helped to solve the problem. The crisis has reappeared now; this new shortage of nurses results from several circumstances.

Because the length of the nurses' professional life has increased (3 to 5 years in 1970, around 8 to 9 in 1989), the health ministry has set, since 1980, a maximum class enrollment in the nursing schools (around 13,600 new student nurses each year) which seemed to meet the real needs. Unfortunately, the development of part-time work, especially in hospitals; the extension of maternity leave; the increase of absenteeism; the development of medical technology which needs more and more nurses in recovery rooms, in palliative care, in care for people with AIDS, and so on have created new needs which have not been covered these past years because of budget cutting. In many wards there is work for one or two extra nurses. Moreover, the growing lack of interest among students for the nursing profession is such that in some nursing schools even the agreed number of students is not reached. For example, in Paris, for 1500 places, 900 student nurses enrolled.

Nurses working in hospitals or in the community are overloaded, physically and mentally, and consider that the salaries are too poor taking into account the length of their training (3 years after the end of secondary school), the inordinate overtime, the responsibility and the constraints of the work (weekend and night duty . . .).

Another reason for the shortage of nurses rests in the poor relationships with the medical profession; nurses should collaborate with the physicians, but most often the real relationship is "dominating-dominated." Too many doctors still think that they have only to obey and execute what is prescribed. Nurses are not partners in the planning of care, although they prepare and implement the nursing care plan. This is no longer acceptable.

The legislation in 1978 gave a new definition of nurse, stressing the specific role of the nurse (called *"role propre"*), which refers much more to caring than to curing, and in 1984 a list of nursing interventions related to caring and curing was defined. But many nurses and most physicians are not at all interested by this specific caring role, and the work load is usually so heavy that the nurses execute first the curing interventions which will be controlled by the doctors, and the others are only provided if they have time. These caring interventions are too often left to the auxiliaries, who in many cases are not competent enough.

The recent and long strike of nurses in France has added stress to all these problems.

GEOGRAPHIC AND RESOURCE ALLOCATION FACTORS VERSUS GOOD NURSING CARE

Because of the large expansion of medical care and hospitals, the priority of the successive ministries of health has been much more to define ratios of nurses for hospitals and to try to educate enough of them than to develop community care. Generally, nurses are much more interested in work in hospitals in high-tech services than in geriatric or long-term wards or in the community. Because of regional and local conditions, we may also find vastly different conditions from one region to another.

The current lack of nurses prevails mostly in the huge cities, be they in the middle, the north, or the south of France. The concentration of the population in these cities is such that the health needs of people are increasing more quickly than the possibilities of caring, although most nurses work there.

The hospitals are so big that the working conditions are depersonalized and worse. Moreover the cost of living (board and lodging) is higher in these towns, but nurses get the same salary and are not given specific allowances.

For the community care too, there are more nurses in the cities than in the rural areas. The organization of community care is much more structured in the towns. In rural areas more than in cities, nurses working on liberal practice are alone, which means that they are always on duty, and a lot of nurses can't accept such working conditions.

In addition, as the social security system allows only the reimbursement of the care prescribed by a doctor, all the educative and preventive interventions have to be done on a benevolent basis on the free time of the nurse, and therefore this type of care, the core of nursing, is not always provided.

REWARDS ALLOTTED NURSES IN REMOTE AREAS

The system of wages is such that nurses all over France are paid according either to the public statutes or to the trade-union agreements in the private sector, accounting for the qualifications, the position, and the seniority to which are added some risk bonus (about 1 percent of the salary).

The nurses on liberal private practice are paid according to a scale defined by the social security system, and the more they work, the more they earn money. No special reward is given to nurses to encourage them to work in rural areas. The only thing to underline that

may attract nurses is that in rural areas the cost of living is lower than in the cities, the working pace is often slower, and the environment more safe, quiet, and pleasant. Sometimes, too, nurses have more autonomy.

PREDOMINANT PROVIDERS OF PRIMARY HEALTH CARE

The concept of primary health care is not new in France, but, for many people, it still sounds rather strange. As in many industrialized countries where the hospital care is very developed, the people working there think they are not concerned with primary health care. However, a lot of health promotion activities have already been, for a long time, implemented in France:

- Health centers for tuberculosis, for maternal and infant protection, immunization.
- Health centers for diagnoses and treatments.
- Occupational health services that include a medical check-up once a year, follow up of sick workers, and preventive measures in all workplaces where people work.
- Medical check-up once a year and preventive activities at school, from the kindergarten to the university. Follow up of sick students and health education.
- Home care, much more developed in these last 10 years, for the elderly and others.

Very often different public and private associations intervene for the organization of prevention and education, but their interventions are not coordinated. Most of these preventive activities are under the responsibility of physicians working with the help of nurses, midwives, and/or social workers.

At the moment because of the project Health for All 2000, huge efforts are being made to develop primary health care. These efforts concern not only the community but also the hospitals and the nurses training in basic and postbasic nursing schools.

The primary health care developed for mothers and children, students, and other workers is provided mostly by nurses, although for the elderly the tendency is to leave them to auxiliaries. Of course these auxiliaries work under the responsibility of a nurse, but the latter can't control everyday decisions.

The training of nurses has always been and is today medically oriented and hospital based. However, for about 10 years nurses have been trained for primary health care delivery, but what they learned was so different from what they found in practice that they did not believe what they were taught was right.

The International School for Nursing in Lyons has, from the very beginning, opened a special section to prepare leaders for the community care and the development of primary health care. Several postbasic nursing schools have also offered a special training to prepare chief nurses to work in the community.

Since 1986–1987, with the huge mobilization of nurses in the Fora preparing the European Conference for nursing in Vienna, primary health care has been a focus, and now many nurses are quite aware of the importance of developing primary health care. Several models have been implemented in different practice settings.

Many nurses have discovered that they were providing primary health care without knowing that they were doing so, but what nurses have to better learn and be aware of is how to help the population to really participate in the organization and development of primary health care, how to help people to be responsible for their health. That is the biggest challenge.

LEGISLATION FOR RECOMMENDATIONS

As mentioned, legislation fosters the practice of nurses, especially in the perspective of primary health care. But the everyday reality is totally different, because the legislation does not give nurses enough power to practice as mandated.

In hospitals, it is difficult for nurses to make decisions on caring, even if that is defined as their specific role, if the doctor does not agree, because the medical legislation says that the doctor is entirely responsible for the patients and the care given to them. In the other fields of practice the complaint of nurses is that they have so much prescribed technical care to administer that they can't provide nursing care.

The recommendations for change follow several lines:

- Put more nurses in places with shortages, in order to give nurses enough time for nursing beside the medical, technical care.
- Don't use too many auxiliaries especially for the care of the elderly, whose needs have to be assessed and answered by well-prepared nurses. Qualified staff are more cost-effective.
- Have the regulatory authorities, doctors and nurses too, understand the importance and the role of nursing.
- Recognize the nurse as a partner in the planning and delivery of care in hospitals and in the community at local, regional, national levels.
- Intensify the nursing education on a high level (university level) to train nurses as leaders and partners in a multidisciplinary team.
- Intensify the possibilities of in-service training and continuing education in hospitals as well as in the community, particularly on subjects related to leadership, management, coping with long-term patients, coping with stress, burn out, self-esteem, and so on.

CLINICAL NURSE SPECIALISTS

For several years the question of clinical nurse specialists has been raised in France. The first needs appeared in very specialized units (neurosurgery, dialysis, oncology, etc.); in these wards the turnover of the nursing personnel was very high, and the chief nurses were always confronted with new nurses who knew almost nothing in the specialty. The in-service training of these newly recruited nurses increased the work load of the senior nurses.

In addition, the evolution of the technical and caring procedures was so quick that nurses with a high level of competency were required to adapt these procedures to the needs of the patients and to teach their colleagues. It quickly became apparent that these so-called clinical nurses have their place not only in the "high-tech" units but also in general medicine and surgery wards to develop care adapted to the patients and based on specific clinical knowledge.

And last but not least, for a lot of nurses who were very interested in caring at the bedside, there was no possibility of being promoted and thus getting better wages. The only possibility they had was to become a head nurse or a nursing teacher. So, in developing this new domain of practice, it would be possible for them to improve their expertise and use it at the bedside to get a better position.

The International School of Nursing in Lyons has for some years developed a 9-month education program for nurses caring for patients with stomas, and a new qualification was born—"enterostomathérapeute" (stoma therapist). These programs are now numerous in France, and we consider that this is a beginning.

In that perspective, the nurse at the ministry level (hospital directorate) has tried to prepare, with a group of nurses, a project to train these clinical nurses and to give them recognition and an acceptable position in the nursing hierarchy. In a parallel direction, some private institutions for continuing education have established a 2-year training, part-time, program to prepare clinical nurse specialists. However, when these nurses go back to work, their expertise is not officially recognized.

Because the regulatory authorities are afraid to have to increase the pay of these highly qualified nurses, the authorities have decided that these clinical nurses were not useful, that all nurses could be, with their diploma, clinical nurses.

ALLOCATION OF NURSES IN PARTICULAR PRACTICE SETTINGS

It has always been difficult to have nurses for particular practice settings, especially long-term care, neurosurgery, or any unit where the patients are very dependent (except the intensive care units).

Presently the shortage of nurses makes this difficulty more acute: 3 percent of budgeted posts are not filled up in the hospitals of Ile de France, but 13 percent of posts in geriatric hospitals of the same region are vacant. In hospitals, when newly trained nurses are recruited, especially those who have a salary or a scholarship during their training, they are often appointed in these settings, but they leave as soon as possible. For some, work in such settings is such a bad experience that they leave the nursing profession.

There is no plan at the national level to address this allocation problem, and at the moment each region's local authorities or each hospital's administration are allocating according to the most urgent needs.

A plan to address this problem should

• Define a percentage of nurses to be appointed in these settings.
• Make these positions more attractive, for instance, specific working time conditions, valorization of the care provided, specific training for nurses in these units and then choice of the best nurses for the posts, giving them a better salary or specific bonus.

Of course these changes would require new legislation, since the working conditions and the salary scale are defined on a national basis for all the nurses. Nevertheless, at local levels some measures could be taken, for example, adjustment of the working hours, payment of part of the inordinate overtime, more days off.

CONCLUSION

For the next 10 years, the nursing profession has to take up the challenge given to them by Dr. Mahler, former director of WHO, in his paper, "Nurses lead the way." Nurses must prove that they can be successful leaders in developing primary health care. Confronted with the growing number of elderly and of people with AIDS, nurses will have to face the ever-growing development of new technologies.

To accept the challenge they will have to cope with all the above difficulties and they will have to cooperate with other health professionals, but also they'll have to take into account and mobilize the major resources which rest in the energy, the willingness, the force of the young nurses who need appropriate guidance to follow the way. Isn't that the task of leaders?

Appendix 15-1

Distribution of Nurses in the Most Important Working Settings

Setting	Total number
Public hospitals	117,708
Private hospitals	39,253
Psychiatric sector	60,947
Liberal private practice	24,429
National-regional level	5,021
Occupational nurses	5,003
Maternal and infant protection	3,691
School nurses	4,448
Health care centers	5,696
Blood transfusion centers	1,096
Home care	1,275
Long-term institutions for elderly	3,468
Institutions for handicapped children and adults	7,172
Nursing schools: teachers and directors	3,183
Postbasic nursing schools: teachers and directors	136
Psychiatric nursing schools: teachers and directors	657
Specialties schools	
• Pediatric nurse	74
• Operating theater nurse	22
• Anaesthetic nurse	54
Others	5,785

Source: Ministère des Affaires Sociales et de l'Emploi—Service des statistiques, des études et des systèmes d'information, S.E.S.I., pp. 110–112, February 1988.

Health Personnel per 100,000 Inhabitants

Personnel	Total number	Percent
Physicians	231.000	418
Midwives[1]	9.725	82
Nurses	233.313	422.1
Psychiatric nurses	60.947	110.3
Physiotherapists	35.746	64.7

[1] Per 100,000 women between 15 and 44.

Source: Ministère des Affaires Sociales et de l'Emploi—Service des statistiques, des études et des systèmes d'information, S.E.S.I., pp. 110–112, February 1988.

Chapter 16

Challenges to Practice in Geriatrics

James Williamson

One basic problem associated with population aging is that we have no precedent to guide us since it has never happened before in human history. Hence we must be prepared to look at new methods and practices since simply offering more and more of what we have been doing can never cope with the problem.

DEMOGRAPHIC CONSIDERATIONS

I shall not attempt to deal with demographic trends in detail but will give only broad outlines. Figures 16-1, 16-2, and 16-3 show population changes in the United Kingdom from 1901 to 2021 for the age groups 65+, 75, and 85+.

Figure 16-1 shows the extraordinary increase in persons aged 65 up to 1981, but it also shows a leveling off reflecting declining birth rates in the interwar years. Figure 16-2 shows a similar steep increase in the over 75s, and this will continue till the end of the century, when it will level off. Figure 16-3 is perhaps the most impressive, since it shows that the steep increase in the 85+ group will continue right into the next century. This age group poses the greatest demands on health and social services since it contains a high proportion of individuals with multiple disability conditions, physical and mental, and these individuals are also more liable to be socially disadvantaged.

In each age group females outnumber males, and this discrepancy increases with age; in the 85+ group there are 5 females to 2 males. This reflects the fact that females outlive males (by about 6 or 7 years in the United Kingdom) because females have an innate biological "superiority" and because males are more likely to die prematurely from a variety

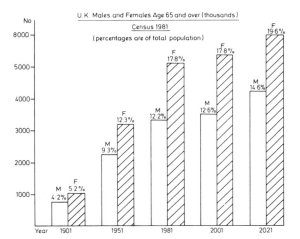

Figure 16-1

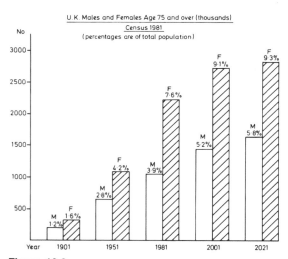

Figure 16-2

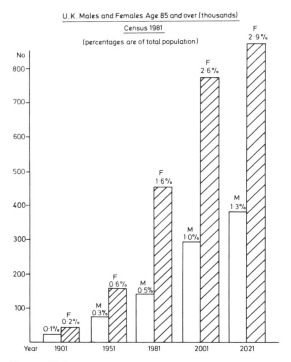

Figure 16-3

of causes (tobacco and alcohol-related illness, accidents, and acts of warfare) in which self-destructive behavior is a factor.

These U.K. figures are very similar to other Western European countries where precipitous falls occurred in infant and child mortality in the nineteenth century due to public health advances and control of the great epidemics and pandemics of communicable diseases. This remarkable achievement ensured that a higher proportion than ever before of those born at that time would survive into adulthood and eventually old age. This together with a continuing high birth rate was responsible for the ''geriatric problem'' of the second half of the twentieth century.

It is noteworthy that, until the last few decades, there was little or no change in the survival time of elderly individuals, who would in general live no longer than their great-grandparents who had reached a similar age. However, in the last 20 to 25 years there has been a significant increase in expectation of life for even the oldest groups. The reasons for this are not clear; probably the main factors have been general improvement in standards of living and better medical care of the elderly and aged both in the community and in institutions.

In the developed world these changes have occurred slowly and over the space of generations with at least the possibility for authorities to make some adaptations (although medical authorities could not claim to have seized this opportunity very avidly). It is most noteworthy, however, that the aging of populations is now occurring most rapidly within the developing world.

Figure 16-4 shows the proportional increase in the over 60s and over 80s in the whole world, the developed and the developing world, in the last 30 years of this century. For both age groups the increases are far higher in developing areas, in which the over 80s will see an increase of about 180 percent. It is perhaps salutary to add that this increase in Latin America will be no less than 215 percent. This startling growth in the most aged group is occurring in countries which are still struggling to cope with the traditional problems of the third world—poverty, political instability, high birth rates, and crippling debts. It is baffling to imagine how this latest problem will be surmounted, and there is a certainty of great misery for many of the millions

who now survive into extreme old age in these territories.

Nor do bare population statistics give the whole picture; while these demographic changes have been taking place substantial social changes have occurred in both developed and developing countries. In the former, increasing numbers of elderly persons live alone, especially females; in the United Kingdom more than half the females aged 75 + now live in single-person households. Average family size has tended to decrease (although this trend was temporarily interrupted by World War II's "baby boom") which means that the average number of family carers has likewise declined. Daughters and daughters-in-law are the traditional supporters of family elders, and we have seen a great increase in the proportion of married females in employment outside the home—in the United Kingdom now about seven out of ten middle-aged married females are so engaged. This trend will surely increase in the years ahead in which recruits to commerce and industry will increasingly be females. Again this trend, however welcome it may be for the emancipation of women, can only mean further erosion of traditional family support for frail elders. In developing regions, parallel social and economic changes are already bearing heavily on the increasing numbers of old people, especially the tendency toward rapid and uncontrolled urbanization which tends to leave the elders unsupported in rural settlements as the younger generations leave for the cities. Even more distressing may be the fate in store for those who grow old in the cities and shanty towns where life is so hard even for young and vigorous persons. The erosion of historical patterns of family and village life and traditional methods of agriculture and husbandry can only make great difficulties for the least adaptable who are the very old. All these changes pose great challenges to the caring professions as we approach the twenty-first century.

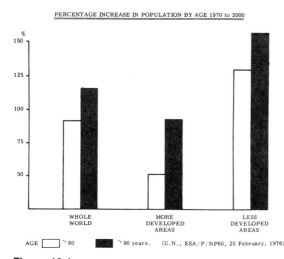

Figure 16-4

UNDERSTANDING THE NEEDS OF THE OLD AND THE AGED

It is true to say that, in many important respects, the medical professions have been slow to respond to the needs of increasingly aged societies, and there has been a tendency to suggest that the answer must be simply to provide more and more of those resources which are now regarded as necessary for health care of younger and middle-aged persons. Although it is true that many old people (especially the "younger old") do need this kind of care, this is certainly not true for the "old old" or the frail elderly who require special management by staff who are trained to understand their special needs.

A series of simple diagrams in Figure 16-5 help to put this concept across. Figure 16-5 shows the traditional relationship of function and age with the customary three phases of development: (1) growth, in which there is a rapid increase in function, (2) maturity, in which there is a brief maintenance of function, and (3) a slide into senescence with a linear decline. Throughout the whole process there is increasing variability.

Modern gerontological research has shown that this is a grossly inaccurate and incomplete picture which provides a generally unjustifiably pessimistic view. The older model was based on misleading data usually derived from cross-sectional studies in which measurements were made on individuals of different ages; modern studies are based on longitudinal studies of representative population samples—measurements on the same individual over long periods. In this way the effects of important secular trends have been eliminated and a much more accurate picture is now available.

Figure 16-6 depicts two functions. Function A could represent visual accommodation, which begins to decrease early as the crystalline lens loses elasticity (usually in early teens). Once the age-related decline starts it continues in a linear fashion, but usually it is not clinically apparent until 45 to 50, by which time most individuals will require reading glasses. Function B could be muscle strength, which does not show age decline until much later (25 to 30 years); once this decline commences, it also is linear.

In complex animals such as humans living in complex societies, such simple rules must be modified. Figure 16-7 shows the effects of behavior on function over time. Adopting unhealthy behavior such as cigarette smoking will lead to a more rapid loss of function (re-

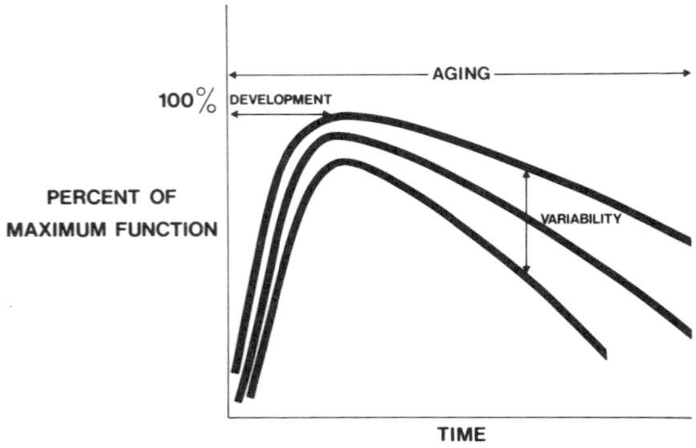

Figure 16-5

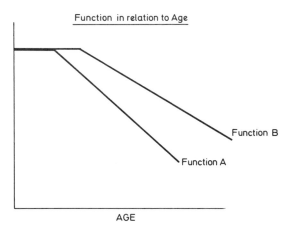

Figure 16-6

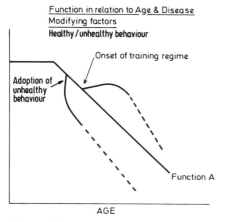

Function in relation to Age & Disease
Modifying factors
Healthy / unhealthy behaviour

Onset of training regime

Adoption of unhealthy behaviour

Function A

AGE

Figure 16-7

spiratory, cardiac, and skeletal), whereas the adoption of a healthy life-style such as regular exercise will improve function. Until recently it was assumed that although these factors might be important in younger individuals, they had little relevance in old age, where functional loss was marked and nothing could be done about it. If we take muscle strength as an example we learn some surprising and important lessons. It is now known that, *at any age,* muscle strength can be increased by 15 percent by taking regular exercise. Hence a sedentary adult will increase muscle power by this amount through a program of exercise. This is obviously of great importance for athletes who seek to wring every extra effort out of their neuromuscular systems; however, for other ordinary younger and middle-aged persons it makes little difference, since their reserves of muscle power are large and a 15 percent loss still leaves them able to do all the things they need to or want to do such as daily work, playing golf, or running for a bus. However for the very old, where reserves of muscle strength are seriously limited, the loss of 15 percent may be crucial. Thus a healthy woman of 80 years living an "ordinary" existence will generally only just have the muscle

power in her legs to enable her to rise unaided from a low armless chair. Should she suffer a period of enforced immobility (after illness or injury for example) she will lose up to 15 percent of this leg strength. She will have then lost the ability to rise from such a chair. Hence the period of inactivity may rapidly result in a state of dependency upon others for help with ordinary living activities. The importance of exercise throughout life is now recognized as being of the greatest practical importance in health promotion in old age and, contrary to common wisdom, the older the individual, the more important exercise is.

In addition to effects of behavior, we have to take into account environmental factors, e.g., the effect of prolonged exposure to coal dust will reduce lung function and presumably so will exposure to cigarette smoke through passive inhalation. Other forms of environmental pollution may have important implications for those experiencing lifetime exposure.

Figure 16-8 shows the effect of acute illness which may lead to rapid and severe loss of function, e.g., myocardial infarction or pneumonia. The degree of recovery will depend on the amount of functioning tissue permanently lost which reflects the severity of the illness and speed and efficacy of treatment.

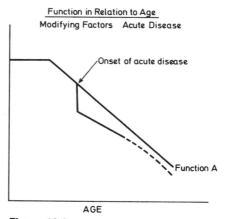

Function in Relation to Age
Modifying Factors   Acute Disease

Onset of acute disease

Function A

AGE

Figure 16-8

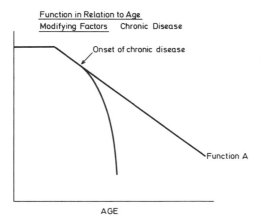

Figure 16-9

Figure 16-9 shows the effect of chronic illness which, of course, may be greatly modified (as in Figure 16-10) by effective treatment and rehabilitation, e.g., in rheumatoid arthritis and Parkinson's disease.

The picture which we witness in an individual old person therefore is infinitely complex and variable, the result of the interplay of four factors:

1 Heredity—some individuals (and some families) appear to age more slowly than others

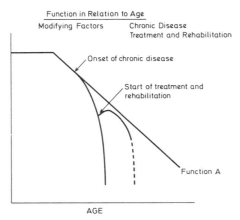

Figure 16-10

2 Age changes

3 Disease changes

4 Effects of behavior and environmental factors

It is noteworthy that modern medicine has tended to concentrate mainly or exclusively upon 3 above with the provision of a pathological diagnosis (localize the lesion and determine its pathological nature). I cannot emphasize too strongly that in old age, especially in the very old, this is an inadequate and incomplete diagnosis, since we must include age effects and effects of behavior. We therefore have to learn to "think beyond the pathology" and consider our diagnosis (it becomes easier if we call it "assessment") in functional terms. The use of problem lists helps in this, and geriatricians were using a problem-based diagnosis long before this became fashionable in the wider field of medicine. Hence we would end our assessment with such items as "difficulty in transferring and dressing lower limbs" in someone with dyspnoea due to obesity and ischaemic heart disease plus osteoarthritis of knees and hips.

The simple model shown in Figure 16-5 is thus seen to be inadequate. In its place we offer that shown in Figure 16-11, which shows four phases of development:

1 Growth, with rapid functional increase.

2 Maturity, which shows function being maintained for much longer than suggested in Figure 5.

3 Senescence which is slower and more "benign" than Figure 5 suggests.

Up to this point the news has been good: the obsolete model was indeed unduly pessimistic, based on misleading cross-sectional studies. Modern longitudinal studies and much ordinary clinical experience show that more and more old people continue to enjoy good health and satisfying lives.

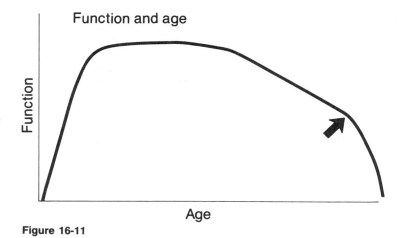

Figure 16-11

4 Now for the bad news! Figure 16-11 also shows that there is a fourth phase which starts at the arrow on the curve. Beyond this arrow, functional loss is accelerated, individuals become frailer with significantly reduced functional reserves.

Figure 16-12 has been provided by Professor Alvar Svanborg (orginator and director of the famous Gothenburg longitudinal study). This shows the four phases referred to above but also shows that, although variability increases throughout phases 1, 2 and 3, it actu-

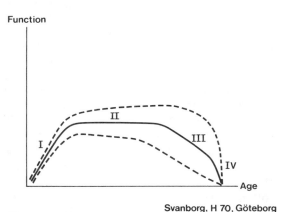

Svanborg, H 70, Göteborg

Figure 16-12

ally decreases in phase 4. Thus, just as we all enter this world with similarly low functional reserves, the increasing numbers who survive into extreme old age experience rapid reduction in these reserves.

This concept of a "fourth phase" is the main reason underlying the need for a specialty of geriatric medicine, since individuals who survive thereto have special needs and require management by multidisciplinary teams of professionals who have undertaken training to understand their needs. A parallel may be drawn with pediatrics, especially as it relates to the neonate and young infants who also require special management because of their meager reserves.

Figure 16-13 shows the same idea in a rather different fashion. Here it is shown that in young adulthood we possess ample reserves and most of us achieve 65 (the official, if largely arbitrary, start of old age) with reserves which are "generally adequate." However, for the increasing numbers who survive beyond 75 there is the prospect of existence with "significantly reduced reserves," and as we move into extreme old age we pass through what I have termed "the zone of geriatric medicine" and approach that theoretical state

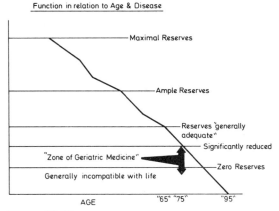

Figure 16-13

where we have no reserves at all, a state incompatible with further survival.

It is important to recognize the existence of this group of increasingly frail individuals within the fourth phase, which has also been called the "terminal phase." I do not like the latter title because it suggests that individuals therein are terminally ill in the way that this term is applied to cancer sufferers. This is not the case; these people are not "dying," although they are more likely to be dead! This paradoxical statement simply reflects that, provided the 95-year-old lady does not fracture her hip or acquire a pneumococcal pneumonia or other overwhelming stress, she may well live for another 6 months or even 6 years despite the precariousness of her homeostatic mechanisms. She is, of course, on the brink of the precipice, since minor stresses, which would not be a danger to persons not at this stage, may be fatal to her.

There are three outcomes of stress for these frail elderly persons, and each has great significance for nurses and doctors who look after them:

1 *Death,* which may be the most desirable outcome in circumstances where the individual has reached a sensible conclusion that the burdens of life are no longer counterbalanced by its pleasures and satisfactions. The task here is to be certain that this is genuinely the case and that there is no factor such as undiagnosed depression or untreated anemia, which, upon correction, would significantly alter the balance.

Where it is decided that death is indeed the desirable outcome, then it should be achieved with dignity and a minimum of discomfort, and this demands high levels of nursing skill. At present about 70 percent of people die in hospital in the United Kingdom, and I cannot believe that this is in the best interests of many, especially the frail elderly who are so susceptible to environmental stresses. Almost certainly it reflects the common view in modern societies that a dying patient always needs the resources of a hospital; clearly this is not the case for many patients who could assuredly die more contentedly in the security of their own homes and among their own folk. This represents an important challenge for community nurses to demonstrate the benefits of terminal care at home and to educate others.

2 *Full recovery,* which in all circumstances is the most welcome outcome for patient, doctor, and nurse. For it to occur, there must be skilled geriatric care and a carefully devised rehabilitation plan. Full recovery does not merely mean the resolution of a pathological process, but it must also imply restoration to the level of function which pertained before the illness (or in some cases to an even higher level). What does it mean if a pneumonia has been "cured" by antibiotics with complete resolution of the chest X-ray shadows and yet the patient remains bedridden and dependent? In such circumstances the patient may well question the significance of the word *cured!*

Achieving this kind of result demands close teamwork in which doctors, nurses, and therapists all work together in setting goals (often quite humble) and in seeing that they are achieved. In this process family and other carers are of the greatest importance, and their wishes and needs must always be considered in the management plans.

3 *Neither death nor recovery,* in which case the patient survives but in a much more dependent state. This may be due to inadequate treatment, late diagnosis, or poor rehabilitation (sadly sometimes *no rehabilitation*) and therefore is preventable. However, even with the best will and the most skilled care, some frail elderly patients will be so afflicted that they will remain in a state of considerable dependency. For them, we must ensure high-quality care. Wherever possible, this should be provided in the patient's home with suitable support from community nurses. Where this is not possible and the patients have a prolonged stay in an institution, then the quality of care should be equally good with special attention to ensuring maximum autonomy and control over their lives. Once again, wherever the patient may be, due respect must be paid to the needs and wishes of family carers.

It is obvious that, in all these considerations, the nursing profession has a vital role to play and this will become more and more important as we move into the next century.

PLANNING COMPREHENSIVE HEALTH CARE OF THE ELDERLY

I have attempted to evolve logical patterns of care for aging populations and here present a simple scheme which purports to indicate where efforts have to be exerted in health care systems.

First of all, I reiterate that the elderly are not homogeneous as regards their health care needs; many require no more (and no less) than the care which is appropriate for younger adults. Thus the 70-year-old man who has a myocardial infarction on the eighteenth tee of the golf course does not require specialist geriatric care. However, the 85-year-old woman found lying on the floor by her home help who is unable to get up, who lives alone, has failing memory and poor postural stability, etc., certainly does need geriatric care; if denied it and admitted to a nongeriatric setting, she will fare very poorly.

The essential elements in planning comprehensive health care for the elderly are quite simple to define, although very complex to execute:

1 A means of identifying the needs of elderly persons and their carers.

2 Resources available to meet these needs in a timely and economical manner.

Implementing these elements necessitates suitable training and education for all the professionals who have contact with the elderly. It also requires a continuum of resources for meeting identified needs. No country that I am aware of has so far succeeded in providing such a continuum in which each service is provided to adequate standards. Most have in fact a marked "discontinuum" in which some services are absent or grossly inadequate, e.g., homemaker services in the United States or overprovision of nursing home care as in parts of Australia. The certain result is that patients will receive inappropriate care which is often inordinately expensive and renders many unhappy and miserable. Thus, where there is a dearth of homemaker and other domiciliary care, old people will find their way into residential care where they may block the entry of persons who need this sort of care. They in turn move into the next level, i.e., nursing home care or long-stay hospital. The end result is that the unprotected underbelly of the system, the emergency room, is invaded by old people who have been denied the kind of care they need. They find their way to the emergency room either by waiting until an acute episode actually occurs or when it is "concocted" by desperate community workers as the family finally signal that they have had enough and refuse to offer more support.

This is commonly described as "family rejection"; in truth it is almost always a manifestation of catastrophic failure of the health system and a dramatic demonstration of the "discontinuum" of care.

FIVE LEVELS OF HEALTH CARE

I have proposed that in planning comprehensive care for the elderly, we should specify five levels upon which to concentrate our efforts:

1 Prevention and case-finding
2 Primary care
3 Specialist geriatric care
4 "Specialist geriatric care" brought into nongeriatric settings
5 Improve care in long-term institutions

Prevention and Case-Finding

It is common to dismiss the idea of prevention in old age because, to prevent disease, one must start in youth or middle age. Certainly this is true of conditions such as tobacco related diseases, e.g., lung cancer, chronic lung disease, and coronary artery disease. Nevertheless many things can improve health in old age such as stopping smoking (which even in old age has benefits and saves a lot of money), moderation in alcohol consumption, and, as already pointed out the continuation of healthy exercise. There is also little doubt that continued active involvement in family and community roles and in recreational pursuits helps to keep old people mentally alert and content. Many of today's old people already know this and live full, useful, and satisfying lives after contributing substantially to the well-being of their families, their neighbors, and wider society. These individuals, unlike many of their predecessors, have rejected the negative image of old age which indicated that not much could be done to mitigate the effects of growing old and when troubles arose it was

pointless to struggle against them. Unfortunately many younger persons (and some older ones) still share this negative view, and it is doubly unfortunate that many health professionals likewise have unhelpful and pessimistic ideas on this matter.

There is thus great scope for education involving members of the public who should realize that growing old does concern them, since there is a high probability that, for the first time in history, the ordinary person will be allowed the privilege of survival into old age. Education must also involve health professionals and planners and politicians who should be helped to understand the importance of keeping old people fit and independent, plus the supreme importance of protecting carers so that they may continue their informal caring roles.

Case-finding is a form of tertiary prevention in which old people with existing problems are sought out and offered help. It has had a chequered history. In the early days it was viewed largely as a matter of "medical" screening, but now it is more logically seen as the detection of loss of function. This must be very broadly based—loss of physical function, of mental function, and of social function. I prefer also to specify loss of family function, since the role of family carers is so vitally important.

Case-finding has two stages: (1) identification of high-risk groups and (2) offering these high-risk individuals appropriate advice and help.

Identification can happen in a number of ways:

1 By the use of predefined groups such as the very old (85 +), those recently discharged from hospital, those recently widowed, or those who have been relocated. Others have added another risk factor—those without a confidante.

2 By opportunistic identification. Over 80 percent of old people have contact with their

general practitioner in any year. The general practitioner (or a nursing colleague) may use this opportunity to inquire about current problems, concentrating on loss of function rather than detection of disease.

3 Use of postal questionnaires. A modification of this is the Edinburgh birthday card scheme.

Once identified, those in high-risk categories, should then be visited by a community nurse who will make a detailed inquiry as to current problems. For many of these problems the nurse will herself seek solutions; for problems of a more "medical" nature she will make referral to the general practitioner.

Slowly, evidence is accumulating that this approach helps in reducing mortality, morbidity, and use of expensive hospital resources. Such an approach has the considerable advantage that it requires no capital expenditure and can be adopted as and when time permits, e.g., during the quieter summer months, community nurses may undertake case-finding which can then be reduced when work increases in winter.

Requirements for successful case-finding include:

Good health education policies and practices given national and local priority.
Good primary care. Well-educated, well-motivated family physicians and community nurses prepared to work closely as team members.
Adequate resources in the community to meet identified needs.
Determined action in the fields of education and health care practice once again at national and local level and by the various professional bodies concerned.

Primary Care

In line with the Alma Ata declaration of the United Nations, good primary care is essential in any health care system.

It has already been emphasized that primary care personnel will be involved in prevention and especially in case-finding, but their main contribution will always be in meeting declared medical need (once again I use the word "medical" in the widest context). This involves the detection of medical need plus social need, since in old age the two are usually inextricably linked. This must then be followed by skilled and expert management and therapy both for patient and involved carers.

The above is a very brief and general description of primary care for the elderly which is an extensive and complex affair. One aspect deserves special mention and that is the management of acute and subacute illness within the patient's own home whenever possible. This is advocated not just with a view to sparing expensive and scarce hospital facilities but also to avoid the hazards of admission as they bear upon frail elderly persons. Among these hazards are:

1 Disorientation and worsening of preexisting confusion, especially where vision and hearing are impaired.
2 The occurrence of incontinence when the "system" within the hospital ward cannot adapt to the urgency of micturition in old ladies with unstable bladder musculature. The demoralizing effect of the first wet bed can scarcely be imagined by the average adult.
3 The ever-present danger of hospital infection acquired after admission.
4 The effects of general destabilization as an old person is removed from familiar, friendly, and reassuring surroundings.

Hence primary care teams should agree on policies to treat simple acute illnesses at home by stepping up their own involvement (mainly a nursing matter) and the contribution of others (mainly from the homemaker service).

Good primary care also requires well-educated, well-trained and highly motivated family physicians working closely with community nurses. Also required is a range of community services in suitable balance and readily available when need is identified. Primary carers must also be able to depend upon the full range of specialist services including the specialist geriatric service immediately available when needed. Obviously these requirements will necessitate a thorough review of training for primary carers, who should receive a good grounding in gerontology and geriatric care plus adequate continuing education in these fields with emphasis on team effort and prevention.

Specialist Geriatric Service

It is of more than passing interest that the United Kingdom is the only country to have opted at an early stage for provision of specialists in geriatric medicine as one way of coping with aging of the population. The history of the development of U.K. geriatrics is interesting, dating from the great visionary achievements of Dr. Marjory Warren through the lean years of the 1950s to the 1970s when demand seemed to grow by the hour while resources remained sparse and recruitment was abysmally poor. Finally, by the late 1970s and the 1980s the light at the end of the tunnel was visible for those stalwarts who had withstood the stress, and the specialty is now the most rapidly expanding in the Health Service, and good doctors and nurses are, in most areas, quite easy to recruit into the specialty.

There is now a national network of geriatric units serving geographically defined populations in every health district and staffed by doctors, nurses, and therapists who have elected to do this as a career (or who wish to gain specialist geriatric experience before going off into another field such as primary care, psychiatry, or orthopedics).

Emphasis is upon multidisciplinary team approach to identifying needs of patients and carers followed by the evolution of treatment and rehabilitation plans for each case.

The first essential is for primary carers (family physicians and community nurses) to be fully aware of the uses and potential of the specialist geriatric service so that they will make appropriate referrals. The family physician acts as gatekeeper by referring at an early stage patients who need the geriatric team approach. Likewise the physicians have to be trained and trusted not to make unnecessary referrals of patients physicians ought to manage themselves or by inappropriate referrals who ought to go to some other specialist. There will always be a shortage of specialist geriatric staff, so it is essential that only patients who need their care are referred.

A good geriatric service ought to offer house calls, day hospital and outpatient service, and inpatient care for investigation, treatment, and rehabilitation. These services should be provided for geriatric patients whether they be acutely ill or suffer from chronic progressive conditions.

An important provision is respite care, which is aimed at sharing the burden of care with family and other informal carers. Every family has limits to the degree of care that it can provide, and an essential task of the geriatric services is to ensure that carers are not pushed beyond these limits; otherwise they will collapse, withdraw support, and what might have been salvaged by short-term admission then may necessitate permanent institutional care. For many aged ladies with family support, a few weeks' admission two or three times per year will enable that family to continue support for the last few years of the patient's life. Once the old lady is dead and gone the family has the solace of knowing that they were able successfully to discharge their responsibilities right to the end.

Specialist geriatric services of this sort require dedicated doctors and nurses who have undergone postgraduate training and who participate in programs of continuing education throughout their careers.

An important aspect of the specialist geriatric service is its educational potential for undergraduates and postgraduates in many fields of medicine and nursing and within continuing education. There is a wealth of difference between the educational impact of a series of lectures to a class and the "come and see us in action" approach. Many medical students, on completing their month of geriatric medicine in Edinburgh, spontaneously remarked upon the enthusiasm of the staff and the obvious enjoyment they obtained from their work. This could not be conveyed in a lecture, however stylishly delivered.

Meeting Geriatric Need in Nongeriatric Settings

This recommendation may be described as an extension of specialist service, since it is aimed at importing geriatric specialist skills and management into areas which may contain "geriatric patients." These "geriatric patients" may have found their way therein for valid reasons, as is the case of the aged lady who falls and sustains a hip fracture, or they may have been sent there for wrong reasons as in the case of the elderly person who has been slowly deteriorating and whose family, driven to despair, demand that "something be done," leading to the inappropriate referral to the emergency room when what ought to have occurred was the patient's referral to the geriatric service, preferably at a much earlier stage long before the family felt under such strain (a clear example of the importance of including carers in the case-finding process).

There are numerous settings into which geriatric patients may stray for good or bad reasons (acute internal medicine, orthopedic surgery, emergency rooms, psychiatry wards). We have shown how regular visits by a geriatrician to an acute internal medicine department will reduce mean stay dramatically, especially for the most elderly patients (mean stay for females over 85 reduced from 49 to 19 days). This involves bringing the geriatric approach to bear upon these elderly pa-

tients; this transcends the usual consultation service, since the geriatrician is not invited to see individual patients but makes regular (biweekly) visits in order to identify "geriatric patients." Similar benefits have been shown to follow from joint geriatric/orthopedic management of hip fracture patients.

We have not been able to prove similar benefits from providing geriatric skills in the emergency room, although studies have shown remarkable benefits for frail elderly randomly assigned to geriatric care compared to controls treated in acute internal medicine settings.

This practice of importing geriatric skills and methods of management represents a most useful development and can, of course, be done at an early stage of development of geriatric services, since it requires only the knowledge and skill of the members of the geriatric team and does not depend on separate capital developments.

Meeting geriatric need in nongeriatric settings necessitates a well-trained enthusiastic geriatric team capable of making speedy, accurate, and comprehensive assessments of need for patients in these settings. Where there is a separate geriatric service with inpatient capacity, such a service must be sufficiently well staffed to allow staff time to make regular visits to these settings. This has not often been feasible, although we have been fortunate enough to be able to do it in Edinburgh.

As emphasized above, this service transcends and complements the customary consultation service which will generally become increasingly superseded as the geriatric penetration becomes more established.

Improvement of Care in Long-Term Institutions

Elderly people who spend long periods, often their remaining months or years, in long-stay hospitals, or in residential or nursing homes can readily become the Cinderellas of health care. They are easily lost sight of, their complex needs are readily overlooked, and staff (nurses and doctors) derive little or no traditional professional satisfaction from looking after them. They are almost invariably suffering from multiple chronic illnesses, often have degrees of dementia, and commonly are on several medications.

Likewise the staff who look after them are often held in low esteem and can readily become professionally isolated. This applies particularly to nursing staff, who not only have to understand and cope with the physical and mental demands from patients but often have to cope with critical, guilt-ridden, and anxious relatives who may take much of their time and leave them feeling unpopular and unloved.

Improving care in long-term institutions will be a complex and demanding task. The first necessity is thorough, expert preadmission assessment to ensure that only patients who cannot be looked after at home will be consigned to long-term care. This may mean admission to a geriatric assessment/rehabilitation unit or a period of attendance at a day hospital. However it may be achieved, thorough assessment must be carried out with treatment of any identified disease and a determined attempt at rehabilitation.

Patients who require long-term care must be looked after by nurses who have special training in and good insight into the needs of this group of patients and their carers. In addition, the accommodation should be of good quality with single, homely rooms for a majority and well-designed furniture and equipment for all.

Interested medical staff must be available who are prepared to visit regularly and preferably are prepared to undergo special training. In the United Kingdom we have the Diploma in Geriatric Medicine of Royal College of Physicians, London, and there is a rather higher qualification now available in the United States.

Is it ever defensible that a nursing home with fifty or sixty residents should have thirty or forty different doctors in charge of patients? How can the nursing staff ever get to know these physicians, and how can they cope with whole ranges of different prescribing and treatment practices? Surely long-term institutions should appoint their own physicians who will meet the needs of these patients and offer appropriate support to the nursing staff.

Acute illness in residents should, whenever possible, be managed on-site, and this requires that doctors are prepared to visit patients and be involved in their care. In a 6-month period in our own ninety-bed long-stay unit, only three patients were transferred to acute care—two with serious gastrointestinal bleeding and one with hip fracture. They were all back within a few days or weeks. This contrasts markedly with the situation in many North American settings, where elderly patients in nursing homes are sent forthwith to emergency rooms for acute admission while all they may need is (often simple) treatment from their physicians plus a few days extra nursing care from their usual nursing attendants.

Needless to say there should be readily available expert advice from the geriatrician and members of the geriatric team. Physicians' extra efforts and skill used for these patients should be reflected in remuneration. Almost nothing could be more wasteful and inhumane than sending an old lady into acute care from a nursing home simply because she has a straightforward RTI or UTI which could very appropriately be treated within the home.

CONCLUSION

Focusing on the five objectives is appropriate for developed countries, whereas in developing countries some of the objectives are not currently relevant. Prevention and case-finding ought to receive priority in all settings, and the establishment of a specialist geriatric service is now essential for any country with 10 percent or more of the population in the elderly category. For developing countries, there is a need for some internists to undergo training in geriatric medicine, and they, together with similarly trained nurses, will provide the shock troops to spearhead the drive to establish better standards and new practices in care of the elderly.

Underlying all these efforts must be a concerted educational campaign aimed at the general public, the elderly and their carers, planners and politicians, and, by no means least important, health professionals.

Resources must be provided in a balanced continuum and be readily and speedily available on identification of need.

Professionals must be taught to appreciate the essential nature of the multidisciplinary team approach and the satisfaction to be had from such working practices.

The question will be raised, "How are we to afford all this?" The answer is that not to plan in this comprehensive fashion will undoubtedly be more expensive as elderly people find their way into inappropriate and costly settings where they will fare badly. Not only is this approach economically sound, it is also sound from every humane point of view.

SUGGESTED READINGS

Exercise and Muscle Strength

Aniansson, A., Grimby, G., Rundgren, A., Svanborg, A., Orlander, J. (1980) Physical Training in Old Men. *Age and Ageing,* 9: 186–189.

Grimby, G. (1986). Physical Activity and Muscle Training in the Elderly, *Acta Medica Scandinavica,* Suppl. 7-11, 233–237.

Young, A. (1986). Exercise Physiology in Geriatric Practice, *Acta Medica Scandinavica,* Suppl. 7-11, 227–232.

Case-Finding

Hendriksen, C., Lund. E., Stromgard, F. (1984) Consequences of Assessment and Intervention among Elderly People: A Three Year Randomised Controlled Trial. *British Medical Journal,* 289, 1522–1524.

Taylor, R. C., Buckley, E. G. (1984) Editors: Preventive Care of the Elderly: A Review of Current Developments. Occasional Paper No. 35, *Journal of Royal College of General Practitioners,* 14 Princes Gate, Hyde Park, London SW7 1PU.

Williamson, J., in Williamson, J., Burley, L. E., Smith, R. G. (1987) Primary Care of the Elderly: A Practical Approach. John Wright & Sons.

Geriatric Consultation Teams

Barker, W. H., Williams, T. F., Zimmer, J. G., Van Buren, C., Vineed, C. J., Pickard, S. G. (1985) Geriatric Consultation Teams in Acute Hospitals. *Journal of the American Geriatrics Society,* 33, 6, 422–428.

Burley, L. E., Currie, C. T., Smith, R. G., Williamson, J. (1979) Contribution from Geriatric Medicine within Acute Medical Wards. *British Medical Journal,* 23: 90–92.

Orthopedic Surgery

Kennie, D. C., Reid, J., Richardson, I. R., Kiamari, A. A., Kelt, C. (1988) Effectiveness of Geriatric Rehabilitative Care after Fractures of the Proximal Femoral Neck in Elderly Women. *British Medical Journal,* 297, II, 1083–1086.

Reid, J., Kennie, D. C. (1989) Geriatric Rehabilitative Care after Fractures of the Proximal Femur: One Year Follow-up of a Randomised Controlled Trial. *British Medical Journal,* 299, II, 25–26.

Section Four

Policy Issues

This section asks the presenters to identify the key policy issues expected to develop from the present to the year 2020. What social policy issues can be expected to have the greatest impact on health policy and the influence nurses, physicians, social scientists and others may have on these developments are discussed. The question of the effectiveness of the health professions in policy development and the preparation necessary for increased effectiveness are unifying themes in these chapters. There is considerable agreement among the various authors, but distinct differences appear between members of diverse disciplines.

Chapter 17

Improving Health Status through Health Policy: An Agenda for Nursing Leaders

David Mechanic

Beginning in the post–World War II period, there have been remarkable reductions in mortality in much of the developing world, largely a consequence of the reduction of infant and child mortality.[1] These advances have occurred more rapidly than might have been expected on the basis of the prior experience of developed countries and despite considerable economic disadvantage in many regions where mortality has substantially declined.[2] Such nations and regions as Sri Lanka, Kerala, Jamaica, Cuba, China, and Costa Rica have achieved levels of health well beyond what their economic positions might have led us to predict and comparable to health indices of more developed nations. In light of this experience, the WHO campaign for health for all has more substance than might be apparent.

WHO's definition of health as a state of "complete physical, mental and social well-being" and its recent inclusion of spiritual well-being might strike the tough-minded as a definition divorced from the tough realities. Despite its utopian character, it gives centrality to two important and incontestable facts: Health is shaped fundamentally by culture, society, and environment, and it is mostly at the margins that medical care makes a difference. Most of the large advances in health status result from basic improvements in education, economic status, nutrition, lifestyles, and the environment. The WHO statement also reminds us that physical illness and psychological discomfort, however influenced by inheritance and biology, arise in no small measure from conditions in the family, at work, and in the community more broadly.

Patients' experiences of illness reflect both responses to noxious influences and ways of adapting to intolerable stresses that tax their capacities and spirit.

In considering how to meet the goal of health for all, there seem to be at least three general pathways. The first involves social and economic development. It is not my intention to examine in any detail the social and political factors that affect the fate of so many of the world's economies except to note the importance of investments in human resources within a nation. There is impressive evidence that schooling has a remarkable effect on the health of populations[3] and that female schooling, in particular, is linked with substantially reduced fertility and lower maternal and infant mortality.[4] In the long range, social policies that ensure schooling and literacy, particularly literacy and participation among women, have great potential to improve health. Countries with a high proportion of females in primary school in 1960 had the lowest infant mortality rates in 1982 and the highest expectation of life at birth.[5] In short, what a nation does to educate its youth, to ensure adequate nutrition, to provide meaningful economic and employment opportunities, and to give people a stake in their society is likely to have major direct and indirect effects on the health of populations.

At the levels of public health and health services, there is abundant evidence that ensuring safe sources of water, appropriate management of waste, adequate sanitation, and aggressive immunization and family planning services are indispensable to promoting health. Moreover, effective organization of prenatal care, safe childbirth practice, appropriate infant nutrition and care, and the expeditious management of diarrhea and bacterial disease are extremely powerful devices for reducing child mortality and increasing longevity in a society. Nations that have committed themselves to a well-developed primary health care system, accessible to all social strata and supported by outreach and educational programs, have been remarkably successful in reducing infant and child mortality. Systems of primary health care, properly balanced in relation to high-cost, technically oriented tertiary care, offer a powerful option for relatively poor countries to achieve health indices comparable to more economically advanced nations. Such countries as Cuba and China, with their emphasis on the local organization of primary care services as a matter of national policy, have made rapid progress. Other countries with less developed and less aggressive public policies concerning accessibility to primary care services have done well also by educational policies that result in a high population demand for appropriate and effective medical services—a product of an orientation that has been called "psychological modernity."[6] Populations that have high levels of psychological modernity and also well-organized primary health care systems do especially well across the range of health indicators.

Alex Inkeles, who coined the concept of psychological modernity suggested that persons with this orientation take on "new transformative roles within their societies and their more immediate social networks."[7] One can debate the best definition of the orientation, but whatever the specific elements, they fall into both cognitive and action dimensions. At the cognitive level, individuals with such orientations are open to new experiences, believe in the efficacy of science and medicine, have ambition for themselves and their children, believe in planning their affairs in advance, and are interested in national and international news and politics. At the action level, such persons are more active in voluntary organizations and politics, practice birth control, are quicker to adopt innovative practices, keep their children in school and encourage technical occupations, and are supportive of social change. The single most important predictor of "psychological modernity" is schooling. Inkeles maintains that much of the schooling effect is not from curricula but results from the structuring of the classroom situation such as ordered sequences of activities and scheduling and to modeling and other psychosocial processes.[8] Factory work is not as strong a predictor as schooling but is believed to have similar effects in developing nations through inducing an orientation to time and scheduling and other types of personal discipline important for adaptation in complex environments. In making these distinctions, it is important to note that even in highly developed nations such as the United States, we have subgroups characterized by "low psychological modernity."

In a paper some 15 years ago,[9] I argued that nations throughout the world were focusing on five basic medical care challenges that had profound implications for the quality of health care and ultimately health:

1 Allocating resources so as to diminish inequalities in health care

2 Developing approaches to link the provision of health care services to the needs of defined communities for which the providers of health care could be held responsible

3 Integrating the fragmented components of health services and linking health with related social and welfare services

4 Overcoming excessive specialization and maintaining the integrity and vitality of primary health services

5 Improving the efficiency and effectiveness of health services and containing the escalation of medical care costs

These challenges seem even more important today as many nations experience increasing economic resource constraints while facing rising expectations, growing numbers of elderly and others with chronic diseases and disabilities, and the seeming imperatives of dynamic biotechnological development. The evidence suggests that social policies that are sensitive to the needs for modernity but also set a framework for access to health care offer their populations the largest health potential. Adjudicating the demands for increasingly sophisticated care by the educated strata against the need for equitable access for all is a source of tension in many societies including the United States and the United Kingdom, requiring firm policy decisions at all levels of government.

There is still much-needed effort in many countries to provide essential public health services, basic primary care, and adequate nutrition. And in much of the developing world, and in subgroups within the developed countries, much morbidity and mortality could be prevented through application of relatively simple public health and basic medical care initiatives. Nevertheless, the developing countries are increasingly experiencing a shifting burden of morbidity characterized by chronic disease, accidents and violence, and a range of social pathologies including substance abuse. The AIDS epidemic, and the spread of HIV infection, particularly in Africa, also pose enormous problems of care and challenges to health education and behavior change strategies. Increasingly, the developing world will have to address such issues as maintaining function, preventing secondary disability, and reducing suffering, problems which loom large on the agendas of developed nations.

FUTURE CHALLENGES

The challenge for all nations is how to truly get value for money expended in the health care arena. Although the wealth of nations is associated with the health of populations, expenditures for medical care are only weakly if at all associated with indices of mortality and morbidity. It seems clear that wealth as it affects the integrity of living environments, basic public health practice, and healthful styles is more important than its enablement of sophisticated biotechnology and tertiary medical care.

The importance of healthful habits and behavior is now well-recognized throughout the world, and the ideas of prevention and health promotion receive increasing attention. It seems self-evident that if we prevent illness we not only avoid a great deal of suffering and disability but also can contain costs. What appears self-evident, however, is not necessarily true; the field of prevention needs much tougher evaluation than has been the norm. Many prevention efforts fail because they are based on poor knowledge and flimsy premises about the causes of disorders and how they might be modified. Other interventions are efficacious and prevent disease and disability but are so difficult to target and must be directed to so many potential recipients, that they are very costly relative to alternative investments. In considering prevention approaches, we have to examine the efficiency of the intervention, the size of the target group relative to those truly at risk, and the costs involved.[10] Some approaches such as immunization may involve an effective intervention requiring a single encounter; others such as exercise promotion involve a lifetime of repeated choices. The area of prevention requires tough thinking not only about the cost-effectiveness of varying approaches but also about the relative value of modifying attitudes and behavior in contrast to regulatory approaches using tax incentives, new technologies, or legal restrictions.

In respect to personal health services, an accessible source of basic medical care services that assumes continuing responsibility for dealing with episodic acute illness and longitudinal monitoring of health needs is an es-

sential component of health maintenance in any society. Central functions include maternal and child care, family planning, treatment of common acute disorders, and management of chronic illness. Depending on finances and priorities, the organization of primary care may involve different levels of personnel with varying preparation and skills. The existing evidence indicates that well-trained nurses can carry out the vast majority of primary care functions, and often perform at levels equal to or superior to medically trained personnel. In many areas of the world, personnel with much less training than nurses carry out these functions and often do a creditable job. In such instances a strong management system is essential that ensures that the range of primary care functions are adequately performed, that the quality of care is monitored, and that treatment personnel receive feedback and opportunities to upgrade their skills. The fact that there are some 37 million uninsured persons in the United States, many without a source of primary care, suggests that maintenance of an adequate system of primary care remains problematic even in some of the most wealthy nations.

Hospital care, of course, is the most expensive component of care in technologically advanced countries, and in many of the developing nations manufactured drugs also constitute a major financial burden. In each case there is compelling reason to use these expensive resources wisely not only to conserve scarce financing but also to avoid iatrogenic illness. In the United States there is extraordinary variation in the use of expensive medical and surgical modalities from one area to another, and most informed observers believe that a significant amount of what is done is wasteful and of little utility. The challenge is how to use these resources more wisely and to balance expensive technical care with accessible basic care and attention to the increasing burden of chronic disease and the prevention of secondary disabilities.

With the extension of longevity and changing demographic structures, every country in the world will have to come to terms with a large aging population and the chronic diseases associated with aging. In 1980, only 250 million of the world's population were 65 years of age or older. By the year 2000, this elderly population is estimated to increase to 403 million, and by 2025 to 760 million.[11] By 2025, 70 percent of all the world's elderly persons will be in the less developed countries. Although the aging of populations is much more pronounced in more developed nations than their less developed counterparts, the growing numbers of elderly throughout the world will pose extraordinary socioeconomic and political issues for all nations.

Many nations striving to develop their economics and improve conditions of life are ill-prepared to respond to the morbidity of the elderly and the growing challenge of long-term care. Many of the less developed countries have relatively traditional kinship structures and norms supporting strong family responsibility for the elderly. Ironically, these traditional forms are being eroded with social and economic development, and the increasing prevalence of older populations will create large social stresses.

The elderly are, of course, a large and heterogeneous segment of a nation's population with needs varying from health promotion and maintenance to long-term care for incapacitating physical and mental disorders. Apart from those limited instances where science and technology have made possible the extension of life and function with quite extraordinary techniques, much of the challenge of care for the elderly is to facilitate people's abilities to perform the tasks of everyday living and to facilitate coping with the inevitable and, at times, irreversible illnesses and disabilities so

as to protect the quality of life, control pain, and preserve support.[12] Such services, in contrast to technologically oriented hospital care, may require different contexts for treatment, a different mix of personnel, and a different philosophy of care. Perhaps, most importantly, such services require a longitudinal point of view, attention to the patient's social context, and a broad view of sociomedical needs. Excellent technical care in a narrow sense must underlie these efforts, but such care must be allied with a range of social supports and other services for facilitating coping.

Given the diversity of social systems, and range of financing mechanisms found around the world, it is impractical to discuss briefly the alternative options available for organizing and paying for long-term care of the elderly or others with serious chronic disease. The United States faces critical problems in responding to present and impending long-term needs, and despite per capita medical care expenditures of $2500 per year, we have yet to develop a viable financial or community framework for organizing and paying for the needed services. The system in the United States is far too medicalized, and institutionally dependent, to be a useful model for other nations or to provide the caring framework necessary for its own people.

There are constraints, however, that apply to all. Given the dynamism of biomedical science and technology, the possibilities for expensive interventions and the extension of life are awesome, and the potentials for imbalance among interventions quite dangerous. In every country, the elite demand the "best" that science and technology make possible, often squandering the resources essential to develop an accessible, equitable, and relatively effective system of care for the whole population. Every nation must confront the scarcity of resources and the need to allocate intelligently to ensure the largest potential effects on health status, function, and quality of life. The pressures to make tough tradeoffs in a context of growing population demands will engage the time and energies of political leaders all over the world.

THE CHALLENGE TO NURSING LEADERSHIP

Nursing has had a strong traditional commitment to public health, maternal and child care, the management of chronic disease, and psychosocial interventions as complements of its traditional technical skills. Thus, it is particularly well positioned for the changing medical care arena and impending policy debates about the allocation of the medical care dollar. These debates ultimately focus on values, and their resolution involves a blend of influences including perceptions of population needs, professional self-interest, and concerns about power and money. Facts and technical studies inform the debate and contribute to its resolution, but major issues of broad public concern are resolved less by scientific inquiry and more by politics.

Nursing has substantial unrealized power in the emerging situation. Long a female profession, subservient to medicine, its assertiveness has been limited both by sex discrimination and the legacy of its religious and charitable history. Both sex and calling have been used to justify the relatively low wages of nurses, their limited autonomy, and their meager powers in setting priorities for health care or in managing health services. Nurses themselves have had less professional consciousness than would be optimal, their alliances tied more to family and local area and hospital than to larger health care agendas or professional assertiveness. When dissatisfied, they are more likely to exit, using Hirshman's useful term,[13] than to exercise a forceful voice in changing their role and the conditions of their work.

The potential political strength of the nursing profession comes from its numbers, its many central roles in health care, and the fact that nurses have the loyalties of vast numbers of patients to whom they provide caring services. This potential, if focused effectively, could be extremely influential in the evolving debates. Focus depends on effective nursing spokespersons, well-informed on the issues, who can command the loyalties of the nursing community but who can also articulate the issues for broader populations.

As a sympathetic observer of the nursing profession and its efforts to upgrade its standing and influence, I have some concerns. Nursing leaders have dealt with the uncertain position of the nursing profession through a number of strategies that may yield some short-term gains but may be costly in the long run. Resenting the dominance of physicians, some nursing leaders have sought niches where they more readily can exercise autonomy. Such niches are almost always in specialties outside the hospital and removed from the most seriously ill. The legitimate resentments of nurses have sometimes resulted in "doctor-bashing" as well, which may be cathartic but doesn't really focus on the real dilemmas of the division of labor in health care. Many important changes are occurring in the larger health arena, with new emphases on prevention and health promotion, but the core of both medicine and nursing will continue to be the care of seriously ill patients. Nursing leaders have to work cooperatively with physician leaders and administrators to develop more appropriate working arrangements that make the best use of nursing skills and offer a rewarding professional experience. Neither escaping into more independent niches nor doctor-bashing confront the central issues. Nursing and medicine are inevitably interdependent.

One central issue is the preparation of nurse

leaders for policy roles in all levels of government and the health care structure and in research. Nurses must be prepared conceptually and scientifically to hold their own in public forums, and some do remarkably well in these contexts. But some confuse nursing rhetoric with carefully considered analysis. These patterns are exacerbated by the growing insularity of nursing as a profession, which seeks to educate emerging nurse leaders substantially within their own domains.

In my experience as a mentor of a number of outstanding nurse researchers, I am troubled by the protectionism that excludes some from nursing faculty positions because they lack an advanced degree in nursing. These are registered nurses with outstanding training who are now excluded from nursing leadership because they have chosen broader, and probably superior, educational preparation to that typically provided by graduate programs in nursing. This exclusionary orientation finds expression in that rapid proliferation of Ph.D. programs in nursing which now increasingly substitutes for the Ph.D. in education and in the basic biomedical disciplines.

I understand and can empathize with the motivations that propel the diffusion of doctoral programs in nursing, but I believe that the proliferation of weak programs can damage future nursing leadership by providing less adequate preparation for talented nurses than is possible. Nurses are increasingly directed into nursing Ph.D. programs and away from the strongest Ph.D. programs in their speciality. Such alternatives to traditional training may prepare them poorly to compete successfully with others no more talented but better trained. If nursing insists, however mistakenly, on the urgency of developing autonomous research training programs, it has a special responsibility to exercise leadership in monitoring these programs and ensuring minimal standards.

In sum, nursing leadership could build on traditional nursing ethics, a clear grasp of the policy issues and dilemmas, and an appreciation of its potential power base. Nursing leaders must be trained as rigorously as possible, developing opportunities to articulate their values and goals in public forums and policy arenas. To successfully alter their professional roles and standing, nurses must learn to function in a range of settings and to forge coalitions with other professional and consumer groups. The particular issues to be addressed may vary from one nation to another and over time, but nurses everywhere share a commitment to promoting the quality of patient function, an appropriate objective for health care in the next century.

REFERENCES

1 N. Birdsall, "Thoughts on Good Health and Good Government," *Daedalus* 118, (1) (Winter 1989), 89–117.
2 J. C. Caldwell, "Routes to Low Mortality in Poor Countries," *Population and Development Review,* 12 (1986), 171–220.
3 David Mechanic, "Socioeconomic Status and Health: An Examination of Underlying Processes," in J. P. Bunker, D. S. Gomby, and B. H. Kehrer, eds., *Pathways to Health: The Role of Social Factors.* Conference held at the Kaiser Family Foundation, Menlo Park, California, March 25–27, 1987.
4 Caldwell, "Routes to Low Mortality."
5 *Ibid.*
6 Alex Inkeles and David Smith, *Becoming Modern* (Cambridge: Harvard University Press, 1974).
7 Alex Inkeles, *Exploring Individual Modernity* (New York: Columbia University Press, 1983).
8 *Ibid.*
9 David Mechanic, "Ideology, Medical Technology, and Health Care Organization in Modern Nations," *American Journal of Public Health* 65 (1975), 241–247.
10 Louise Russell, *Is Prevention Better Than*

Cure? (Washington, D. C.: Brookings Institution, 1986).

11 P. M. Hauser, "Aging and Increasing Longevity of World Population," in H. Hafner, G. Moschel, and N. Sartonius, eds., *Mental Health in the Elderly: A Review of the Present State of Research* (Berlin: Springer-Verlag, 1986), pp. 9–14.

12 David Mechanic, "Health Care and the Elderly," *Annals of the American Academy of Political and Social Science* 503 (1989), 89–98.

13 Albert O. Hirschman, *Exit, Voice and Loyalty* (Cambridge: Harvard University Press, 1970).

Chapter 18

Health and Social Policy in Australia: The Role and Professionalism of Nursing

Paul Gross

Australia is a nation of 16.6 million people. Its demographic profile is not dissimilar to the United States and Canada, a political system that is based on "federalism" (viz., a federal government sharing powers and tax revenue with seven state and territory governments), a national universal compulsory health insurance system (Medicare) that is partly funded by a 1.25 percent levy on taxable income (with the poor paying no levy), an oversupply of acute hospital beds (5.3 acute beds per 1000 population which are used at the rate of about 1500 bed-days per 1000 population), an oversupply of doctors, a shortage of nurses (about 140,000 nurses, or 94 per 10,000 population) and a growing awareness of the social and economic impact of chronic illness as the proportion of persons aged 65 years and over increases from 11 percent in 1989 to 16 percent in 2015. In 1989, total national health expenditures will exceed A$23 billion, roughly A$1500 per person—and the health sector will consume about 8 percent of gross domestic product (GDP).

In 1989, the medical profession in Australia has been effectively "balkanized" by the 1985 doctors dispute in New South Wales, the enmity between the Australian Medical Association (AMA) and the Royal Australian College of General Practitioners over the two-tier free system introduced by the federal governnment in August 1989, and the apparent inability of the AMA to either handle the needs of a burgeoning number of medical specialties or overcome the reluctance of a large number of young medical graduates to join the AMA.

The nursing profession in Australia is only slightly happier. The conversion of basic nurse education programs from hospitals to colleges of advanced education is taking place at the same time as inadequate roles, salaries, and conditions of service cause an exodus of trained nurses from hospitals to occupations other than nursing. The resultant shortage of nurses comes when the complexity of case mix in acute hospitals and nursing homes is increasing as a result of government policies affecting both areas. Domiciliary nursing services, while available, are used at a annual rate that is about 25 percent of the current U.S. rates for home health care (Gross, 1989).

MAJOR HEALTH POLICY ISSUES TO THE YEAR 2020

Australia's health and social welfare system is at yet another watershed due to changes in government policies affecting the funding of acute hospitals, nursing homes, hostels (which offer accommodation for the aged and chronically ill), home and community care, and retirement benefits. The major health policy issues affecting the evaluation of health care to the year 2020 have not been addressed systematically by national inquiries or by a consensus of the major interest groups in health care. Some selected issues to which nursing inputs could make a critical contribution are summarized below; although this chapter's focus is mainly on Australia, some of the conclusions and tables may have relevance in other developing nations. The chapter's focus on specific types of "high-tech" medical technology in Appendix 18-1 make it less relevant to the emerging needs of developing nations.

Health Outcomes: The Roles of Individuals and Governments

Australia's health profile—and the subsequent use of resources to change that profile—is heavily influenced by the preponderance of the diseases of modern civilization (heart disease, stroke, cancer, and accidents). Compared with 1985, 500,000 extra persons over the age of 85 will see the year 2015 and most of them will be affected by chronic illnesses that are disabling. Increased longevity will probably affect the demand for services associated with acute illnesses. There has been very little

debate between or within the major political parties or amongst the general public about the sharing of responsibilities in the achievement of an improved health status for all Australians. For example, a recent study for all Australian ministers of health (Gross and Taylor, 1988) found that three risk factors (smoking, high blood pressure, raised cholesterol) were responsible for about 25 percent of all the healthy days of life "lost" by Australians in 1986. These three risk factors are amenable to change, but others affecting the incidence of chronic illness are not as easily manipulated. The truth is that we do not yet know (1) how many Australians have a chronic illness due to disease, birth injury, injury, or aging, (2) whether these chronic disorders are preventable by the actions of individuals through self-care or national programs of prevention of chronic illness and disability, (3) whether these disorders are better treated by alternatives to the "medical model," and (4) whether Australia yet has in place (or in planning) the services that are needed to treat the profile of health disorders anticipated in the year 2020.

The potential effects of early intervention through primary care and of better compliance with established treatment are evident in the recent U.S. study of uninsured patients admitted to District of Columbia (D.C.) hospitals in 1987 (Levin / ICF, 1989). In that study, 24 percent of all uninsured admissions (36 percent if obstetric cases and trauma cases are added) might have been medically preventable with better primary care or better compliance with medical advice. Although this study is a guidepost to the potential effects of primary health care on hospital costs, it is also a useful indicator to the nursing profession that nurses can carry out such studies better than most other health professions. In addition, nurses have the potential to improve health outcomes through at least three other interventions:

• In the nurse's role in *policy analysis* and formulation within peak organizations affecting the planning of service needs for curative and preventive services for the year 2020

- In the nurse's role as a *primary health care practitioner* in preventing major disorders or in the modification of risk factors
- In the nurse's role as *researcher/analyst* of the costs of disease, the costs of health care, and the costing of strategies to reduce the effects of chronic illness and other risk factors

Outcomes in Health Care: Better Value for Money or More Money?

Any health system that consumes 8 percent of GDP is a visible target for cost containment for as long as expenditures on health care have

a 10 to 15 percent annual growth rate. In the past decade the three driving forces behind these increases in health expenditures have been population growth and composition (10 percent), the prices of goods and services and the wages of health personnel (60 percent), and the increased per capita use of health services and the increased intensity of use per contact with health services (30 percent). The effects of aging in these expenditures is evident in Table 18-1, drawn from a recent study by OECD (1985). The entries in the table for Australia do not reveal the full effects of an aging population on government or private household budgets. For example:

Table 18-1 Breakdown of Health Expenditure Increases in OECD Countries (Compound annual growth rates 1960–1984)

	Nominal expenditure	GDP deflator	Health prices	Relative prices	Real expenditure	Demography	Utilization/ intensity per person
Canada	12.5	6.1	5.6	−0.5	6.5	1.4	5.1
France	15.3	7.5	6.9	−0.6	7.9	0.8	7.0
Germany	10.1	4.3	5.6	1.2	4.2	0.4	3.8
Italy	17.6	10.5	10.5	0.0	6.5	0.5	5.9
Japan	16.8	5.7	6.0	0.3	10.2	1.1	9.1
United Kingdom	13.1	8.7	8.3	−0.4	4.4	0.3	4.1
United States	11.8	5.1	6.2	1.0	5.3	1.1	4.1
Big 7 average	13.9	6.8	7.0	0.1	6.4	0.8	5.6
Australia	13.7	7.2	9.5	2.2	3.8	1.6	2.1
Austria	11.3	5.1	8.3	3.0	2.8	0.3	2.5
Belgium	11.8	5.4	6.3	0.9	5.2	0.3	4.9
Denmark	14.1	8.2	8.2	0.0	5.4	0.5	5.0
Finland	15.4	8.8	8.1	−0.6	6.8	0.4	6.3
Greece	18.3	10.3	9.3	−1.0	8.3	0.7	7.5
Iceland	34.8	27.4	30.2	2.2	3.5	1.3	2.2
Ireland[a]	18.2	10.3	10.0	0.3	7.5	0.9	6.6
Netherlands[a]	13.7	6.2	8.4	2.1	4.9	1.0	3.9
Norway	14.5	7.1	8.4	1.3	5.6	0.6	5.0
Spain[b]	21.8	12.1	13.0	0.8	7.7	1.0	6.7
Sweden	13.7	7.3	6.0	−1.2	7.3	0.5	6.8
Switzerland[c]	12.1	5.0	6.7	1.7	5.1	0.9	4.2
13 country average	16.4	9.3	10.2	0.9	5.7	0.8	4.9
20 country average	15.5	8.4	9.1	0.6	5.9	0.8	5.1

[a] 1960–1983
[b] 1964–1984
[c] 1960–1982

Sources: Measuring Health Care 1960–1983, Paris, OECD, 1985, and OECD Secretariat estimates for 1984.

- 23 percent of all expenditure on health care by the federal government in 1984–1985 was directed at the 3.8 percent of the population aged 75 years and over.
- 17 percent of all federal government expenditure on medical services and 48 percent of expenditure on pharmaceutical benefits went for the care of persons aged 65 years and over (11 percent of the population), and the figures are 7 percent and 21 percent, respectively, for persons aged 75 years and over.
- 40 percent of all acute hospital bed-days are used by the 11 percent of the population aged 65 years and over.
- 95 percent of all nursing home bed-days are consumed by the same age group.
- In 1984–1985, the total per capita allocations by commonwealth and state govern-

ments for health care varied from $322 for persons aged 0 to 15 years to $1573 for persons aged 65 to 69 years to $4325 for persons aged 75 years and over. The mean per capita expenditure for all age groups was $716 (Table 18-2).

Australian policymakers have not reacted as quickly as U.S. legislators to conspicuous evidence that Australia has a surplus of acute beds that are overused, because economic incentives do not exist for doctors, administrators, or patients to find less costly, equally effective, and equal-quality services. Comparing the use of hospital services in two nations whose age composition is similar, Table 18-3 indicates the average length of stay in acute general hospitals (public and private)

Table 18-2 Government Outlays by Age, 1984–1985 ($ per capita)

	Age group										All age groups
	0–15	16–24	25–39	40–49	50–54	55–59	60–65	65–69	70–74	75*	
Social security and welfare											
Commonwealth	600	773	570	565	935	1353	2704	3682	4042	4546	1119
States	92	48	3	4	6	10	71	154	193	205	55
Total	691	821	573	568	941	1363	2776	3836	4234	4552	1174
Health											
Commonwealth	145	193	243	281	382	438	688	924	1091	2526	386
States	178	199	212	236	365	380	504	649	946	1799	330
Total	322	393	455	518	747	818	1192	1573	5027	4325	716
Education											
Commonwealth	392	821	179	76	46	17	16	7	7	7	280
States	1386	374	69	46	38	18	24	10	10	10	434
Total	1779	1195	248	122	84	35	40	17	17	17	714
Employment											
Commonwealth	5	231	60	46	34	26	5	—	—	—	59
States	—	—	—	—	—	—	—	—	—	—	—
Total	5	231	60	46	34	26	5	—	—	—	59
Total of Above											
Commonwealth	1142	2018	1051	968	1397	1834	3413	4613	5139	7079	1845
States	1656	621	284	286	409	408	600	813	1150	2015	819
Total	2798	2640	1335	1254	1806	2242	4012	5426	6289	9094	2663
Total relative to the average for all age groups	1.05	0.99	0.50	0.47	0.68	0.84	1.51	2.04	2.36	3.41	1.00

Source: EPAC: Economic effects of an aging population. Canberra, Economic Planning Advisory Council, Council Paper No. 29, January, 1988, p. 68.

Table 18-3 Costs of Compliance with Government Regulations

Relevant costs	Focus of regulations	Examples of costs affecting health care
Extra costs of administration	Standards; assessment forms	Costs of a DRG-like system of hospital reimbursement
Extra costs of production of services	Quality assurance	Extra costs of staff in a quality assurance system for hospital accreditation
Extra capital costs	Good manufacturing practice	Costs of extra equipment required to meet standards of good manufacturing practice for drugs and medical devices
Extra research and development costs	Alterations in equipment and procedures	Costs of research to meet government specifications for occupational health and safety
Extra costs due to loss of competitive position or sales because of regulation	Health insurance funds	Costs of compliance with government regulations not affecting other funds or foreign firms
Extra costs of uncertainty	Occupational health and safety	Costs of overcoming uncertainties in enabling legislation or costs of dealing with regulatory delays
Extra costs of delays in government approval of capital projects	Certificate of need	Costs of interest payments on borrowed capital for major hospital equipment
Extra costs of aborted projects	Certificate of need; drug approval	Costs of extended regulatory delays or revised standards that cause projects to be aborted
Extra costs of lost innovation	Health workforce licensure	Costs of regulations that specify the category of health personnel to be used rather than the standard of care to be provided, leading to the loss of incentive to fund more efficient methods
Costs of misallocation of resources	All forms of regulation	Allocation of resources to the equipment and personnel required to meet standards rather than to increased production efficiency or employment

in New South Wales and U.S. acute general hospitals *circa* 1986–1987. One can only surmise that a combination of policies not yet implemented in Australia (e.g. a DRG-like hospital reimbursement scheme, HMO-like methods of financing, and variants of "managed care") might reduce the average lengths of stay in Australian hospitals to levels that are now experienced in U.S. hospitals.

Such policies are likely to increase the complexity of case-mix in acute general hospitals and increase the share of the wage bill paid to nurses in a time of nursing shortages. It is fairly obvious to all but the myopic that new processes of industrial relations, budget formulation, cost control, and decision making are required as we move from an era where hospital budgets were assumed to be as nondebatable as the original tablets of stone given to Moses to an era in which there is more accountable management of all uses and users of resources. For nurses, the debate about whether we need cost containment or additional resources for health care is critical to their future roles and responsibilities as managers, planners, financial analysts, and researchers in health care.

New Medical Technology: Changing The Balance of Institutional and Non-Institutional Care

It has been estimated that "medical technology," *per se,* is associated with about one-third of the increase in total national health expenditures in the past 10 years. Although the precise impact of medical technology is difficult to estimate, the introduction by governments and the medical profession of formal processes of technology assessment in health care has been a significant development in most nations in the 1980s (Gross, 1989). The three major objectives of technology assessment are to identify emerging technologies that seem likely to influence the patterns, costs, and effectiveness of health care; to assess established technologies; and to disseminate information on emerging and established technologies that would facilitate their more effective diffusion and use in different types of health care.

The identification of an *emerging technology* is an embryonic art. In an era where many emerging technologies are moving care outside the hospital walls or enabling self-care, health workforce planners face some major challenges in estimating future health workforce demand and supply requirements, the complementarity of roles and responsibilities of different health personnel, and the basic and postbasic educational requirements of different types of health personnel when many emerging technologies reduce the demand for surgical and nursing procedures.

Appendix 18-1 summarizes some of the emerging medical technologies that seem likely to influence current patterns of hospital, medical, and nursing practice in most developed nations in the next 2 years. (A longer time horizon would produce a much larger list of examples, and a similar listing for a developing nation would produce a different list of technological imperatives that justify urgent attention.) Most national governments have not yet been persuaded to include nurses on national advisory panels for technology assessment in health care, which may say more about the relative power of the medical profession than about the qualifications of nurses to participate in technology assessment. Since most emerging medical technologies will affect the demand for and supply of the nursing profession, to not seek the appointment of the nursing profession to national advisory panels is a serious tactical error of the nursing profession.

Paying for Health Care: Reconciling Equity and Efficiency

The third health policy issue—an issue that dominates the policy landscape of most nations—is how to pay for health care in the 1990s in the face of rising government expenditures, a weakened international and national economy, changing patterns of risk factors and health disorders, and the inability of many citizens to afford health care without government subsidy. Three sets of issues are yet unresolved in Australia despite the existence since 1984 of a national universal compulsory health insurance scheme (Medicare). The first issue is whether Medicare is sustainable from its two major sources of revenue and the current coinsurance rates of 15 to 25 percent for medical services. At current trend rates of use of medical services and public hospital services, the answer is negative unless the federal government is prepared to increase the tax levy, increase the current subsidies from general revenue, or increase patient coinsurance rates for medical services. The second issue is whether the private health insurance funds should again be permitted to offer insurance for medical services. Medicare, for which no medical insurance can be offered by the funds, does not create positive incentives to reduce specific risk factors or the per capita use rate of medical services (currently about eight visits per person). A recent study (Gross and Taylor, 1988) identified how risk factor reduction may be achieved with alternative forms of health insurance and with modified community rating. The third issue relates to the high cost of changing in modern society, and to an unanswered question: How much should we be spending on dying patients? This particular question is often ignored by nurses who are unduly concerned with another issue, the apparently high correlation between the supply of new medical technology and the high costs of health care in the last year of life. In the U.S. Medicare program (which is a federal government program for the aged), 4.9 percent of Medicare beneficiaries who died in 1978 accounted for about 28 percent of Medicare expenditures; 30 percent of all such Medicare expenditures occurred in the last 30 days of life (Lubitz and Prihoda, 1984; Sutovsky, 1984). It should be noted here that the expenditures on the Medicare program are not the total expenditures on health care in the United States and that these percentages of Medicare expenditures are for the elderly population of the United States, who are obvious at higher risks of dying than the nonaged population and whose costs of care are also likely to be higher than those of nonaged persons.

If nurses are to influence the financing of health care to achieve specific goals for society, they need to identify accurately the causes of increases in expenditures on health care. A recent analysis of U.S. health expenditures from 1929 to 1980 (Berk, Monheit, and Hagan, 1988) identified some factors that are

directly relevant in the debate about the use of scarce resources and national policies for health care. The analysis suggested that there are at least two polar positions on cost containment, which will still be needed to ensure efficient use of all resources even if nurses want to argue that a higher share of GDP should be invested in health care. One school of thought believes that traditional types of health insurance do not provide the appropriate signals to either providers or users of health care, and financial incentives are required to discourage any inappropriate use of services. The other school believes that new medical technologies have caused a disproportionate share of available resources to go to the very sick, particularly the elderly (see for example Riley et al, 1986; Callahan, 1987). The major concern of this school is that as the nation ages, the share of society's resources required to sustain life will increase rapidly.

The U.S. analysis puts to rest a number of bogeymen. Using a wide range of data sets from 1929 to 1980, it finds that

• The top 1 percent of the U.S. population accounted for 26 percent of health expenditures in 1970, 27 percent in 1977, and 29 percent in 1980, the stability of these percentages suggesting that ". . . the diffusion of health care technology during this period had little impact on the concentration of health expenditures" (p. 51, emphasis not in original).
• "The contention that medical expenditures for high cost illnesses were escalating faster than other expenditures during the 1970s is not supported" (p. 51).
• The growth of "major medical" health insurance coverage . . . " may have contributed to the increased concentration of expenditures between 1963 and 1970" [and] ". . . the stability in expenditure distribution since 1970 is likely to reflect the relatively smaller growth in major medical and other health insurance coverage between 1970 and 1980" (p. 52).

• "The diffusion of certain types of medical technology (e.g., open heart surgery, coronary care units, intensive care units, electroencephalography)" . . . also may have contributed to the increased concentration of expenditures between 1963 and 1970" (p. 53).

• "The most noticeable difference in the high-user population is that it is getting older" (p. 54; of the highest 1 percent of users, 32.1 percent were elderly in 1970, 40.1 percent in 1977, and 43.4 percent in 1980).

• "The poor are twice as likely as the general population to be represented in the high-cost population, while the elderly are four times as likely to be in the high-expense group" (p. 56).

• Overall, ". . . almost half of all Americans account for less than 5 percent of total expenditures" (p. 58).

These findings are significant in the future design of equitable and efficient methods of paying for health care in the United States and other nations which have similar groups of high-users, particularly elderly high-users. If catastrophic health insurance is proposed (i.e., health insurance coverage begins once a certain "catastrophic" limit of expenditures has been exceeded in a given period), such insurance seems to increase the concentration of high-cost expenditures in all expenditures, so cost containment efforts are still required even with a catastrophic health insurance scheme. Second, the authors indicated that ". . . unless society is willing to devote more resources to health care or can markedly improve the efficiency of health care delivery, increased access to both preventive and catastrophic care will not be achieved" (p. 58).

For nurses, the cumulative messages of this U.S. study are quite profound. First, nurses can and must be involved in debates about health care financing and assessments of what cause of expenditures to increase. Second, health financing policies that assume either that medical technology is the "villain" behind the rise in national health expenditures or that aging will not affect the concentration of such expenditures are unlikely to benefit the nation's health.

Third, the use of inaccurate statistics to emphasize the shortfalls of modern medical technology is unlikely to lead to an increased share in total wages for the nursing profession or to a real increase in total national health expenditures. A policy of blanket denigration of medical technology is as mindless as a policy of blanket endorsement of all medical technology. The sustained involvement of nurses in the assessment of medical technology is long overdue, as indicated further on. Fourth, the U.S. analysis emphasized that "cost containment efforts that target the use of average consumers will not have as large an impact on health expenditures as a policy which concentrates on the high cost users." Such a conclusion leads to policies such as "managed care" which actively promote high-quality but lower cost alternatives to traditional (institution-based) care. Nurses will surely seek a major role in managed care, particularly in the management process of such care. Fifth, the U.S. analysis identifies some potential problems in the funding of prevention programs if the concentration of high-cost users is not reduced. Nurses aleady have an active role in health promotion and prevention in primary health care, and they cannot be oblivious to the future problems of paying for health care if the usage of high-cost users is not resolved by interventions such as managed care.

The health financing issue directly affects the roles and reimbursement of the health professions. In Australia, Medicare allows only the patients of medical practitioners, psychologists, and optometrists to receive rebates of the charges made by these health professions. The patients of private nurses cannot attract rebates for home nursing services or for other screening services, and nurses receive most of their reimbursement from four sources: salaries from government hospital and primary health care services and private hospitals, fees for private domiciliary nursing services based on negotiated schedules with the Department of Veterans Affairs, payments made by private home health care patients, and salaries received from large domiciliary nursing services (mainly funded by state governments with some federal government subsidy) in the major capital cities. The concept of a nurse practitioner is not well developed in the urban areas of Australia, although rural nursing services obviously benefit from the large number of nurses who perform services normally carried out by medical practitioners. Although community-based nurses are actively involved in health promotion and prevention, the major constraints on an expanded clinical role for nurses in curative services are legislative provisions. Unlike other nations, those legislative restraints on professional licensure have not been relaxed by governments. In other nations, nurses are reimbursed for "advanced practice," although action taken by the U.S. Health Care Financing Administration in New Mexico in late September 1989 will discontinue payment for nurse practitioner services, forcing rural clinics to retrench nurse practitioners. The reimbursement of health services in rural areas promises to be a contentious battlefield unless national governments recognize that reimbursement policies that are designed mainly for urban health services may have counterintuitive effects in rural areas (U.S. Senate, 1988).

Regulation of Health Care and The Health Professions

A fourth health policy issue involves an expanded role for the private sector (a concept loosely and often inaccurately labeled as "privatization") and the potential effects of a less regulated health care environment. As in many other nations, Australia has not yet come to grips with the many dimensions and ramifications of "privatization" or "procompetitive" policies. Much of the furor in the embryonic debate has occurred in New South Wales—where the state government has encouraged the private sector to construct and operate private hospitals on the same grounds as large public hospitals. The NSW government has also indicated its intent to follow the U.K. initiative of contracting with the private sector for the provision of some hospital services (e.g. cleaning, laundry, and linen), but it does not expect the resultant savings to exceed 10 to 15 percent of the current costs.

The potential effects of "privatization" in its many forms are reviewed elsewhere (Gross, 1987), and the effects of procompetitive policies on the use of medical technology and the roles of different health professions have not been reviewed extensively in Australia. Studies by OECD (OECD, 1982) indicate that (1) the privileges of the established health professions are being challenged to eliminate restrictive practice, (2) there is very little effective competition between the public and private sectors, (3) government restrictions on advertising by certain professions may increase the costs of health care to consumers, and (4) the current monopolies of some professions should be further limited by changes in professional licensure requirements and easing of advertising restrictions on fees and qualifications. A study by the Office of Technology Assessment of the U.S. Congress (OTA, 1982) identified other aspects of "competition" that might affect the diffusion, use, and costs of new medical technologies. Obviously there are many unknowns affecting policies for privatization and competition (see for example Langwell, 1982; Langwell and Moore, 1982; GAO, 1982; Pauly and Langwell, 1983; Weisbrod 1981), and the effects on health expenditures of "privatization" and "competition" *per se* in Australia or other nations are far from self-evident

(Logan, Green, and Woodfield, 1989). Nursing organizations have not always been visible in the resolution of some of these debates on paying for care.

SOCIAL POLICY ISSUES AFFECTING HEALTH POLICY

Social policy in Australia is not always in harmony with health policy—which in the past decade could be more accurately described as policies for health care financing. First, thanks to the work of the Better Health Commission, there is a partial national consensus on appropriate goals for "health" and how to improve health status. Second, until April 1988 there was no agreement between federal, state, and territorial ministers for health about priorities for a concerted attack on modifiable risk factors through prevention. Third, there is still no agreement within the relevant federal ministries on the preferred methods of linking social security benefits for the aged with tax and health financing policies. Fourth, although isolated papers have discussed the likely impact and needs of an aging society (e.g., EPAC, 1988), there is very little consistent evidence that governments, opposition parties, or the public at large yet recognize that some major social issues affecting health policy are unresolved. For example:

• What is Australia's potential role in the emerging Asian economic zone? What are the implications of our current economic linkages and dependencies for future trade investment in the health sector and the assurance of essential medical supplies; the implications for appropriate goals for "health" and foreign aid responsibilities, migration policies, and related health services needs?
• In a multicultural Australia, what specific health care needs are not being met by established health services, and what are the implications for future workforce training of policies for self-development, self-care, com-

munity care, and ethnic-specific alternatives to mainstream medical services?
• What are the specific needs for extra resources for health care in urban and rural areas, and do existing policies adversely affect the health of rural Australia?
• What are the implications of an aging society for the ability of governments to sustain their existing commitments in health care, to meet the new needs associated with a higher incidence of chronic disease, and to link alternative types of home and community care to both the formal and informal caring networks (the informal caring network of friends and relatives provide about 80 percent of the care needed by the aged and chronically ill in Australia)?
• In a just society, what are the responsibilities of individuals, taxpayers, governments, and corporations in providing for the financial and health care needs of retirement? How can essential health care and related welfare services be made available to meet the needs of the aged and chronically ill at an affordable cost? What will be the tax revenue base in the year 2020, given variable unemployment rates, an increasing dependency ratio and marital breakup, and smaller family size? What is the desirable mix of public and private effort? What incentives should governments provide to ensure greater personal effort where such effort is feasible and desirable? What safety nets are required for those who cannot provide for retirement through savings during the working life or related retirement benefits?

One fundamental dilemma of an aging, multicultural society such as Australia is to reconcile the needs of all age groups in social justice. The fundamental economic dilemma is evident in Table 18-2, which reveals that across four major areas of social policy (social security and welfare, health, education and employment), per capita government outlays vary widely by age group. What the table does not show is that as the nation ages, the per capita allocations increase significantly in the older age groups, reflecting the demands of the aged. Australia has of yet addressed two related issues: whether subsidies to the aged will have to be contained in fairness to taxpayers and other age groups, and whether there are alternative methods of providing essential health care at a lower per capita cost, e.g., through variants of "managed care"? Any evolution toward managed care of the aged and chronically ill has profound implications for the roles of different health professions, particularly nursing. Although not discussed further here, the prevalence of chronic illnesses of all major origins (congenital condition, accidents, and disease) requires alternatives to the traditional medical and social models of care (based mainly on "cure"), which would mean that variants of managed care in Australia are not likely to reduce the costs of chronic illness in Australia. Current cost containment policies in Australia and our traditional preoccupation with acute treatment discriminate against persons with chronic illness. Australia is not the only nation to offend in this regard, and nurses have not yet directed the public debate on chronic illness to emphasize how the strengths of nursing actually lie in a model of prevention of chronic illness, which refocuses attention on (1) the patient as a person and (2) "professionalism" in an era of chronic illness.

INFLUENCING HEALTH AND SOCIAL POLICY: STRATEGIES AND ROLES OF HEALTH PROFESSIONALS AND SOCIAL SCIENTISTS

The roles and influence of different health professions in policy analysis and implementation have not attracted widespread study in Australia. In health policy making, many nations, including Australia, have seen the emergence of the economist as a major force. Located within Prime Minister's Department, Treasury Department, Economic Planning Unit, and sometimes in ministries of Health, the economist has assumed much of the influence formerly exerted up to the mid-70s by medical advisers within ministries of health or other

related national advisory structures. If this view of the movement of power and influence is valid, a corollary is that the health professions are currently not as effective in policy formulation or policy analysis as they were up to the mid-1970s. Another corollary is that many academic advisers have also lost their former positions of influence in policy formulation, mainly because the policy "solutions" required these days are acutely tuned to the economics of government budgets, the requirements of financial institutions who underwrite investments of the private sector in health care, and the need to shift some of the costs of health care from government budgets to private households, private employers, or private health insurance funds. Most advisers from disciplines other than economics and cost accounting are poorly equipped to advise in this environment.

In Australia, consumers have emerged as an influential force in health policy making. The federal government has provided generous funding for the support of Consumer Health Forum, the Health Issues Centre in Victoria, and community health councils in some states. In the area of health care technology assessment, the federal government has recently announced its intent to appoint a consumer representative and a trade union representative to the National Health Technology Advisory Panel (NHTAP), which does not yet have a representative of the nursing profession.

The medical profession is a diminishing influence on health policy making in Australia. Because of the continuing fragmentation of the political inputs of medical practitioners in major policy issues, the medical profession has not satisfactorily resolved a number of challenges: the oversupply of doctors, the emergence of new health professions, and / or the more active involvement of established professions (e.g., pharmacy) in community health care; the overt policies of government to fragment the political and professional roles of the medical associations and some of the royal colleges of medicine; constraints by governments on the fees and charges of the medical profession as part of cost containment of medical services; and the actions of the federal and state governments (through NHTAP) to restrain the diffusion of high-cost medical technologies by limiting their use to teaching hospitals in which evaluations of the technology can be undertaken prior to decisions to pay Medicare benefits for the use of the technology.

In at least three substantive areas of health policy, the inputs of the health professions and social scientists have been conspicuous by their absence. First, unlike the situation in nations such as Netherlands and the United States, hospital medical specialists and other specialists in the medical profession have not set up their own formal processes of health care technology assessment. They have not had the same influence on government decisions affecting the diffusion of medical technology as have organizations such as the DATTA program of the American Medical Association or the ACEP program of the American College of Physicians. Nursing organizations have not yet developed formal processes of technology assessment built around extensive and politically astute nursing inputs, although there have been some isolated attempts to develop the capacities of nurses in technology research in other nations (e.g., University of Texas Health Science Centre).

Second, there has been no conspicuous effort by the health professions to assess the benefits and costs of the major regulations now influencing the roles, responsibilities, supply, and costs of major health services. Not satisfactorily resolved are a number of challenges: the oversupply of doctors, the emecent years, the effects of regulation on

nursing roles and practice (see for example Styles, Storey et al.). In some nations, using an astute political education program, the nursing profession has achieved significant changes in the regulatory constraints affecting its roles, responsibilities and representation (e.g., Cyprus).

The traditional focus of early reforms of the regulations affecting the health professions has been on the *credentialling process* and the exclusionary effects of licensure on professional incomes, fees, and the costs of health care (e.g., Gaumer, 1984; Cohen, 1973). Very little research has gone into the critical area of the efficient regulation of *consumer information* on health care (e.g., Beales, Craswell, and Salop, 1981). In other areas of public concern, the focus has been on economic evaluation of the *costs and benefits of particular types of regulation* (see, for example, Weidenbaum, 1974, 1975). Any regulation affecting society or groups in society has a number of economic costs (see Table 18-3). Economic impact statements can provide convincing arguments to policy makers if appropriate costing methods are used to determine the costs and benefits of regulatory processes affecting health care. Economic assessments without political education campaigns are unlikely to change the regulatory processes now impeding nursing practices, hospital practice, community care, and cost-effective prevention of the future costs of chronic illness.

In formulating an agenda for policy reform for the nursing profession, an assault on regulatory processes retarding professional roles, growth, and remuneration is not the only priority. Table 18-4 summarizes a wider agenda for review by nurses. Obviously since the priorities of the nursing profession will not be similar in every nation, the listing in Table 18-4 is indicative rather than comprehensive. The list is biased toward policy reforms that require an economic perspective, but other disciplines (e.g., political science, sociology,

Table 18-4 Policy Issues for Extensive Review in the 1990s by Peak Nursing Organizations

Policy issue	Type of review required
Aging and disability in society	Changing patterns of aging and health disorder The care requirements of acute and chronic illnesses The roles of different health professions in prevention, cure, and rehabilitation under alternative models to the "medical model" Likely effects on health care expenditures of alternative roles of the health professions The overlapping roles of social security, taxation, and health systems in the care and housing of the aged and chronically ill The role of self-care and the informal caring networks The particular roles of nurses in enhancing the health and functional status of the aged and chronically ill Regulatory barriers affecting the potential contributions of nurses in alternative roles
Consumer information on risk factors, health and effective use of services provided by selected health professions	Estimated effects of particular risk factors on the health status of the nation Identification of types of information required by consumers to modify risk factors or health status Potential roles of related health professions (particularly nursing) in providing the required information Identification of vehicles for linking information needs to use of health services (e.g., data bases maintained by third-party insurers or financing organizations) Assessment of the cost-effectiveness of using nurses to convey IEC in different settings (primary health care, inpatient and outpatient services, vertical health programs, long-term care, national risk factor reduction programs for special target groups—MCH, heart disease, cancer, stroke, disabled)
Regulatory reforms adversely affecting the roles of health professions, particularly nursing	Costs and benefits of existing regulations for credentialling (registration, certification and licensure) of the health professions and effects on occupational choice; provider incomes, fees, and health care costs; career mobility and productivity; advertising restrictions and ethical practice; quality of care; professional competence Costs and benefits of other regulations affecting institutional accreditation; hospital admission privileges; third-party reimbursement of hospitals and other services; peer review; malpractice costs and sequellae
Technology assessment in health care	Roles and responsibilities of governments, private sector providers, third-party payers, and the health professions in health care technology assessment (HCTA) Adequacy of current methods of HCTA for emerging technologies, established technologies Potential models of HCTA involving the health professions in a proactive role Potential contribution of the nursing profession in different forms of HCTA: international forums (WHO, UNICEF, UNDP, World Bank etc.), national organizations, professional organizations Educational requirements of nurses involved in HCTA and possible pilot projects linking education and HCTA processes Political education programs required to ensure greater involvement of nurses in HCTA in selected nations and in international organizations (e.g., WHO)

Table 18-4 *Concluded*

Policy issue	Type of review required
Financing health care to achieve goals of equity and efficiency	Assessment of existing use of financial resources in paying for health care
	Assessment of equity of current allocation of resources to health care
	Assessment of economic efficiency of major health services including estimates of unit costs, staffing patterns, and technology
	Assessment of alternative methods of paying for care, including new sources of revenue (privatization, user charges, private health insurance, social security taxes) and alternative methods of reimbursement of providers of services and institutional care
	Assessment of the role of health and life insurance funds in risk factor reduction and health promotion
	Assessment of the needs of nurses for training in health economics in basic and postbasic educational programs in a curriculum covering at least: financial planning, financial management information systems, financial controls and monitoring, procurement and stores management, economics of institutional and equipment maintenance, economics of regulation of health services, disease costing, clinical costing in major services (hospitals, PHC, vaccination programs, breastfeeding and family planning, child survival strategies), cost-effectiveness analysis in health care
International health	Feasibility of achieving the goals of Health for All by the Year 2000 (HFA 2000) and other major international programs
	Feasibility of achieving the goals of PHC at affordable costs
	Prevention of major health disorders (Hepatitis B, AIDS, malaria, worms) by cost-effective strategies
	Contributions of nurses in future organizations (WHO, UNICEF, UNDP, World Bank, other development banks)
	Forecasting in health care and the role of nursing organizations
	The likely demand for nurses and nurse-substitutes under changing patterns of payment or other changes in government policy or private household income
	The likely requirements in supply for nurses and nurse-substitutes under alternative assumptions about medical technology, technology transfer, productivity, and reimbursement methods

ethics, and epidemiology) have equally valid claims to provide offsetting or complementary perspectives.

LINKING CONSUMERS AND HEALTH PROFESSIONALS

The involvement of consumers in the search for affordable health care is never-ending. Although the goal is admirable, the reality of consumer involvement and effective empowerment is that the effective collaboration of consumers, governments, and the health

professions is not necessarily achieved by increasing the proportion of consumer representatives—or of the health professions—on national advisory structures.

However, if self-care and health promotion are to be rendered more effective, the task of communicating essential health information to a sufficiently large cadre of consumers requires more effective techniques of information, education, and communication (IEC) tied to specific objectives for the improvement of health status and quality of life. The cost-ineffectiveness of many forms of health education is mute testimony to the fact that because we communicate a health message, the message may not necessarily be received or acted upon.

Nurses have a special place in health care and the development of improved forms of IEC for consumers. Nurses are involved in all facets of health care in a variety of locations in the home, community, office, and institution (diagnosis, cure, prevention, and rehabilitation), they are generally in contact with patients for longer periods than any other health professional, and they have a very high approval rating as a profession. Consumer empowerment does not stop with an IEC program. Changing the pattern of resource allocation in health care is fundamentally a matter of changing the power structure that advises on or makes policy decisions. At some time in the process of consumer empowerment to sustain self-care and achieve better health, the sensitive task of forming coalitions to achieve political goals assumes a particular importance. Nurses need to develop particular skills (e.g., in coalition building, media education, and political education) to achieve particular health goals involving consumers.

In the rush to assess the economic effects of new policies, the preeminent goal of achieving "better health" is often forgotten. Consumers and governments both need to have health goals, and nurses are in a good position to help them develop those goals and achieve them. It is now time to develop a new cadre of nurse policy analysts in different nations to change some of the public debate that often masquerades for informed decision making. It is now time to apply the tools of economics and politics in regulatory reform and in the promotion of policies which enhance consumer health and professional status in all areas of health care from "low tech" health promotion and primary health care to high-tech practice in major referral hospitals.

REFERENCES

Beales H, Craswell R, Salop S C (1981). "The efficient regulation of consumer information," *Journal of Law and Economics* XXIV (December), 491–544.

Berk M L, Monheit A C, Hagan M H (1988). "How the U.S. spent its health care dollars: 1929–1980," *Health Affairs* (Fall), 46–60.

Callahan D (1987). *Setting limits: medical goals in an ageing society*. New York, Simon and Schuster, 1987.

Cohen H S (1973). "Professional licensure, organizational behavior, and the public interest," *Milbank Memorial Fund Quarterly / Health and Society* 51 (Winter), 73–88.

EPAC (1988). *Economic effects of an ageing population*. Canberra, Economic Planning Advisory Council, Paper No. 29, (January)

Gaumer G L (1984). "Regulating health professionals: a review of the empirical literature," *Milbank Memorial Fund Quarterly / Health and Society* 62 : 3, 380–416.

Gross P F (1987). "Health sector financing study: Government of Pakistan." Working Paper No. 3.

Gross P F (1989a). "The economics of health care in Australia: The inevitability of increased use of home health care and self-care," *Medical Observer* (forthcoming).

Gross P F (1989b). "Technology assessment in health care in Australia," *International Journal of Technology Assessment in Health Care* 5, 137–153.

Gross P F, Taylor R (1988). *The total economic cost of disease in Australia and the contribution of smoking, high blood pressure and cholesterol 1985/86*. Sydney, Institute of Health Economics and Technology Assessment, Health Economics Monograph No. 17 (August).

Langwell K M (1982). *Research on competition in the financing and delivery of health services: A summary of policy issues*. Washington D.C., Office of Health Research, Statistics and Technology, National Center for Health Services Research, U.S. Department of Health and Human Service, NCHSR Research Summary Series PHS-83-3328-1 (October).

Langwell K M, More S F (1982). *A synthesis of research on competition in the financing and delivery of health services*. Washington D.C., Office of Health Research, Statistics and Technology, National Center for Health Services Research, U.S. Department of Health and Human Services Service, NCHSR Research Report Series PHS 83-3377 (October).

Levin / ICF Consultants (1989). Indigent Care Project, Parts I–IV, Washington, D.C. Levin / ICF and DC Hospital Assoc., 25 October, mimeo.

Logan J, Woodfield A, Green D G (1989). *Healthy competition*. Sydney. Centre for Independent Studies and the New Zealand Centre for Independent Studies, CIS Policy Monographs 14.

Luitz J, Priha R (1984). "The use and costs of Medicare services in the last two years of life," *Health Care Financing Review* 5: 117–131.

OECD (1982). *Competition policy and the professions*. Paris, OECD.

OECD (1985). *Measuring health care 1960–1983*. Paris, OECD.

OTA (1982). *Medical technology under proposals to increase competition in health care*. Washington D.C., OTA-H-190 (October).

Pauly M V, Langwell K M (1983). "Research on competition in the market for health services: problems and prospects," *Inquiry* 20 (Summer), 42–161.

Riley G et al. (1986). "Changes in the distribution of Medicare expenditures among aged enrollees." *Health Care Financing Review* (Spring) 53–63.

Scitovsky A A (1984). "The high cost of dying: what do the data show?" *Milbank Memorial Fund Quarterly/Health and Society* 62: 591–608.

Storey M, Roemer R, Maglacas A M, Riccard E A P (1988). *Guidelines for regulatory changes in nursing education and practice to promote primary health care*. Geneva, World Health Organization, Division of Health Manpower Development, Report WHO/EDUC/88.194.

Styles M M (1985). *Report on the regulation of nursing: Report on the present, a position for the future*. Geneva, International Council of Nurses, (June).

U.S. Senate (1988). *The rural health care challenge: staff report*. U.S. Senate, Special Committee on Aging (October).

Weidenbaum M L (1974). *Government - mandated price increases: Neglected aspect of inflation*. Washington D.C., American Enterprise Institute.

Weidenbaum M L (1975). "The case for economizing on government controls," *Journal of Economic Issues* 9:2 (June), 205–218.

Weisbrod B A (1981). *Competition in health care: a cautionary view*. Madison (Wisconsin), Institute for Research on Poverty, Discussion Paper DP 678-81.

Technological Change in Health Care: Increasing the Demand for Noninstitutional Care in Australia

Developments in medical technology have moved—or will soon move—much of the care once provided in hospitals and institutional care outside the hospital walls. In planning the future of home health care services, it is necessary to anticipate some of those technological developments which will affect five general classes of patients:

• Patients discharged earlier from acute care and requiring minimal nursing care
• Patients discharged from acute care following trauma or other conditions which require rehabilitation
• Patients who want palliative care provided within their own homes or within the homes of their informal caring network (including AIDS and cancer cases)
• Elderly persons who require minimal care
• Persons with chronic illnesses requiring services which enhance their capacity for independent living or their quality of life

The following illustrate some of the technological breakthroughs that will reduce the demand for hospital care and increase the demand for home health care in Australia.

Intravascular balloon embolization (IBE) is now used in the treatment of intracranial aneurysms. Of the 40,000 to 50,000 Americans who suffer brain hemorrhages each year, 15,000 to 20,000 intracranial aneurysm surgeries are performed, each requiring 7 to 10 days of stay costing US$25,000 to 50,000. IBE offers several advantages over surgery. It requires a 2 to 3-day hospital stay; it eliminates the costs of operating room, recovery room, and ICU—and thus eliminates a cost of US$6,000 to 10,000; it allows greater preservation of the patent blood vessel; and it has a 6 to 7 percent mortality rate. It is currently experimental in the U.S. and used only for patients who have failed surgery or who are poor surgical candidates.

For males with benign prostatic hyperplasia, open or transurethral surgery has been the preferred treatment in the U.S., requiring 3 to 4 days of hospitalization and 3 weeks of recovery. The costs include the fees of the surgeon and anaesthetist and the costs of operating rooms and pharmacy charges, leading to an overall cost of about US$10,000 in both U.S. academic and private hospitals. About 25 percent of all males require the surgical procedure, and its side-effects include high rates of infertility in younger males and retroejaculation. In NSW the procedure requires an average length of stay (ALOS) of 10.7 days in public hospitals and 6.7 days in private hospitals. One new technology is **retrograde balloon urethroplasty** with a balloon catheter, recently evaluated in a recent trial on nine patients in Minnesota. The trial results suggest that it decreases medical costs; it is a 30-minute outpatient procedure costing US$120, followed by prophylactic antibiotics initiated prior to the procedure and continued for 7 days. It has minimal expected morbidity and no mortality. It has an 88 percent success rate in men with side-lobe enlargement (the most common condition) and a 50 percent success rate in men with middle-lobe enlargement.

The rapid development of **freestanding vascular disease centers** in the United States is a symptom of the rapid movement of traditional diagnostic services outside the hospital walls. These units will offer noninvasive ultrasound or 3-D Doppler blood flow studies instead of angiography. With start-up costs of roughly US$350,000 per center, the first units in Florida expect to test 100 patients per month at an average charge of US$225. Of the 500,000 cardiac catheterization procedures performed in the United States in 1987, even if only 15 percent had been performed on an outpatient basis, the annual savings in catheter-related expenditures would have been US$51 million, ignoring other benefits such as improved patient satisfaction, more personalized medical care, less work loss, and avoidance of the stress of hospitalization (NEJM, 10 November 1988, p. 1251).

Other technological advances seem likely to accelerate the relocation of some cardiovascular services from hospital inpatient services into ambulatory care or home care. In early 1989, an elderly man in Florida became the first patient in the United States to receive a home-based trans-telephonic defibrillator, linked to Sacred Heart Hospital in Pensacola. Although the device can defibrillate a patient effectively and accurately in controlled trials, there are still many logistical problems to be solved with such devices, including methods to minimize any panic by the family/carer supposed to activate the device in an emergency. This is a technology where the human interface with the machine is not yet optimal but where it may be possible to avoid the costs of hospitalization for maintenance therapy for individuals with arrhythmias.

Thrombolytic therapy in peripheral vascular disease has now reached a point where a new procedure, pulsed spray pharmacomechanical thrombosis, is in use in two hospitals in California, and a commercial machine and catheter will be available late in 1989. About half the new procedures require 1 ampoule of urokinase (250,000 units) and the other half require 2 units, both significantly less than conventional thrombolytic therapy using 8 or more ampoules. The new therapy requires 3 to 4 hours in an angiography suite compared with 18 hours in an ICU with conventional thrombolytic therapy. Cost savings include bed costs, about US$1,000 per day, plus the savings in drug costs. The procedure has been used successfully in 96 percent of patients with complete blood clot blockage of dialysis grafts, arterial bypass grafts, and peripheral arteries.

Percutaneous transluminal coronary angioplasty (PCTA) is now accepted as an effective long-term therapy for angina. In the United States it is now achieving event-free survival rates of 61 to 69 percent at 25 months, with patients requiring no further PCTA, medical, or surgical intervention. Total 3-year survival rates at the Thorax Center (Rotterdam) were about 96 percent. Restenosis rates of 30 percent suggest that PCTA will not completely replace coronary artery bypass surgery (CABS), and it may in fact increase the number of surgical interventions as many interventions involve patients who would not have received any procedure before PCTA arrived. In a recent comparative trial in Atlanta (USA) the range of average length of stay for PCTA was 3 to 25 days, compared with 7 to 65 days for CABS. Total 1-year charges for PCTA were 52 percent less than for CABS (US$11,100 versus $22,860), and there is a lack of compelling data to show that the quality of patient care has decreased in U.S. hospitals with PCTA.

The national debate on the implications of an aging population has not really affected surgeons to date, but it is hard to see this quarantine continuing. In one recently reported study in the United States the ALOS for hip fracture fell from 21.9 days in 1981 to 12.6 days in 1986, due largely to the hospital reimbursement scheme (DRGs) introduced in October 1983 (NEJM 1988; 319: 1392–1397). Australian hospitals are likely to soon experience a similar reimbursement scheme. The U.S. experience has shown that DRGs leave the sicker cases in the hospital beds, discharge many more to nursing homes (we do not have extra places available in Australian nursing homes), and the number of patients remaining in nursing homes 1 year after hospitalization increased by 200 percent. More intensive outpatient rehabilitation programs and home healh care are justified if we are to compensate for reduced ALOS in hospitals and diminished quality of life.

In Australian hospitals in 1985, the ALOS for cholecystectomy was 10.6 days for females (range 9.3 to 11.9 days) and 12.6 days for males (range 10.9 to 13.5 days). Two emerging technologies seem likely to reduce the demand for surgery by patients with gallstones. First, nonsurgical treatment of gallstones is already possible using either extracorporeal shockwave lithotripsy (ESWL) or gallstone dissolution therapy. In some situations, bile salt therapy (using chenodeoxydilic and ursodioxydilic acid) has been used 1 week before ESWL and up to 3 months after the total disappearance of gallstones was confirmed by ultrasound. The ALOS for this new procedure is 2 to 3 days, and the additional costs include the bile salt therapy required for up to 24 months where there are small diameter gallstones. In 1989, a team at the Pittsburgh Laser Center reported the effects of laser cholecystectomy on ALOS. One recent report of 79,782 U.S. patients indicated that the ALOS for cholecystectomy was 10.6 days (roughly the same as NSW public hospitals). In the hospital in which the laser device was used, the ALOS for cholecystectomy had been 5.3 days (range 3 to 9 days). The average cost of nonlaser cholecystectomy patients was US$3699, compared with US$2643 for laser cholecystectomy patients, a reduction of about 25 percent in hospital costs. These patients will still require some home health care if they are discharged earlier.

Applied to Australian patients the reductions in expenditures on cholecystectomies would not be trivial. For example, the total number of these patients in Australia in 1985 was 14,000. The total days of their hospital stay in 1985 were:

$$(10,053 \times 10.6) + (3693 \times 12.6)$$
$$= 106,560 + 49,934$$
$$= 156,494$$

The projected total days of hospital stay if laser cholecystectomy was used are $14,000 \times 2.4 = 33,600$ days. Theoretical reduction in bed-days possible with the new procedure is $156,494 - 33,600$ or 122,894 bed-days. Theoretical cost savings at A$400 per day (1989 prices) are $122,894 \times 400$ or $49.2 million.

Other developments in dialysis, antibiotic therapy, incontinence therapy, pain management, parenteral nutrition, and chemotherapy will reduce the demand for institutional care. New developments in laser surgery for blocked arteries will further reduce the ALOS and increase the demand for home health care. It remains to be seen whether Australian households yet recognize the potential value of home health care, or whether they can be induced to use such care more extensively if it reduces the taxes they pay for Medicare.

Chapter 19

The Case for Nursing's Preeminence in International Health

Pamela J. Maraldo

Health care in America is in trouble. And the most casual examination of industrialized as well as developing nations around the world will find most either in a similar predicament or fraught with the makings of a similar predicament as a result of one or more of these factors:

- The aging of the population
- The overutilization or inappropriate utilization of costly hospitalization and extremely costly medical technology
- The cost of treating AIDS patients

Many nations around the world who are feeling government pressures to reduce cost, realize greater effectiveness, and spread access to primary health care services, have systems which bear a very striking resemblance to the U. S. system of care.[1]

Indeed, all industrialized nations are faced with rapidly greying economies,[2] and increasingly high rates of health care inflation.[3] Our inflation in the United States is intolerably high, and health care is consuming an ever-increasing share of GNP, with no substantial improvement in the quality of care or the overall health of the nation to show for it.[4] Many health care sectors in industrialized countries, once very charitable and philanthropically oriented are now, of necessity, becoming very businesslike and bottom-line oriented. In many developing nations as well, the effects of a market-driven economy—such as the Philippines—are just as apparent. Poverty, gross social and economic inequities, high prevalence of infectious disease, and inaccessible, uncoordinated, inadequate health services are highly prevalent in the Philippines.[5]

From this perspective many nations around the world are headed in similar directions, experiencing similar problems in health care despite wide variations in the political and cultural fabrics of the nations.

New York City feels like a third world country: one out of every three admissions to Bellevue Hospital is crack related, 25 percent of the AIDS victims in the nation are in our shelters and health facilities, almost 2 million New Yorkers have incomes below the federal poverty line ($11,611 for a family of four); about 1 million people are on New York City's welfare rolls, and half of them are children.[6]

In the United States, health status and economic indices are worse than other nations. Health care expenditures, for example, both in absolute terms and relative to gross domestic product, continue to increase, as does the gap between U.S. expenditures and those in other major industrialized countries. Total health expenditures as a percentage of gross domestic product (GDP) in the United States is 11.1 percent.[7]

In 1986 public health expenditures, as a percentage of total health spending, ranged from 40.8 percent in the United States to over 90 percent in Greece (94.8 percent), Luxembourg (90.7 percent), Norway (97.3 percent) and Sweden (90.9 percent). Australia has an OECD average (Organization for Economic Cooperation and Development) of 76.7 percent, and Australia, spending 73.0 percent of total health expenditure on public health.[8] However, although OECD average has stabilized since 1980, the U.S. ratio is still increasing, and the gap between the United States and other countries continues to widen. In fact, most of the other six major OECD countries have exhibited stability in their health-to-GDP shares over the past three years.

Canada has been stable at 8.5 percent since 1984; France has increased slightly from 8.4 to 8.5 percent; Germany has been stable at 8.1 percent; Italy has increased slightly from 6.6 to 6.7 percent; Japan has been stable at 6.7 percent; the United Kingdom has been stable at 6.2 percent; the United States has increased from 10.5 to 11.1 percent.[9]

Likewise, per capita spending is the highest in the United States, exceeding Australia by 120 percent; Canada, by 41 percent; France, by 85 percent; Germany, by 87 percent; Italy, by 152 percent; Japan by 131 percent; and the United Kingdom, by 171 percent. The average per capita expenditure for Canada, France, Germany, Italy, Japan, and United Kingdom was $1033 in 1987; U.S. expenditures were $2051.[10] The gap (percentage difference) between the United States and each of these other countries continues to grow.

On average, nominal health expenditures increased by 10.1 percent per year in industrialized nations; overall prices increased by 6.1 percent; health care prices increased by 6.9 percent; health care price inflation *in excess* of overall price inflation increased by 2.9 percent; population increased by 0.5 percent; and utilization per person increased by 2.5 percent.[11]

Despite the U.S. lead in health spending, trends in most westernized nations and some developing nations are similar: Health care inflation is rising at a considerably greater rate than inflation in the general economy, populations are aging, and the rate of utilization of services is rising very substantially.[12]

Substantial health care expenditures notwithstanding, in industrialized as well as developing nations access to care is not what it should be, long waiting lists preclude attention to much badly needed health services, hospitals face serious financial difficulty and quality of care is increasingly inadequate.[13]

The impact of all these factors threatens to eventually eat away at the very social fabric of our nations. The twin epidemics of drugs and alcohol are ubiquitous in developing as well as industrialized nations. Meanwhile delivering high-quality affordable health services to all who need them is a thing that seems to elude most countries around the world.

And the question remains, in the context of the worldwide movement launched by the WHO at Alma-Ata in 1978, to achieve health for all through the primary health care approach, how can nurses around the world—in the face of divergent political, economic, and cultural situations—strive to maintain a professional commitment to meet the health needs of people in light of constrained economic circumstances as well as an extraordinary demand for greater access to health care?

To fulfill the WHO goal to improve the public health of all nations, to launch national health care policies that will provide affordable basic health care for all, nurses must be used as primary care providers in nations throughout the world. Over a decade of research and serious experimentation in the United States provide evidence that nurses as providers of primary care are in a key position to exercise leadership to achieve such a goal.

In every way in industrialized and developing nations, health care delivery is ripe for reform, away from the technological "fix it" model and ripe for reform by nurses toward affordable community-based systems of care. For example, in Nicaragua, a nation clearly limited in economic capacities, the national health system functions mostly through community-based primary care outposts. In spite of the country's war-torn climate, the nation has achieved remarkably high levels of health status of several key indices. The rate of infant mortality has declined 50 percent in the past 10 years, and the incidence of many communicable diseases has also decreased.[14] Such models of primary care could be replicated using nurse providers and could clearly have similarly far reaching results in the United States and other countries around the world.

If one looks back over the past 5 years at the U.S. example, when health care in the United

States experienced fairly major changes, moving to prospective payment financing, we can gain some insight into the problems and the solutions we need. During that period, U.S. health care witnessed a period of change fundamentally. After literally decades of trying to get some handle on soaring health costs, major change began when the Reagan administration tried to fix the problem and rectify the ills of a system built on the assumption that resources would be unlimited. So, a prospective system of payment to hospitals was enacted, and hospitals are now given a certain amount for diseases they treat. This new method of payment has thrust the U.S. system of health care into a highly competitive mode, just like the airlines or banking or communications industries.[15]

There have been political shifts under the new DRG payment system. Physicians who have always been the captains of the health care ship are incredibly threatened, because they now have businesspersons monitor their costly practice patterns and ask them to alter their behavior if spending excesses persist.

There has been tremendous turnover among hospital management in recent years, under increasing pressure to maintain a health revenue stream in the face of a federal policy directed at reducing costly acute care and in the face of increasing competition from new provider arrangements (PPOs, HMOs, CNOs). MDs and hospital administrators are fighting because hospital administrators are forced to control medicine's costly behavior. To make matters worse, the entire industry is caught in the middle of the worst nursing supply crisis it has witnessed since World War II.[16]

Well, you might ask, was there any advantage to moving to a system of prospective payment based on diagnosis? Many U.S. health policy makers, upon considering resources expended compared to improved levels of health status, would answer in the negative. Many Americans have referred to the DRG system as "rearranging deck chairs on the Titanic."[17] However, other informed observers would acknowledge some positive effects of the changes in financing.

The United States is on the verge of developing a true health care marketplace, but the crux of the change can be summed up thusly: The centers of power have shifted from the traditional providers of health care (doctors and hospitals), to those who pay the bills (consumers)—primarily in the form of the purchaser of care, business, third-party payors, and the federal government.

In addition, with so much emphasis on the *cost* of health care, lawmakers and administrators have begun to take a more careful look at what nurses have to offer. And indeed one of nursing's greatest strengths is their ability to achieve cost savings and increase access. In fact, competition and diversification into new forms of health care has created a climate more receptive to payment for nursing care.[18]

However, despite a shift in the locus of decision making and a greater receptivity toward competition among providers, the ability of the United States to support the primary health care approach to health care delivery continues to be constrained by political and economic factors.

A comparison with the Canadian system, which has managed to achieve comprehensive coverage of people and services, makes clear that it is the funding system which is critical. In Canada, the universal public insurance programs in each province, which reimburse all hospital and medical costs (through direct budgetary allocation and fee-schedule negotiation, respectively), make expenditure control, not easy, but possible.[19]

Despite much ado about prospective payment policies and cost containment rhetoric, in real terms the United States has not reduced health care costs at all. As a nation the United States will spend $620 billion in 1989;

in 2 more years, that figure will surpass the $2 billion dollars a day mark.[20] A recent issue of *Fortune* magazine referred to health care costs as the "killer cost stalking the business community."[21] Many businesses incurred a 30 percent rise in health care costs last year—an absolutely untenable rate of increase in economic hard times.[22]

Recent national surveys report that it's not just business that is suffering from the cost of care. The survey reported that two-thirds of Americans failed to receive the health care they needed because of financial constraints.[23]

The United States is at a juncture where many Americans cannot afford to be sick, and many believe that some form of rationing health care is likely if the factors that continue to fuel the growth in health care expenditures are not addressed.[24]

With all due respect to the serious problems we face as a society over the cost of care, the most difficult problems we face are not just cost related. We have at present many grave inadequacies and failures. We are, in fact, currently at a point where our entire system of health care is in jeopardy, and we have a huge medical industrial complex that can no longer respond to people's health needs or socioeconomic imperatives. If the U.S. experience is relevant, much can be learned and mistakes averted by studying the U.S. state of affairs. U.S. investment in sophisticated technology is enormous when compared with other nations. America's per capita availability of medical interventions from magnetic resonance imaging to open heart surgery exceed the capacity of other industrialized nations by as much as 500 to 1. Some industrialized nations, most notably Canada, have set national goals for the availability and distribution of costly technology; the U.S. competitive health care industry makes such national level planning extremely difficult to conduct.[25]

Yet as a society we are witnessing the limits of medical science. We have unmistakable evidence that emotions, lifestyle—psychosocial factors, if you will—have an infinitely more far-reaching effect than the medical community is willing to acknowledge in its activities.[26]

Meanwhile, it is patently clear to many and especially policy makers that the old ways are not working, and evidence of the inadequacies of the medical model, which is the basis for our current emphasis on acute care, is everywhere:

• Despite all our strides in medicine and technology in this country, the United States has one of the highest infant mortality rates in the developed world.[27]

• Second, more than half of the Americans living in poverty with no access to health care are children.[28]

• Huge amounts spent on Medicare notwithstanding, almost half of what the elderly spend for their health care is out of pocket.[29]

• Consensus is growing that half the coronary bypasses, most cesarean sections, and a significant proportion of many other procedures such as pacemaker implants and hysterectomies are unnecessary.[30]

• With all due respect to the strides we've made in longevity, the majority of Medicare dollars are spent on life-sustaining technology in the last year of life in individuals over 80 years of age.[31]

• The leading causes of death in the United States, and indeed throughout much of the globe—heart disease, cancer, stroke, chronic obstructive pulmonary disease, cirrhosis of the liver—are, in large part, preventable. The U.S. Bureau of the Census reported in 1987 that the largest difference in mortality rates among countries can be attributed to circulatory diseases (yet only 1 percent of the U.S. health care dollar is spent on prevention).[32]

• It has been estimated that over 81 percent of the strides we have made in decreasing the incidence of heart disease is attributable to dietary and lifestyle changes; that is, as a society we have stopped smoking and cut down on fats. The other 9 percent has to do with cardiovascular drugs and surgery—not a very substantial return on our investments.[33]

• In limiting the causes of infectious disease in many ways we're far from victory. Obvious examples are legionelosis, or legionnaires' disease, related to air conditioning open vents; genital herpes, a sexually transmitted virus which is related to sexual mores; and, of course, the most frustrating and frightening of all to date, Acquired Immunodeficiency Syndrome (AIDS).

• Finally, the quality of health care Americans receive is increasingly unsatisfactory and, at times, borders on hazardous. The media carries daily messages that cite episodes of poor quality. Recently, *American Health* magazine with a readership of 1 million, warned its readers that "Hospitals are dangerous places and should only be used as a last resort."[34] *Boardroom Reports,* which goes out to CEOs of *Fortune* 500 companies, carried the same message—"Stay out of hospitals if you can."[35]

Peters and Waterhouse, in the widely read bestseller, *A Passion for Excellence,* also drive home a typically critical public perspective on the matter of care in hospitals in their passage entitled "Poor Dumb Patients," which elaborates on the actual disdain health care workers seemed to have for patients.[36]

Quality has been declared a number one public policy problem by the U.S. Health Care Financing Administration, and the situation is destined to worsen. Just as concerns over cost prevailed during the past two decades, concerns over quality will be predominant in the late 1980s and 1990s.

At the root of the quality problem and other pressing problems in our health delivery system is the U.S. system of financing, which provides strong incentives toward high-technology medicine and the "fix it" model of cure.[37] The extraordinary investment of resources in high-technology medicine has created a situation where the medical paradigm prevails as a practice and as a culture and creates a political inability to alter our patterns of care to accomodate the changing needs of society.

A striking depiction of the problem can be found in a situation described by former Governor Lamm of Colorado: "What chance is there that she will leave this unit alive?" asked Governor Lamm. The group of physicians looked annoyed a this question. They were all clustered around the bed of a 91-year-old woman, a patient in the intensive care unit for 2 weeks, kept alive by a web of tubes and hoses. The attending physician swallowed his personal resentment and responded, "Very small, but every once in a while someone survives. But medicine must do everything possible as long as there is a chance."[38]

The United States has approximately 87,000 intensive care beds, far more than any other country. An intensive care bed is the most expensive medical setting possible, usually staffed by one to one and one-half nurses per bed and surrounded by hundreds of thousands of dollars of high-technology equipment.

These units *do* save some people who would have been previously lost, but at a tremendously high cost to other important priorities in society.

Once people get into the health care system, we will spend fantastic amounts exploring a small chance of survival for them, yet 33 million Americans do not have basic health insurance, and 30 percent of our children have never seen a dentist.[39] We have seemingly unlimited resources for patients in the system but painfully few for citizens outside the system. Our health care spending is reactive and reflexive rather than reflective.

In practically every town in the United States, the best building is the hospital (40 percent empty). The highest paid professionals are physicians, the lowest paid are nurses. We spend more than other industrialized nations on health care, both in total dollars and percent of GNP devoted to health care, yet we do not keep our citizens as healthy as they do.[40]

Moreover, in meetings with the Japanese, the Soviets, the Chinese, the Canadians, it is all too apparent that other nations are drifting toward the U.S. approach and are unfortunately all too eager to follow the U.S. obsession with technology and cure at the expense of other models and approaches to achieving a healthy society.[41]

The basic dilemma of U.S. medicine is that we have invented more medical care than we need or can afford to pay for and more than we are willing to evaluate in terms of its outcomes and effectiveness. Health care has become a fiscal black hole that can absorb unlimited resources. We have the finest technological means in the world, but all too few are asking, "To what end?"

The heart of the matter is that the medical model of disease, which is the foundation of entire health delivery systems, is built on, grew out of, and was most appropriate to the infectious disease era. In this simpler world diseases had causes (germs), and the task of the bioscientific enterprise was to identify the cause and to devise an appropriate and specific cure. The success of this approach, for its time, has been dramatic. We've seen a 99 percent reduction in the frequency and severity of infectious diseases such as smallpox, typhoid fever, syphilis, polio, tetanus, and diphtheria.[42]

Now our most pressing and unrelenting national health problems are mostly chronic in nature and will simply not succumb to direct application of the medical model. They require primary nursing care just as acute disease states have required primary medical intervention.

The social and psychological roots of the

current problems run deep, and our system and patterns of care must shift to address these new imperatives.

So we are at a juncture in health where the limits of the present system are becoming apparent. At one time we all believed as a society that eventually medical science would know all that there is to know. But now it appears that's not the case. So the question is, what are the implications for the nursing profession around the world? Nursing, as a profession, knows from the U.S. experience that building sophisticated biomedical enterprises throughout the globe is not the answer to achieving a healthy citizenry. We know that societies that fail to take care of their people, to provide a basic sense of security for their people in matters such as health care, are potentially in jeopardy.

Nurses as a collective of professionals around the world have the power to exert leadership; to direct and refocus a badly needed transformation. Nurses have the power to change the face of things in health care, to fulfill the Alma-Ata goal to provide primary care to all. But to achieve this, in order to fully function as professionals in a worldwide system badly in need of nursing care, a politically sound, viable strategy is essential.

Laying the groundwork for such a strategy requires some basic assumptions. First we shall assume that if the U.S. experience is relevant and we can observe close parallels, then it is likely that industrial nations will witness:

- Continued financial pressures
- Sicker patients with shorter lengths of stay
- Shift in the demand for care from acute care in hospitals to primary care in the home and in community-based settings
- Increased use of technology in the home and community and outside of the hospital

- Subsequent decrease in the need for acute care hospital beds
- An increase in the population of elderly persons—which will mean an increase in chronic illness
- An increase in the rate of infectious disease
- Increased numbers of the population with no access to care
- Increased need for prenatal care and prevention services.

Developing nations will experience:

- Poverty
- Inadequate nutrition
- Increased need for primary care
- Increase in the population with no access to care
- Increase in the need for prenatal care and preventive services
- Increase in the number of elderly persons—which will mean an increase in chronic illness.

The cornerstone of a nursing strategy for international health policy—key to setting health policy back on the right track—will reside in the ability of nurses around the world to shape and advance policies that will reduce the inordinate and costly bias toward expensive inpatient care and costly technology, and to place a new and unprecedented emphasis, in industrialized and developing nations alike, on (1) prevention and primary care services, (2) long-term care, and (3) the need to develop high-quality community-based systems of care.

In each of these areas, nursing has a rich history of experience and much to offer in terms of new directions, new solutions.

And indeed, many have observed that these are areas in which nurses are well suited to provide solutions, to offer leadership and give direction to badly needed reforms in the health care delivery. To achieve these goals, a five track strategy is offered.

First, nurses around the world have the responsibility to vigorously seek full professional status and positions of independence, authority, and accountability that goes with it. Positions in senior management, chief executive officers, and positions in government will advance nursing paradigms and badly needed nursing models of care.

There must be relentless pursuit of higher education for nurses. Always a tool for advancement of minority status groups, education is vital to nursing's future progress.

Our nations are demanding more and more nurses to supply increasingly technical, increasingly complex care. As a result, nursing education has reached a critical juncture. Education must reach out to students more than ever before through innovative, flexible education options while making sure students have a broad array of skills, abilities, and humanitarian values required in today's variety of health care settings.

In general, nursing education programs have been slow to recognize the need for change and to implement the changes required to prepare today's graduate for the world of health care. And the nursing education community has not managed to project the excitement and tremendous rewards that derive from a career in nursing over a lifetime.

Now of course, enrollments in the United States have steadily declined since 1984. Baccalaureate programs in general have been hard hit—down 10 percent for the 1985–1987 years and preliminary data for 1988 show a drop of 8 percent.[43]

These trends are, at least in part, a striking reflection of the need for a more relevant and responsive system of nursing education, one in which faculty are more clinically adept and can serve as clinical role models as well as scholars and researchers, one in which students graduate with a deep knowledge of the political and economic factors governing today's health care delivery system, one in which students are inspired by the leadership in the university to go out and realize their fullest potential to make the world better through better health care.

Many of these qualities are all too rare in undergraduate nursing education programs. There is much work to be done to transform nursing to better equip it to meet the challenges of today's rapidly changing health care delivery system.

Schools of nursing could serve as community resources through the establishment of community nursing centers of home health agencies linked to schools of nursing. Just as academic medicine has been the beacon of scientific advancement and has provided leadership for the biomedical enterprise, academic nursing should take the initiative wherever feasible to offer guidance and health services to communities and populations in need.

But, to be fair, and to put things in perspective, a great deal in nursing education should be cherished and preserved. When one considers that medicine has not changed its model of medical education since 1910 and the essence of the reform is now calling for a broader liberal arts base, nursing's progress and, indeed, superiority is apparent—medicine had developed an awareness that psychosocial factors ultimately have a profound effect on the health status of the individual.[44]

It's encouraging and progressive that the medical community has come to this realization, of course, but the truth is nursing models of education have always been predicated on developing a deep and abiding knowledge of human behavior in all its facets. And at present nursing models are what our health care delivery system needs most.

The second strategy calls for direct payment for nursing services in and out of hospitals and in all types of delivery settings to provide full access to nursing care throughout the world settings. To address the cost and access issues that are plaguing us, consumers and purchasers of care need direct access to nursing services.

As primary care providers and clinical specialists, with payment for our services, nurses should become the new gatekeepers of the system. Why should MDs continue in the gatekeeper function if the medical model is no longer achieving effective results? Nurses should always be working to acquire financial independence, admitting privileges, to eliminate the need for doctors' orders to practice nursing. Changes of this nature could really help restructure the workplace and alleviate the worldwide shortage of nurses.

The third track in the strategy will require a fundamental restructuring of nursing's jobs in and out of hospitals—to render professional accountability and control over nursing practice—as well as adequate remuneration for education and experience. And the worldwide shortage of nurses provides the perfect vehicle to launch this strategy.

The key to resolving the nursing shortage is not numbers but utilization. As pointed out in testimony before the Select Committee on Aging, the ''widget'' approach to nurse staffing is not only inefficient, depriving the public of the vital capabilities and resources nursing has to offer but also demoralizing to nursing staff. This approach creates the ''stature'' gap that deters potential entrants into the field.[45] It is only through proper utilization that the health care delivery system's insatiable need for nursing resources will be met. And if nurses are appropriately positioned as full professionals with complete accountability and authority over their work as clinical specialists, primary care providers, and case managers, new entrants will assuredly be attracted into the profession.

Restructing nurses' roles using one of these models—the case management model, clinical specialist model, or a group practice model—and giving nurses the authority and responsibility to truly make decisions about patient care and to truly be accountable would inevitably have a marked effect on cost and quality in clinical settings.

If the nurse is strategically positioned to control the case, she or he should be able to direct and monitor laboratory, EKG, pharmacy, and so forth to eliminate duplication, inefficiencies, lack of coordination, etc. In an arrangement of this sort, the nurse would be empowered to manage the case as case manager or as the clinical specialist in charge of the cases with assistive nursing personnel or, in a group arrangement under contracts, to perform technical functions. If delivery systems foster this model effectively, patients will benefit because the providers with the closest proximity to patients, nurses, would be empowered to address issues that most frustrate patients and are most important to patients.

At present, vital decision making in the current health care delivery system is too removed from the patient to be effective, flying in the face of a basic tenet of management: Give the authority directly to the people on the front lines. Putting central responsibility for managing and coordinating the case in nursing's hands provides much greater continuity and coordination, because the nurses' proximity to the patient allows nurses to see things through the same lens as the patient.

The fourth strategy calls for nurses in every nation to lead the way to make prevention an overarching priority. An international disease prevention policy that would be aimed at drug abuse, alcohol abuse, teenage pregnancy, infant mortality, and so on is essential, and such a national policy on prevention should have teeth in tax incentives, in employee benefit packages, and in the financial structure of the health care system.

Not only would national policies aimed at prevention accomplish the obvious—that is, improve the health and welfare of the nation at hand—they would also reap tremendous benefits in reducing the cost of health care.

From the cost perspective, prevention is unalterably essential—because the cost to the public of sickness, ignorance, neglect, dependence, and unemployment over the long term exceeds the cost to the public of preventive investment in prenatal care, immunizations, and health education in the short term.

In the United States it costs an average of $47 for a complete set of immunizations for a child (the nation saved an estimated $1 billion in the first decade of measles immunization efforts).[46] In the United States it costs an average of $40 to provide a child the needed preventive checkups for an entire year under Medicaid. An average $2000 daily is charged to hospitalize a child for an illness that could have been diagnosed and treated without hospitalization if there had been a routine preventive check-up.[47]

Our commitment to help the neediest children has been increasingly fragile in recent years. During the last 2 years the improvement in our national infant mortality rate—already nineteenth among industrialized nations—has stopped. Between now and the end of 1990, nearly 17,000 United States babies will die because of low birth weight. We can prevent many of these deaths by providing their mothers with prenatal care.[48]

Finally, in addition to providing incentives to prevent illness, the need to reshape our public financing programs to provide an adequate system of long-term care that will address chronic illness is fast becoming a critical issue around the world. Although most elderly families in the United States have annual incomes of $11,554 or less, general nursing home costs average about $22,000—and that's if you're willing to put your mother in one at all![49] Yet, to increase the supply of nursing home beds, or to muddle along with the current financing systems as they currently exist, is not the answer. The U.S. financing system pays only for acute-care-oriented medical services inappropriate for chronic or posthospitalization patient care needs, which require, by and large, nursing care that can be delivered much more inexpensively and com-

passionately at home. Payment incentives in the public and private sectors for care at home and in high-quality nursing homes are essential.

Policy makers, insurers, consumer groups, everybody knows that the problem of developing an adequate system of long-term care in the nation is one of the most pressing problems we face as a society. Yet, not much has been done. Good proposals never seem to get past the talking stage.

The mounting of an international effort that includes strong nursing leadership is the challenge before us. The failure to act, the failure to chart a new clear direction, will not and should not be acceptable. This five-track strategy should be launched to consume the majority of our resources as a profession. Independence and education are vital to nursing's ability to offer solutions to the current challenges in health care.

The strategic implementation of an international plan shaped around these guiding principles is critical. A well-conceived international health plan, sponsored by nurses, will necessitate the most highly and well developed of political strategies. Such a strategy would be linked primarily to the formation of powerful consumer allies—state and national consumer organizations should be identified and targeted for support. Educating and acquiring a network of strategic relationships would provide a broad international base to establish a preeminent position for nurses as mainstream providers of health care. Next steps would be, of necessity, based on the political and economic situations of particular nations.

REFERENCES

1 Whiteis, D., & Salnon, J.: The Proprietarization of Health Care and Underdevelopment of the Public Sector. *International Journal of Health Services,* 17, 1, pp. 47–65, 1987; U.S. Department of Health & Human Services Public

Health Service; *Health United States 1988,* DHHS Pub. No. (PHS) 89–1232, U.S. Government Printing Office, March 1989.

2 National Center for Health Statistics: *Proceedings of the 1987 Public Health Conference on Records & Statistics.* National Institute on Aging, U.S. Bureau of the Census, July 13–15, 1987.

3 Schieber, G., & Poullier, J.: Datawatch: International Health Care Expenditure Trends: 1987. *Health Affairs,* 8:3, pp. 169–178, Fall 1989.

4 *Ibid.,* p. 172.

5 DeBrun, S., & Elling, R.: Cuba and the Philippines: Contrasting Cases in World-System Analysis. *International Journal of Health Services,* 17:4, p. 681, 1987.

6 New York City Department of Health: *Health of the City.* Report to the Mayor and Citizens of New York. March 15, 1989, pp. 84, 92, 105.

7 Schieber, G., & Poullier, J.: Datawatch: International Health Care Expenditure Trends 1987. *Health Affairs,* 8:3, pp. 169–178, Fall 1989.

8 *Ibid.,* p. 174.

9 *Ibid.,* p. 176.

10 *Ibid.,* p. 177.

11 *Ibid.,* p. 179.

12 Organization for Economic Cooperation and Development: *Health Data Bank,* 1987.

13 Blendon, R., & Taylor, H: Datawatch: Views on Health Care. *Health Affairs,* 8:1, pp. 149–158, Spring 1989.

14 Braverman, P., & Siegel, D.: Nicaragua: A Health System Developing Under Conditions of War. *International Journal of Health Services,* 17:1, pp. 169–179, 1987.

15 Prospective Payment Assessment Commission: Medicare Prospective Payment and the American Health Care System: Report to the Congress, 1989. Washington, D.C., U.S. Government Printing Office, 1989.

16 U.S. Department of Health and Human Services: Secretary's Commission on Nursing Report on the Shortage of Nursing Personnel. January 1988.

17 Shortell, S.M., & Hughes, F.X.: The Effects of Regulation, Competition, and Ownership on Mortality Rates among Hospital Inpatients. *New England Journal of Medicine,* 318, 19, pp. 1100–1107. 1988.

18 Sovie, M.C., Tarcinale, M.A., Vanputee, A.W., & Stunden, A.E.: Amalgam of Nursing Acuity, DRGs and Costs. *Nursing Administration,* p. 42, March 1985.

19 Palley, H.: Canadian Federalism and the Canadian Health Care Program: A Comparison of Ontario and Quebec. *International Journal of Health Services,* 17:4, pp. 595–617, 1987.

20 Mechanic, J.: "Medicare Costs to the Year 2000: Who Will Pay?" *Health Affairs,* 8:2, Summer 1989, p. 39.

21 Loomis, C.: The Killer Cost Stalking Business, *Fortune,* pp. 58–67, February 27, 1989.

22 Freudenheim, M.: A Health Care Taboo Is Broken, *New York Times,* May 8, 1989.

23 Enthoven, A.: A Cost-Unconscious Medical System, *New York Times,* July 13, 1989.

24 Kramon, G.: Employers Cut Health Costs by Bargaining with Doctors, *New York Times,* May 15, 1989.

25 Canadian Hospital Association: Ottawa, Ontario, 1988: Der Bundesminister fur Jugent, Familie und Geseundht, *Gesundheitswesens in der Bundersrepublik Deutschland,* 1988; American Hospital Association: *Hospital Statistics,* Chicago: AHA, 1988.

26 Fagin, C.M., & Jacobsen, B.J.: The Economic Value of Nursing Research: A Critical Review. In Werley, H. (ed.): *Annual Review of Nursing Research.* vol. 3, New York, 1985, Springer Publishing Co., pp. 215–238.

27 Wegman, M.E.: *Annual Survey of Vital Statistics in Pediatrics 1988,* vol. 82, pp. 817–827.

28 *Ibid.,* p. 818.

29 Farnham, A.: No More Health Care in the House. *Fortune,* p. 71, February 27, 1989.

30 Leape, L.: Unnecessary Surgery. *Health Services Research,* p. 352, 24:3, August 1989.

31 Califano, J.: Billions Blown on Health. *New York Times.* April 12, 1989.

32 National Center for Health Statistics. National Institute on Aging. U.S. Bureau of the Census: *Proceedings of the 1987 Public Health Conference on Records and Statistics,* July 1987.

33 U.S. Department of Health and Human Services: *Health United States 1988,* PHS 89–1232, March 1989.

34 Tynan, K.: New Warnings about Hospitals. *American Health,* p. 42, March 1987.

35 Problems Cited in America's Hospitals. *Boardroom Reports,* p. 3, April 1987.

36 Peters, T., & Waterhouse, P.: *A Passion for Excellence.* New York: Dow Jones Publishing, pp. 85–89, 1986.

37 Heaney, R.: Human Choices and the Technological Imperative: Values in Conflict. The Dean's Distinguished Lecture Series, University of Pennsylvania, 1987.

38 Lamm, R.: Saving a Few, Sacrificing Many at Great Cost. *New York Times,* August 2, 1989.

39 Koop, C. Everett: My Turn. *Newsweek.* August 28, 1989, p. 10.

40 *Ibid.*

41 Relman, R.: The Prospects for National Health Insurance, *NEJM,* 315: 402–425, 1986.

42 Schroeder, S., Academic Medicine as a Public Trust. *Journal of the American Medical Association,* 262:6, 803–811, August 11, 1989.

43 National League for Nursing: *Nursing Data Review 1989.* New York Division of Research, p. 36, 1990.

44 Schroeder, S.: Academic Medicine as a Public Trust.

45 U.S. House of Representatives, Proceedings of the House Select Committee on Aging, April 1988.

46 Strauss, A., & Corbin, J.: *Shaping New Health Care Systems.* San Francisco: Jossey Bass, 1988.

47 "Fallible Doctors." *The Economist,* December 17, 1988, pp. 19–21.

48 Brooten, D., Kumar, S., Brown, L., Finkler, S., Butts, P., Bakewell-Sachs, B., Gibbons, A., Delivoria-Papadopoulos, M.: A Randomized Clinical Trial of Early Hospital Discharge and Home Followup of Very Low Birthweight Infants. *NEJM,* 315:1986.

49 Weissert, W.G.: Seven Reasons Why It Is So Difficult to Make Community-Based Long-Term Care Cost-Effective. *HSR* 20, 4:424, 1985.

Chapter 20

Political Challenges for Nursing in Latin America: The Next Century

Esperanza de Monterrossa
Ilta Lange
Roseni Rosangela Chompré

Policies concern the expression of the interest of hegemonious groups in a determined historical, political, and social moment; policies produce priorities for the society as a whole and/or for specific groups.

In recent years in Latin America the predominant policies, committed to the interests of hegemonious groups, have not contributed to the solution of the social needs and demands of marginal groups of the population. The participation of nursing in policymaking for the health and education sectors is still very limited.

Nurses constitute a group with low social prestige in Latin America, due to multiple factors among which the following stand out:

• It is a profession which is predominantly female and which constitutes about 50 percent of the labor force in the health sector.

• In current Latin American society, nursing students come from the lower social classes.

• Due to the process of selection within the educational system and because of their social origin, nursing students have poor elementary and high school preparation.

• Nurses as a social group have limited or no participation in social and political movements.

On analyzing the practice of nursing and its relationship to the role of women in Brazilian society, Mendes (1989) affirms that the predominance of women in itself compromises and limits the prestige of any group of which they belong. Women's groups suffer because

An earlier version of this chapter appeared as "Nursing in the 21st Century in Latin America: Part III—Policies," in *International Nursing Review*, vol. 37, no. 4, 1990.

of their ideological values, the historical role of women who work, and their contemporary role in Latin American society. Silva (1986) perceives that the work of nursing is not limited in prestige because it is done by women but rather it is done by women because it lacks prestige. These arguments may help explain why nursing in Latin America has not participated in an effective way in the processes of general policy determination.

Even so, it cannot be said that there is a total absence of nursing policy. In recent decades, the participation of women in the labor force has changed their role in society, especially in those countries which are oriented toward industrial production. Nursing as an eminently female profession has benefited from the impact of these changes. This can be demonstrated by the greater participation of nurses in significant positions and activities within the health services. It can also be deduced by:

• The gradual increase in numbers of nurses in some Latin American countries and the growing number who obtain master's and doctoral degrees.
• The strengthening of representative bodies of nurses who are beginning to play an important role in society through collaborative projects with representative bodies of other professions
• The presence of nurses in leadership roles in sectors of health and education, including directive posts at a state level

Although progress can be recognized, nurses as the largest group of workers in the health sector are still timid and not very active. Consequently, they have little presence in the determination of policies for the health and educational sectors.

Policies in health and education are determined by the interests and social priorities of the existing economic powers of each country. In this sense the policies are defined according to the political interests of the macro system, which finally attends to the interests of national and international power groups.

POLICIES FOR THE HEALTH SECTOR AND FOR NURSING

In the middle of this century, a health policy was established in Latin American countries through which the coverage of health services was extended to broad sectors of the population. Implementing this policy required an increase in the physical resources for health care delivery and the hiring of a great number of health workers. This had the following repercussions for nursing:

• The incorporation of a large number of nursing personnel without adequate and specific training for practice
• An increase in duties delegated to the nurses and to the rest of the nursing personnel
• Few positions available for nurses in outpatient clinics, reducing their participation in primary health care
• Lack of regulations that support or protect the nurses while carrying out delegated duties
• Lack of a policy that deals with human resource development in nursing, with consequent lack of short- and medium-term goals at the undergraduate, graduate, and continuing education levels
• Lack of a policy on science and technology to stimulate the development and incorporation of appropriate technology in the extended health services
• Lack of an administrative policy regarding personnel issues such as salary regulation, working hours, and schedules that are acceptable and adequate for the model of practice
• The lack of mechanisms to ensure community participation in the decisions concerning the health services

Carillo (1985) states that the health movements in Latin America in past decades were characterized by their critical questioning concerning health, by their search for ways to humanize health care delivery, by taking into account the great needs of the world's population, and by expressing the philosophical principle that health is one of the rights of humanity. The policies creating an increase of health services allowed a quantitative increase in nursing personnel but gave no consideration to the qualifications of the nursing labor force that was incorporated into the health sector. The incorporation of great numbers of unqualified health workers was rationalized by the scarcity of prepared nursing personnel and the need to have low-cost health services. Because of their scarcity, nurses were not incorporated as part of the work force in primary health care and community work.

The evolution of these programs and the reorganization of health services have demonstrated the importance of the inclusion of the nurse as a *strategic* professional in the organization, management, and offering of services at the primary health care level. During the sixties, the health policies favored health care delivery at the hospital level; nurses' functions were recognized and reaffirmed by the policies and norms of these health institutions as well as by their own regulations. As an example, the law of professional practice in some of the Latin American countries demands that all hospitals have nurses directing the nursing services.

The last decade has seen important progress in the organization and functions of the national health services of the Latin American countries. The governments have defined priorities and strategies for ambulatory health services giving emphasis to a new technological composition. In this context the human resources are presented as a priority both qualitatively and quantitatively.

EDUCATIONAL POLICIES FOR NURSING

Nursing is a social practice, determined by the economic, political, and social process of society. The present policies in Latin America for the educational sector have influenced nursing in many ways:

- The incorporation of nursing programs into the university
- The creation of specialization courses and graduate programs at a master's level in several countries and recently at a doctoral level in Brazil
- The lack of policies in many countries for the preparation of nursing personnel at medium and/or basic level
- The lack of directives for continuing education programs for nursing personnel in the service institutions
- The lack of policies which foster change in the nursing curricula and programs that currently are very traditional and predominantly oriented toward patient care at the hospital level

The policy that included nursing at the university level permitted the preparation of nurses at graduate levels in countries of Latin America. In the great majority of the Latin American countries, the educational system provides easier access for the more privileged classes of society and excludes the low-income population, limiting their access to public as well as to private educational services. This situation has had important repercussions for the development of the nursing profession.

The preparation of nurses at a graduate level has had, in the last years, an important impact; some nurses have outstanding roles within national associations, health services, educational institutions, and international organizations. Yet some might argue that it would have been better if advancement had been advocated for the preparation of all levels of nursing personnel.

All in all, progress has been made in nursing education policies in Latin America. Highlights include:

- The constitution of nursing schools in Latin America at the beginning of the century (especially during the first decade), with the help of English, Canadian, and U.S. nurses with support of the Rockefeller Foundation

• The sponsorship of the W. K. Kellogg Foundation during the fifties, first to prepare nurse educators in master's and doctoral programs, and later, for institutional development of nursing schools

• The important contribution of Pan-American Health Organization (PAHO) in the elaboration of a model of nursing education in Latin America. Souza and Manfredi (1982) analyze the role of PAHO and its impact on nursing education in Latin America from 1940 to 1980, demonstrating important improvement in the preparation of nurses in the majority of countries in the region

• The national efforts of groups of nurses to create professional associations that are represented in health departments and ministries and that participate in the determination of general education, health, and nursing policies

These efforts have made possible the establishment of nursing education models that point out the real needs for the next century. To fulfill the health needs of the twenty-first century, nurses must become more aware and have a greater participation in the social and political movements of their countries. Hopefully in doing so, they will have these policy goals in mind:

• Access for all to the formal educational system
• Distribution of educational resources without distinction of race or purchasing power
• Free elementary, secondary, and university education for all as a state responsibility
• The determination of nursing by teaching and service institutions using modern, educational technology and considering the strategy of teaching-service integration

POLICIES ON HUMAN RESOURCES

Within the general policies of wages and working conditions, nursing has not had the capacity to mobilize and to organize itself; nursing has not claimed its rights. Due to their marginal condition in the sector, for historical and social reasons, nursing workers have had a passive and submissive attitude regarding working conditions, salaries, and other policies.

It is hoped that the process of democratization, which the majority of Latin American countries are experiencing, will be felt among nurses, inspiring them to participate in determination of wages, schedules, and workload policies. Here, again, certain goals can be identified:

• Workload and working hours compatible with the physical and mental capacity of the worker, guaranteeing the quality of care, and considering the nature and complexity of each job
• Structuring of positions and salaries so that nursing personnel can ascend to higher categories, through an educational process
• Salaries that consider tenure in the institution, complexity of the work, and potential risks
• Assigning value to nontraditional work sites through increased salaries and benefits for nurses in such places as rural areas, factories, schools, and marginal communities
• The establishment of processes to evaluate the quality of health care, and especially of nursing care
• Selection and recruitment of nursing personnel in public and private institutions by tests and/or proven competence for the function
• Regulations for multidisciplinary work that guarantee the participation of nursing personnel in primary health care

REGULATIONS

In the majority of the Latin American countries, nursing has advanced with the establishment of nursing associations which regulate legal aspects of the profession's practice. The work of the International Council of

Nursing reinforces the work of the national associations in the Latin American countries. Much still is to be done in the regulation of nursing practice, in supporting, guaranteeing, and broadening its action in primary health care as well as in ensuring adequate universal, risk-free, comprehensive, high-quality nursing care for the population. The effort of the international organizations in recognizing the need to improve these regulations is confirmed in the second WHO report (1986): In 1977, the thirtieth World Health Assembly approved a resolution in which nurses and midwives are recognized as of great importance in the primary health care team. In 1978, the Declaration of Alma Ata defined a new track in the organization of community health services, with extensive opportunities for action in nursing.

The current health policies in Latin America broaden the concept of health, identifying the relationship between the process of illness and economic and social factors. This broadening of the concept of health increases the range of nursing actions and supports the need for a new order of regulations. This new order requires that nurses take a new ideological approach to their work as members of a society which is preparing for the challenges of the twenty-first century.

New regulations should consider nursing as a social body committed to scientific and technological progress and to the liberty of humans in its fullest sense. Nursing must be seen as having the capacity to solve the health and illness problems of the present society and to anticipate and control the risks of the next decades.

Nursing regulations for the coming decades should consider the production of nursing services within institutions and also in autonomous work. Regulation must incorporate the activities already recognized as inherent in nursing and should increase the actions related to illness prevention, control and elimination of environmental risks, control of working conditions in the home and industries, and, in general, of preventing vulnerabilities to which great population groups are potentially exposed.

Regulation should be the expression of the practice, supporting the professional role and guaranteeing its extension according to the needs and demands of society.

COLLABORATION OF THE W. K. KELLOGG FOUNDATION IN THE DEVELOPMENT OF NURSING POLICIES IN LATIN AMERICA

The W. K. Kellogg Foundation has contributed to the development of a model for preparation of nursing leaders based on identification of the nursing needs in each country. The Foundation has given support to leadership development in different ways:

- Providing exchange among groups of nurses and institutions of nursing education, through meetings, traveling seminars, and networking activities
- Offering fellowships for graduate studies at a master's and doctoral level and scholarships for short periods of concentrated studies
- Stimulating and supporting the participation of nursing schools in multidisciplinary and teaching-service integration projects
- Supporting and establishing networks among projects at schools of nursing, for example, the Centers of Educational Technology, and more recently, the Poles of Development

All these efforts have contributed to the preparation of nursing leaders in education and in practice, leaders who have assumed important positions in their institutions. The efforts also have resulted in exchange and collaboration among programs in Latin America.

The participation and support of the W. K. Kellogg Foundation for nursing projects has also contributed to the recognition of the profession and the determination of policies, including the following:

- The maternal-child projects of the Pan-American Health Organization, in which nurses have important participation
- The project of the International Council of Nursing which supports nursing associations in Latin America to develop regulations for the profession
- The effort to create and support the Latin American Nursing Association (ALADEFE)

All these mechanisms have contributed to making nursing schools "open" for dynamic preparation of nursing leaders through a dialectic process of learn-act-reflect-act. Only in a society which is truly democratic can policies be determined that attend to the interests of the population, based on the principles of equality and justice. To achieve these ends, nursing personnel should participate in associations, political parties, and other organizations in civil society. Meleis (1988), affirms that "if nursing wants to have an international impact, this is the moment to do it, because of the number we are and the point of view that we have. There are seven million nurses in the world. Just think of what seven million people can do if they put their minds to it, if they have common goals and basic knowledge." Maglacas, Ulin, and Ships (1987) affirm that we have the number, and the number may be converted into power if we have the sensitivity, the organization, the policies, and if we mobilize ourselves to develop knowledge.

Finally, the efforts of PAHO/WHO in establishing collaborating centers for nursing in the regions of the Americas must be recognized. Presently these are five centers, three of which are located in the United States: University of Illinois, Chicago; University of Pennsylvania, Philadelphia; and University of Texas in Galveston. In Latin America there are two centers, one in the University of Sao

Paulo in Riberao Preto, Brazil, and one in the Colombian Association of Nursing Schools in Bogota, Colombia.

Each center proposes one line of work in the area of international collaboration. According to Souza (1988) the University of Illinois' priority for international collaboration is related to nursing practice. This collaborating center will also act as executive secretary of the Network of Collaborating Centers. The purpose of the collaborating center at the University of Texas is to integrate nursing education and practice at an undergraduate and graduate level. Riberao Preto will be a reference center in the area of research, and Colombia will work in the area of nursing education. The most important aspect of the work carried out by these centers is the base being built in the concept of bilateral exchange and in the principles of collaboration and cooperation.

CONCLUSIONS

This analysis of politics in nursing in Latin America is based on the background which has determined the current nursing situation. The analysis permits identification of the most important factors that will condition the development of nursing in the twenty-first century. Among the critical factors are the following:

- A greater awareness by citizens of their rights and duties
- The effort of the Latin American countries to open the doors so that the population can participate in decision making
- The financial crises and social and technological progress that require health services to be more accessible to the population, with greater response to problems of costs, keeping health within the reach of the various sectors of society
- Women, as a discriminated-against group, needing to overcome the current situation through mechanisms of organization and par-

ticipation, with a broad view of their rights as women and as citizens

• The need to adopt strategies which reply to the health needs of large population groups by creating innovative models in nursing education and practice

• The need to construct peace based on the principles of equality, justice, and solidarity

Nursing in Latin America is aware of its possible achievements and limitations and of its role as protagonist in contributing to health in the twenty-first century. In spite of the present and future social, political, and economic challenges, nursing must complete this role. A series of problems emerge for nursing in responding to this directive:

• How to establish mechanisms for coordination and collaboration among developed and developing countries within a bilateral framework?

• How to reduce the obstacles which the social heritage has imposed on nurses, such as low status and the lack of a research culture; how to place the nurse in equal status with other professionals; and how to participate in the scientific and technological progress of the next century?

• How to establish intercountry and intercontinental programs which will promote nursing leadership worldwide?

• How to make the profession more attractive for the youth of next century? By raising salaries? Improving the education of nurses? Extending their role to primary health care? Incorporating a high level of technology into professional practice?

The challenge is ours. The social policies of any nation must be considered within an historical context; they must be analyzed as an articulated whole within an integrated plan of development. Nursing must make its voice heard in this process as it evolves in Latin America.

REFERENCES

Carillo, G. (1985). *La situación de la Enfermeria en América Latina*. En: La Enfermeria en Latinoamérica. Estrategia para su desarrollo. Memorias de la Reunión de Lideres de Enfermería. FEPAFEM, Caracas, Venezuela. 121–127.

Maglacas, A., Ulin, P., Ships, C. (1987). *Health Manpower for Primary Health Care: The Experience of the Nurse Practitioner*. WHO/University of North Carolina, Chapel Hill.

Meleis, A., (1988). *Nursing Research: A Need or a Luxury*. Paper presented at Global Nursing Conference, Galveston, Texas.

Mendes, Dulce de Castro. (1989). *Assistencia de Enfermagem e Administracao de Enfermagem: A Ambiguidade Funcional do Enfermeiro*. Rev. Bras. Enf. 38 (314):257–265.

Silva, G. (1986). *Enfermagem Professional: Análise Critica*. São Paulo, Brazil, Cortez, 143.

Souza, A. et al. (1988). Estudio de Tendenciá de la Investigacíon sobre la Práctica de Enfermeria en Brasil.

Souza, A. M., Manfredi, M. (1982). *Perspectivas para la Educacíon de Enfermeria en América Latina frente a la menta de Salud para Todos en el Año 2000*. PAHO.

Chapter 21

The Future Role of Nursing in Health Policy-Making in Colombia

Jaime Arias

Most policy decisions in the health field in Colombia are made by politicians, health officials of high rank, and the medical profession, depending on the issue and the technical level of the matter. Very seldom are nurses called, and only when decisions involve very specific topics which relate to nursing practice. This chapter proposes some ways to increase nurses' participation in the decision-making process so that nurses can be more active in setting policies and norms related to primary health care, a topic of paramount importance in the country.

SUBJECTS OF HEALTH POLICY DECISION

The most important decisions in the public health field in Colombia in the last few decades have had to do with the legal structure of the National Health System, the assigning of financial resources from the national government to the provinces, the number and type of human resources, administrative decentralization, and with the direction of maternal-infant programs, planned parenthood, and infant survival programs, and with the construction and equipment of health facilities throughout the national territory.

In the next few years the discussion will be focused around the following major topics: redesign of the public health system to give greater power to the localities; the movement toward greater participation of the private sector in the provision of medical care; support for drinking water projects and environmental improvement; financing of hospitals and the system in general; technological and scientific development; programs of care for the elderly; services for degenerative pathology; quality control of services; and the extension of coverage by means of primary health care.

Around the aforementioned major subjects, many other topics will arise that involve technical policy decisions, such as the production and type of human resources, technological absorption, production and sale of medicines, and quality standards.

WHO DECIDES ON HEALTH?

In Colombia, as in many other countries, the discussion and making of health policies involve a series of institutions. In the case of major policies and of subjects that imply modifications of legal norms, the predominant actors are high government officials, the political parties, and the Congress, with technical consultation and agreement with the bureaucracy and with certain professional groups, almost always directed by medical doctors.

If the themes of the policy in question have a more technical character, the debate and design of policies and the development of these into norms involve technicians of the health bureaucracy, the medical organizations, sometimes the academic institutions, and very rarely, paramedical or nursing professionals. At the level of technical norms for medical care, the participation of doctors and the other professionals is much greater.

In almost all the cases of policymaking, nursing professionals are absent, with the exception of subjects which directly involve nursing practice or which involve nurse functionaries not because of their profession but rather because of their labor position in the bureaucracy or in the medium-range ministry or government. At the level of some service institutions, nurses are listened to with respect on technical and administrative decisions but almost never have the last word.

FUTURE PARTICIPATION OF NURSES IN HEALTH POLICY DECISION MAKING

It is lamentable that in Colombia a profession so involved both in ambulatory and hospital clinical services and in field work has been so separated from the most important decisions in the sector. Because of its small number in relation to other health professions, of its weak union organization, and because of its lack of access to command positions within the system, the country has been deprived of the assistance of professionals that have a clinical, administrative, and community vision that surely could make very important contributions to health policy. The question is whether nurses are prepared as a social group to assume the responsibility of greater involvement with the complex process of policy making and whether they have interest in participating in the decision process.

In countries such as the United States, in the last decade the nursing movement has looked for a place for nursing in the decision-making process. In contrast, in countries such as Colombia the medical profession and some high-level social administrators (for some more time) will maintain a certain predominance in the decision-making process of the health sector, with the technical assistance of economists, attorneys, administrators, technicians, and scientists. But in any society which tends to open its policy-making process, the access of a more extended range of professionals and occupations to the policy decisions of this sector will be encouraged.

As the nursing profession receives technical and professional recognition, improves its union organization, increases its size, assumes more specific and complex functions in institutions, and takes the leadership in certain camps, the possibilities of major influence in the political-normative level increase.

NURSES AND PRIMARY HEALTH CARE

Primary care in the health field has sprouted in Colombia as a good alternative for the extension of coverage to the entire population in a short time and at rational costs. At this time the coverage reaches only 80 percent of the population, but the last governments have agreed about the need to support the strategy of "health for all" as a realistic goal for the year 2000.

In addition, there is a Latin American movement to strengthen the local services systems, which in the case of Colombia has been represented in policies that place the municipality and the small localities, either urban or rural, in the center of the operational decisions of many public services such as health, education, and housing.

Nurses have played and can play a crucial part in the development of primary care, and in this way, they could become a very valuable resource, both technical and professional, for the formulation of health policies, without excluding other strategic positions in institutions where nurses perform critical tasks. The nursing group has in primary health care an important responsibility either in the community or in clinical work. Community nurses and public health nurses participate as directors and work with families and with the community. Clinician nurses work in triage, in health promotion and specific prevention, in care of the sick and the healthy patient, and in clinical tasks. Auxiliaries and nurse assistants and the health promotors or community health workers have field and institution responsibilities.

With the support of the Kellogg Foundation and Michigan State University, a primary health pilot program has been conducted in the last 3 years in the west of Bogotá; this pilot program has been organized through community sections, where 400 families are assigned to the health community worker called a "promotor"; each promotor is responsible for a section. The sections are grouped to form a module of ten, which is directed by professional nurses, including community, clinical, and hospital nurses. Similar programs are beginning to be implemented in various cities of the country under the leadership of nurses.

We have used the field of primary health care as an example because there is a national policy which supports its development; nevertheless the complementary policies of technical and administrative support haven't yet been developed. Because of nurses' capacity, knowledge, and experience, they could become a critical element in the formulation of policies on primary care in Colombia and other countries.

What we have said of nurses applies to other professions as well, which so far have been excluded from participation in the policy-making process in the Colombian health sector. As in the political arena, democratization can be anticipated, so that more participants are included in decisions about orientation of health services. If those new professions involved in policy making prepare themselves for this important task, a great contribution can be expected.